Community
Health
Nursing

Joan G. Turner RNC, DSN

Associate Professor
University of Alabama at Birmingham
School of Nursing
Birmingham, Alabama

Katherine H. Chavigny RN, MSN, PhD, FACE

Associate Professor of Nursing
University of Portland
Portland, Oregon
Director of Nursing Affairs
American Medical Association
Chicago, Illinois

Drawings by Stephen Kass
Chicago, Illinois

J. B. LIPPINCOTT COMPANY

Philadelphia

London
Mexico City
New York
St. Louis
São Paulo
Sydney

Community Health Nursing

AN EPIDEMIOLOGIC PERSPECTIVE
THROUGH THE NURSING PROCESS

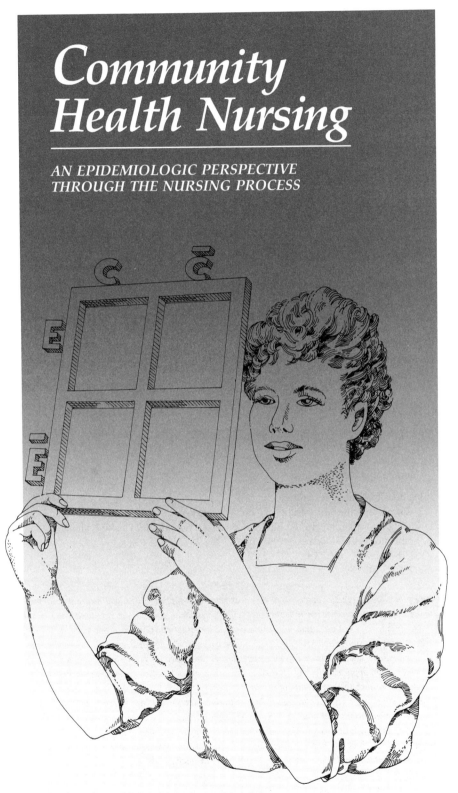

Acquisitions/Sponsoring Editor: Nancy Mullins
Manuscript Editor: Helen Ewan
Indexer: Catherine Battaglia
Design Coordinator: Anita Curry
Cover Design: Anthony Frizano

Designer: Tracy Baldwin
Production Manager: Kathleen P. Dunn
Production Coordinator: Kenneth Neimeister
Compositor: TSI Graphics
Printer/Binder: R. R. Donnelley Sons Company

1   3   5   6   4   2

Library of Congress Cataloging-in-Publication Data

Turner, Joan G.
   Community health nursing.

   Includes bibliographies and index.
   1. Community health nursing.   2. Epidemiology.
I. Chavigny, Katherine H.   II. Title.   [DNLM: 1. Community Health Nursing.
2. Epidemiologic Methods.   3. Nursing Process. WY 106 T948c]
RT98.T87   1988   610.73'43   87-21432
ISBN 0-397-54658-0

Any procedure or practice described in this book should be applied by the health-care practitioner under appropriate supervision in accordance with professional standards of care used with regard to the unique circumstances that apply in each practice situation. Care has been taken to confirm the accuracy of information presented and to describe generally accepted practices. However, the authors, editors, and publisher cannot accept any responsibility for errors or omissions or for consequences from application of the information in this book and make no warranty, express or implied, with respect to the contents of the book.

   Every effort has been made to ensure drug selections and dosages are in accordance with current recommendations and practice. Because of ongoing research, changes in government regulations and the constant flow of information on drug therapy, reactions and interactions, the reader is cautioned to check the package insert for each drug for indications, dosages, warnings and precautions, particularly if the drug is new or infrequently used.

*T*his book is written for the undergraduate community health nursing student using an epidemiologic perspective or framework to guide the beginning level staff nurse in community health nursing practice. Archer and Fleshman state that specialized areas of nursing practice may be defined as a synthesis of nursing theory and the theoretical framework of the science or art used for specialization. The model chosen for the specialty area of community health is the public health model consisting of interactive constructs used to preserve the health of aggregates such as levels of prevention of disease for community well-being. The nursing process is used as the basic model for generalist practice in the community. The purpose of the text is to guide the application of public health principles for nursing services to promote the welfare of populations through the use of epidemiologic methods.

Authors' Foreword

Epidemiology brings to community health nursing a dynamic and exciting perspective. The process of epidemiology adds methods of hypothesizing new problem-solving techniques to the nursing process for practice in the community. Epidemiology formulates new relationships and new associations between nursing and public health. Today we live in challenging, provocative times; epidemiology assists nurses to improve practice and meet changing community needs using methods and tools that are held in common with all members of the multidisciplinary team. This common language improves interprofessional communication and trust. At the same time, the unique attributes of nursing as a profession can be maintained and displayed within the framework of epidemiologic methods and theory.

The public health science of epidemiology is not new to nursing, but its use has been sporadic and its power for analyzing problems in public health has remained unexploited by the nursing profession. In the past, however, epidemiology has not been ignored. Exhortations to use epidemiology for delivery of nursing services and to include it in the curriculum for nursing education appeared in the literature as early as the mid 1960s. In 1975, the Pan American Health Organization (PAHO) pointed out that epidemiology had developed brand new approaches, updated for a modern world with complex needs. No longer was the public health science of epidemiology confined to the solving of problems for communicable disease, but it had become an indispensable method of evaluating health care services and investigating cause and the effects of interventions for the prevention and control of chronic diseases. The era of conserving epidemiology for nationwide studies had given way to mini-epidemic investigations and the solving of problems for small groups.

In 1976, a panel of nurse educators, nurse epidemiologists, and nurse administrators met to implement the goals of the PAHO report. The group of experts recommended the application of epidemiologic methods for nursing education. They also supported the use of epidemiologic perspectives for intramural communities, such as infection control in hospitals. Since then, there is an increasing interest in the nursing community in applying epidemiology to nursing practice and to nursing research. In spite of some discussion on the relative merits of epidemiology for undergraduate and graduate nursing education, epidemiology must be seriously considered to meet the increasing need to validate nursing's impact on the health of the community.

In the 1990s, nursing care of the elderly, the chronically ill, and the stable, acutely ill will be delivered in the community by multidisciplinary teams. The escalating epidemic of AIDS will require an understanding of epidemiologic principles. As competition creates an environment of encroachment on the nursing profession, the need to establish the effectiveness of community health nursing services becomes imperative. The use of interprofessionally accepted, quantified methods makes the teaching and application of epidemiology, by and for nurses, a professional necessity. This book has been written to address this need and to guide faculty in presenting the broad principles and language of epidemiology to staff nurses in community health.

The perspective of epidemiology is unique and provides an understanding of the community that is difficult to equal. It provides a framework that requires the utilization of all nursing skills and sciences. Under the auspices of epidemiology, all basic sciences such as microbiology and all the behavioral sciences such as sociology can be integrated. But the epidemiologic perspective is more than this; it promotes a change in attitude and change in the way the world is perceived by the nurse. Within an epidemiologic context, health policy may be viewed as a community intervention. Accurate documentation of nursing observations includes exposures to risk factors not merely for the individual but for the well-being of the community. Case finding is seen within broader implications as possible hazards to the total community or as implications for delivery of nursing services to aggregates. Cases in epidemiology are defined as instances of recidivism, problems of compliance with medical and nursing therapies, or lack of mobility to accomplish the activities of daily living. These outcomes are the concern of nursing; the epidemiologic perspective converts these concerns into community issues for nursing care.

Epidemiology provides a new vision for the role of the community health nurse. It familiarizes the nurse with a common language for communication with other public health disciplines and for clients and patients receiving community care. The epidemiologic perspective provides the nurse with a special orientation to deliver enhanced care to the sick and well for the prevention and control of disease and the promotion of health in populations.

Community Health Nursing represents an effort to introduce and elaborate upon the basic scope and nature of contemporary community health nursing practice. When nursing and public health art and science are juxtaposed, the areas of commonality provide a substantial conceptual framework to guide community health nursing. Epidemiologic principles and methods are used to accomplish the goals of public health. The nursing process on the one hand and the epidemiologic method on the other provide an explanatory and predictive basis for inquiry, acquisition of knowledge, and practice.

Preface

Although we recognize the vital role that advanced community health practitioners play in health care delivery, this book is intended to help prepare the beginning or entry level nurse to function as a quality health care provider to diverse client populations. When enriched with classroom and clinical applications, this text should provide the serious student with a basic understanding of community health nursing parameters, as well as with knowledgeable approaches to practice derived from epidemiologic orientation.

Perhaps the most unique feature of this book is provided by its subtitle, the epidemiologic approach. The intent is that entry level nurses be competent with quantitative as well as qualitative measures of population well-being. Additionally, as a consumer of research, the bachelor's level nurse should be familiar with research and problem-solving approaches. As depicted in this work, community health nursing at the most basic level requires mastery of specific nursing and public health sciences, a high level of technologic nursing skills, sound nursing judgment, and an appreciation for the interplay between human populations and health phenomena.

Section 1 focuses on the interrelationships of community health, epidemiology, and nursing. Epidemiology as a community health science is discussed, followed by a historical overview of health care. The public health model is followed by the natural history model, and both are presented so that the relationship between public health epidemiology and nursing knowledge can be visualized. For example, epidemiologic concepts embodied in the natural history model are utilized to facilitate conceptualization of the importance of strategic nursing intervention modalities embodied in the levels of prevention.

The emphasis of Section 2 is nursing of groups or population aggregates such as the family and the community. Epidemiologic rates and demographics as quantifications for the well-being of populations are introduced and applied as are various qualification assessment approaches. Sociocultural dynamics of communities are presented in an effort to build upon the student's basic knowledge of sociology, anthropology, and group behavior. Pica as an example of cultural behavior and kuru as an example of utilization of epidemiologic investigation are discussed to enrich the content on culture.

In Section 3, the delivery of community health services, the structure and organization of community health agencies, and characteristics of quality assurance programs are addressed. Health services research and program evaluation are discussed as guides to ensure delivery of quality nursing services. Various definitions of epidemiology are offered, and guidelines for graphs and tables that are representative of population dynamics are offered.

In Section 4, basic epidemiologic research designs—descriptive, analytic, and intervention—are included. The applications of methods to actual community health problem are made throughout. Contemporary community health nursing roles in extramural and intramural settings such as schools, industry, hospitals, and home health are discussed from a community viewpoint.

Health problems in contemporary populations, such as family violence, substance abuse, and communicable diseases, are explored and applied to community health nursing practice in Section 5. The AIDS phenomenon is presented, both from a public education and primary prevention aspect as well as from a tertiary prevention point of view. Family violence, substance abuse, and the newer communicable diseases are viewed in light of their impact on the family and the community, and nursing interventions based on the levels of prevention are elaborated.

Section 6 focuses on community health nursing services in a changing health care system. Health policy and issues such as care for the growing elderly population and the overall trend toward health care delivery in the home are presented. Discussions such as the home visit versus home care are designed to provoke thought and further exploration of the evolving role of the community health nurse.

The advantages of using an epidemiologic perspective for the nursing of aggregates are summarized as follows:

- Epidemiology provides a framework within which basic sciences and behavioral sciences can be used for community nursing practice.
- The nursing process is extended through application of epidemiologic methods to describe community needs and evaluate nursing services.
- Public health principles of family as the unit of society, prevention and control of disease, and health promotion are activated and quantified through the epidemiologic approach.
- Epidemiology provides an interdisciplinary language to promote interprofessional communication and trust.

- An epidemiologic perspective provides a method of extending the relationship of family problems to community welfare.
- The epidemiologic model promotes understanding of the relationship between the environment and agents that expose susceptible populations at risk of impediments to health.
- Epidemiology provides a time-honored method of quantifying nursing outcomes such as recidivism, lack of compliance, and activities of daily living to promote and improve the quality of nursing care in the community.

Joan G. Turner, RNC, DSN
Katherine H. Chavigny, RN, MSN, PhD, FACE

▍ *Acknowledgments*

To my students—past, present, and future. Joan G. Turner
To my children, who enrich my life. Katherine H. Chavigny

Contents

CONTENTS

CONTENTS

CONTENTS

Community
Health
Nursing

Interrelationship of Community Health, Epidemiology, and Nursing

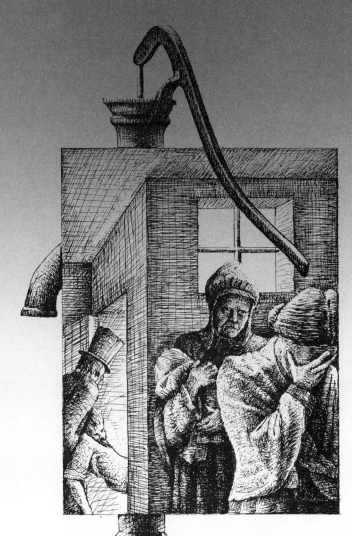

*Now I think
nothing is more
absurd than to
talk even of the
possibility of the
overeducation of
the trained nurse.
That it is possible
for a nurse to
know too much,
to be too highly
qualified on the
practical,
scientific and
intellectual side
of her profession
seems to be highly
absurd.*
—W. H. Welch

Historical Overview of Health Care: Origins of Community Health Nursing

LEARNING OBJECTIVES

After reading and understanding the content of this chapter, the student will be able to:

1. Define community health nursing and state its overall characteristics.

2. Trace the historical evolution of health care and identify the origins of community health nursing.

3. Outline the association between the formation of various military forces and the growth of nursing as a profession.

4. Compare and contrast causes of death in 1900 with current causes of death in the United States.

5. Identify the major contributions of nursing pioneers such as Nightingale and Wald.

6. Explain the relationship between the industrial revolution and the roots of public health sciences such as public sanitation and community health nursing.

7. State the relationship between the 1965 Medicaid and Medicare legislation and the growth of the home health care industry.

8. Trace the origins of issues like the role parameters and educational preparation of community health nurses.

Introduction

*B*efore providing a historical overview of community health nursing, it is important to briefly define this entity. Community health nursing is simplistically defined as a field of nursing practice that blends knowledge and skills from both the nursing and the public health sciences and applies them to the promotion of optimal health for the total population. Community health nursing practice may occur in any institutional or communal setting, so long as the sciences of nursing and public health provide the framework from which the client population is viewed.[1] Community health nursing focuses on populations, that is, the client is always viewed in terms of the larger family and community.

Nurses from other specialities now practice in the community, while some community health nurses, such as discharge planners and infection control nurses, work in hospitals. Consequently, community health nursing is not defined merely by setting, but rather by the presence of an acquired and applied base that consists of a functional union between nursing and public health concepts. The purpose of this chapter is to explore the origins and evolution of various public health principles and their role in the prevention of disease and promotion of health over the years. The chapter identifies the roots of community health nursing and the origins of many contemporary issues that concern this nursing specialty.

▌ *Early History Through the Middle Ages*

Largely through the efforts of paleopathologists, it is known that most primitive people suffered from a number of illnesses and accidents such as pneumonia, kidney stones, tuberculosis, and skeletal fractures. The earliest form of nursing was practiced by family members as they attempted to soothe and cure the sick and injured with a variety of notions and potions. The first types of public health practices probably took the form of sanitation measures such as the burying of human excreta and removing the dead from the living. Actually, it is unknown whether these two practices were related to survival needs or to superstition and early peoples' attempt to deal with supernatural forces.

In ancient Egypt (about 3000 B.C.), therapeutic methods were based largely on the rituals of worship, sacrifice, and purification. Great public halls were erected and designated as healing temples. The sick and afflicted might travel on foot for many days to reach one of these temples to obtain comfort and healing from the gods. Temple priests (sometimes called "nursing priests") endeavored to intervene on the patients' behalf by using various incantations or herbal remedies. Another priestly function was to bathe and refresh the ill and injured and to monitor their relative physiologic state by taking peripheral pulses. Nothing was known at that time about the circulation of blood, and the pulse rate was not counted. Instead, the priests assessed the general strength and quality of the pulsations. Because they valued personal cleanliness highly, the Egyptians also developed a web of drainage systems to route clean water away from wastes.[2]

The Hebrew Hygienic Code (1500 B.C.) was, in effect, a prototype for personal and community sanitation. Not only did the code outline specific dietary omissions and preparation guidelines, but it also set forth the idea that bodily cleanliness was a requisite for moral purity. Garbage and excreta were disposed of outside the city or camp, people with contagious diseases were quarantined, and unhygienic practices such as spitting were outlawed. The Hebrews, like the Babylonians before them, believed that illness was God's punishment for individual or collective sin. Unlike their Egyptian predecessors, the priests of Israel avoided medical interventions and instead concerned themselves with the observance of health rules regarding food, cleanliness, and quarantine. In Old Testament accounts, the nurse appears at times to be a combination servant, companion, and helpmate.[2]

The Greeks (100–400 B.C.) are credited with many contributions to medicine and are considered to be the first people to become conscious of the need for trained nurses. As with the preceding societies, the Greeks believed that personal hygiene and diet contributed to one's overall well-being.

The Romans (300 B.C.) may have initiated organized military nursing. They built hospitals in different regions where wounded Roman soldiers could be treated. These hospitals reportedly comprised wards, recreation areas, baths, and pharmacies. Each Roman legion had a physician and several nurses to treat soldiers on the battlefield or at a nearby post. All Roman soldiers were taught first-aid and were required to carry bandages as a part of their standard equipment.[2]

Even though the Greeks are credited with being the first civilization to recognize a need for nurses, the Romans actually expanded that notion by developing specialized attendants for the sick. Nearly 2000 years would pass before nurses would be recognized for their ability to promote health instead of merely to restore health. Even though these early "nurses" were probably slaves, at least they began to function as specialists separate from medicine or religion.

During the early Middle Ages (A.D. 300–1500), personal hygiene was neglected and refuse and body wastes accumulated amid rudimentary living quarters in overcrowded cities. Health care of any kind existed only for the wealthy few, and public health problems were addressed minimally and ineffectively. Under these dismal conditions, epidemics of cholera, leprosy, and smallpox killed large segments of society on a recurring basis. For instance, bubonic plague, or "Black Death," killed 43 million people—half of the population of the known world in the mid-1300s.[1] Despite the lack of interest in personal or environmental hygiene, medieval people felt a philosophical devotion to the sick and subsequently established many early hospitals and religious nursing orders. During this era, nursing took place largely within the walls of hospitals or monasteries. The first organized home nursing service was established through the efforts of Saint Vincent in the 1600s, resulting in a nursing order devoted to visiting the sick in their homes.[2]

▋ *Early Immunization*

In the later Middle Ages (A.D. 1500–1800), many discoveries changed the way people lived and the way they viewed the world. The New World had been discovered, Newton's observations became known to the informed of the era, and written communication became more widely available because of new paper-making and printing techniques. In medicine, William Harvey accurately described the circulation of blood in humans, and the introduction of variolation, or inoculation with true smallpox, constituted the first rudimentary form of active immunization. However, variolation was done without the benefit of any notion of asepsis, and severe bacterial infection or even death sometimes followed the procedure. For these and other reasons, variolation was not quickly accepted, and most people were actually infected with the smallpox virus during childhood or young adulthood. In fact, an unpocked face was a rarity in Europe during the 18th century; the disease affected almost everyone, although there were survivors.

In 1798, an American, Edward Jenner, demonstrated that it was safer and more effective to inoculate with the cowpox virus instead of live smallpox virus. His inoculation for smallpox with cowpox was the beginning of an effort that ultimately eradicated smallpox from the world 170 years later. Although an effective vaccination for smallpox existed, it was not available worldwide for several years.

Infectious diseases continued to be the leading cause of death through the 18th and 19th centuries. Further, because world explorers carried these diseases to virgin shores, people in newly discovered lands were exposed, for the first time, to measles, syphilis, cholera, typhus, plague, and smallpox. Ironically, the transmission of these diseases to the natives played a role in weakening their resistance to colonization. By the time the Pilgrims landed at Plymouth in 1620, the infectious diseases introduced by previous expeditions had greatly diminished the native American population. Later on, in the southern colonies of North America, smallpox, yellow fever, and malaria outbreaks were introduced by way of the slave trade.[3]

The upheaval in Europe caused by the French Revolution (1789) and the Napoleonic Wars which followed inflicted both injury and illness on the European population. By the time Napoleon I retreated from Moscow, it is said that typhus and dysentery were his chief opponents. In fact, although he was able to raise a new army of 500,000 men in 1813, infectious diseases reduced his force to 170,000 within a few short weeks.[4]

The Industrial Revolution

The Industrial Revolution began in England in the middle of the 18th century and spread to the United States and much of the rest of the world during the next two centuries. Workers, including women and children, labored 12 or more hours a day under very poor conditions that can only be imagined today. No thought was given to the safety and well-being of the worker. In fact, employees were viewed by factory owners as largely disposable or very easily replaceable. Both the environment and the people showed the effects of overwork, lack of sanitation, and a prevailing value system that placed products above human health and life. In short, as the 19th century began, England presented a dismal picture in matters regarding public health and humane treatment. The situation was ripe for reform, and when that reform came, it served as a model to the rest of the world.

Early public health legislation in England occurred in 1837 and provided for some sanitation measures as well as a National Vaccination Board. This Vaccination Board mainly concerned itself with prevention of smallpox, since that was the only disease for which a vaccine was available at the time. A more definitive improvement was made in 1848 when Edwin Chadwick published the "Report on an Inquiry into the Sanitary Conditions of the Laboring Population in Great Britain," which resulted in the establishment of a General Board of Health. Subsequent legislation addressed management of the factory worker, child welfare, and care of the aged and mentally ill. Additionally, the report resulted in environmental improvements such as the installation of fireplugs and the establishment of a safe water supply for the population.[3]

Home Health and Occupational Health in England

William Rathbone (1819–1902), a wealthy merchant in Liverpool, England, reportedly came to realize the value of home nursing from personal experience when his wife became ill. In 1859, Rathbone employed a nurse to care for the sick at homes in a poor section of Liverpool. Two years later, at his own expense, he tried to expand the service to other districts but could not find nurses who were suitably trained. At that point, Rathbone wrote to Florence Nightingale, who had established a training program for hospital nurses in London. Unfortunately, in that year of 1861, Nightingale was deeply involved with the Sanitary Reform Commission for the British Colony in India and was thus unable to give Rathbone's request her full attention. Nevertheless, she responded to his request in a letter in which she said that nurses would have to be specially trained to function effectively in a home setting. Following Nightingale's suggestion, Rathbone established a training school that would prepare nurses for hospital work as well as for district or home nursing. The resultant Royal Liverpool Infirmary Training School was the first in the world to prepare nurses for work in nontraditional settings such as the home. The training program successfully produced nurses who functioned outside of hospital walls. In fact, by 1867, the Liverpool district nursing service had grown from one to 18 districts. In addition to functioning in the home setting, these nurses also contributed to health reform within industrial settings through their interactions with workers and management.[5]

Indicative of her highly evolved social consciousness, Nightingale realized that it would be impossible to improve workhouse conditions without political involvement and legislative change. In 1865, she proposed a bill that would further the occupational health reform begun a few years earlier by Chadwick. That original bill met with considerable political resistance, and the bill was rewritten in 1867. The rewrite became known as the Hardy Bill and contained many of the same features as Nightingale's original one; however, it failed to emphasize the role of nursing in the reform movement as initially intended by Nightingale.[5]

Nightingale wrote extensively about nursing roles outside the hospital and seemed to feel that training programs should be established to train nurses for nonhospital roles. She correctly perceived that district or home health nurses would need special skills and knowledge to be effective, and she identified at least three areas in which such nurses should be proficient. First, Nightingale said that district nurses would have to be good teachers in order to teach family members to provide appropriate health care measures and preventive techniques. Second, she said that the district nurse would have to understand the nature of poverty and "pauperization." Third, Nightingale felt these nurses must understand the importance of preventing disease.[5] Her concern for prevention is illustrated by the following quote from 1894: "Preventable diseases should be looked on as a social crime—it is cheaper to promote health than to maintain people in sickness."[6] While this statement itself would not be considered profound today, the fact that Nightingale was thinking in preventive terms almost 100 years ago is very impressive indeed.

In summary, Nightingale saw the role of the 19th century visiting nurse as one that required an understanding of the human–environmental interaction, social and political processes, and basic sanitation and cleanliness, as well as techniques of disease prevention. She also identified one of the basic tasks of the home health care nurse, which is to teach skills that promote health and prevent disease.

■ *Developing America*

As noted earlier, infectious diseases spread by early explorers probably played a role in lessening the physical resistance of the North American natives to early European settlers in America. In fact, diseases such as typhoid, typhus, plague, and tuberculosis were the undisputed leading causes of death in the United States and remained so well into the 20th century.

Before the late 1800s, public health legislation in America existed mostly in the form of local responses to specific dangers or public nuisances, such as a 1701 Massachusetts law requiring ship quarantine and isolation of persons infected with smallpox. The United States Constitution, adopted in 1789, did not refer directly to public health, nor was the federal government active in health matters at that time. Instead, it was the responsibility of each sovereign state to manage its citizens' health affairs.[1] Before any initial step toward sanitary reform could be taken in the United States, there had to be the realization that a health problem existed. That recognition came slowly. Around 1820, both the size and the number of American cities began to increase dramatically. Between 1820 and 1830, the number of towns having more than 8000 inhabitants doubled and nearly doubled again 10 years later. But the greatest growth of all occurred in large eastern cities. By 1860, New York City had about one million people, the population of Chicago went from 5000 to 30,000, and Philadelphia's population had passed the half-million mark. This rapid growth literally outran the forces of law and order.[7] Because the population was mushrooming, it was impossible to provide sufficient basic services like police and fire protection. With the citizens fearing for life and limb, little thought was given to public health measures.

Even though most large American cities had so-called boards of health as early as 1830, these boards were considered largely ineffectual and were most often ignored. However, by the next decade, the slum districts of the larger cities had become so objectionable that the collective social consciousness was raised. Besides the obvious depravity and stench of the slums, word of the English health laws also stimulated the public health movement in the United States.

The final factor believed to have favorably influenced public health reform in America was the need to know and record vital statistics such as births and deaths.[7] In 1842, Massachusetts enacted a compulsory registration law, which required that events such as births and deaths be systematically recorded. Except for New York, other states were slow to establish this practice. Individual cities such as Philadelphia and New Orleans had recorded births and deaths as early as 1815, and even though these records were crude, they nevertheless showed an escalating rather than a declining death rate.

■ The Shattuck Report

Alarmed by the inadequacy of recording vital statistics, in the mid-1800s the Massachusetts Medical Society appointed Lemuel Shattuck as chairman of a committee charged with drawing up a sanitary survey of that state. Although a layman in health matters, Shattuck was said to be a student of sanitary reform. He went about his task promptly and submitted his findings to the legislature in 1850. He reported that unsanitary conditions were prevalent throughout the state and that nearly 50% of all deaths were unnecessary, since those fatalities resulted from environmental factors that could be eliminated with state-of-the-art sanitary and medical technology. Shattuck's report also addressed matters of water supply, sewage, ventilation, vital statistics, burial grounds, garbage disposal, and housing and plumbing requirements, as well as isolation of persons with contagious diseases. He indicated that a state board of health was a desirable mechanism for implementing and evaluating reforms. And although it can be said that every facet of his report was eventually incorporated into later health programs, 20 years would pass before any of Shattuck's recommendations actually would be implemented.[7]

Thus, the Shattuck Report of 1850 did nothing to improve environmental conditions immediately. Even though the report was well researched and well written, Shattuck failed to arouse the emotional compassion and political support of the American people and their political representatives. Whereas the English reformers, like Nightingale and Chadwick, appealed to human emotion, the Shattuck Report "appealed to the mind rather than the heart."[7] Regardless of its immediate impact, the report was significant in that it illustrated an early and systematic concern for public health problems in America.

■ The Post-Civil War Era

By the end of the Civil War in 1865, several predominant issues pervaded American life and ultimately affected the initiation and development of community health nursing. As industrialization grew, so did the cities and the disease-infested slums. Health conditions, especially in the crowded tenements, were deplorable. The average life expectancy nationwide was 41 years. Causes or etiologies of diseases were unknown, and hospitals were looked upon as places where people died.[8]

At the same time, the evolving democracy created a need for educated people. Although the prevailing sentiment was that the female's place was in the home, women's involvement in issues like abolition was actually the beginning of the feminist movement. The public school system was in its formative stages and by post-Civil War days, women were accepted as the teachers of both boys and girls.[8]

When the transcontinental railroad finally linked the East and the West in 1869, people and goods became more mobile. The steel and iron industry became vital to feed the miles of track and the coal-powered train engines. Printed material became more readily available and subsequently people became better informed. New discoveries like electricity, the light bulb, the telephone, and the typewriter changed the way Americans lived and worked. Even farming became mechanized and allowed a much more efficient means of providing more farm products to a greater number of people.

Products and people grew in number and diversity while millions of new immigrants arrived, causing the population to swell. Despite the short life expectancy, the United States population doubled between 1870 and 1890, growing to 76,303,387 before the turn of the century.[9] Most Americans, including nurses, were poorly educated, but there was evidence of progress as the number of high schools rose from 500 to over 6000 between 1870 and 1900.[10] Still, in 1890, less than 10% of the total population attended high school.[11] Technologic advances such as the sphygmomanometer, the hypodermic needle, and the concept of asepsis as well as improved preoperative and postoperative management helped to create demands for better-educated nurses. During this time, and for many years afterwards, education for nurses took place in hospital-based training programs designed to prepare nurses to work in a hospital. By 1893, there were 225 schools of nursing in the United States.[12]

Just as technologic and conceptual advances created a need for hospital nurses, those same advances combined with society's concern for health helped to validate the need for organized home health care for all socioeconomic levels. Prior to the late 19th century, home health care was provided to upper- and middle-class families by private duty nurses who had been trained to work in the hospital setting. These nurses boarded with the family and were treated as servants who should be available 24 hours a day.[12] Lower class families who were unable to pay for home nurses depended on neighbors and family members.

▮ *Organized Home Health Care in America*

Although the charter dates vary for the different district nursing associations in the United States depending on the source consulted, according to Jacques, the first formal role for public health nurses began in America in 1886 with the formation of organized district nursing associations.[13] In fact, two district nursing associations were begun that year: one in Boston and one in Philadelphia. Both were reportedly organized by American women who had been inspired initially by the work of William Rathbone in England. It was because of Rathbone's influence that the title "district nursing" came to be used in home health care in America. Since the district or visiting nurse did not live with the family as did her predecessor, the private duty nurse, the district nurse enjoyed a slightly higher status and considerably more flexibility in her job. In addition, the district nurse's home visits were both curative and preventive in nature—the first formally sanctioned preventive activities in American nursing.

Lillian Wald and a friend, Mary Brewster, established a district nursing service in New York City in 1893. Instead of establishing an office in a district and living elsewhere, Wald chose to live among the people she served. Wald was said to possess considerable personal wealth. Through numerous personal contacts, she was able to raise the money necessary to support the wide range of activities at what became known as the Henry Street Settlement. Because of Wald's social influence, the settlement benefited from her numerous personal relationships with wealthy and influential people like Theodore Roosevelt, Helen Keller, and John D. Rockefeller, Jr. Clients and their families also made periodic donations to the Settlement. Wald's flair for fund-raising brought the annual budget to a phenomenal $1 million by 1933.[14]

The Henry Street Settlement was unique for a number of reasons. First, the nurses were not associated with any religious group but were aligned voluntarily with the New York City Board of Health. To eliminate the stigma of charity, clients were charged according to their ability to pay. Clientel consisted mostly of immigrants and other poor people who lived in the tenements. Wald and the other nurses visited and cared for the sick in their homes and taught their clients various preventive and health maintenance strategies. The influence of the Henry Street Settlement nurses was not limited to New York City. Over the years, these nurses visited numerous countries of the world where they either initiated or assisted in establishing visiting nursing services.[14]

Wald called herself and the other Henry Street Settlement nurses "public health nurses." The basic idea behind their enterprise was that the nurse's peculiar introduction to the patient and her residential relationship with the neighborhood constituted the starting point for universal services to the area. From the beginning, Wald and her colleagues strived to have both the community agencies and representatives from every religion work toward an improved social and health environment in the community.[14]

Not only did Wald establish the title "public health nurse," but she was also an innovator of specialty roles within public health such as public school nursing. Not long after establishing the Henry Street Settlement, Wald offered the services of one of the public health nurses to the New York City school system as a demonstration of what a nurse could do to reduce the high absenteeism rate due to illness among schoolchildren. Her point was well taken because the school system subsequently placed that nurse on the city payroll, and out of that small beginning came the New York City Bureau of Child Hygiene and the whole notion of school nursing.

In 1909, Wald suggested to officials at the Metropolitan Life Insurance Company that hiring a nurse on their staff could actually save them money because the nurse's activities such as prenatal teaching would help to decrease mortality rates. Wald must have possessed a powerful sense of persuasiveness for as a result of her suggestion, Metropolitan Life established a visiting nurse service for policy holders.

By 1900, public health nursing and its specialties were in a state of rapid expansion. District nursing organizations were emerging in the large cities, and public health nurses were beginning to take on a number of innovative roles. For instance, in 1897, a nurse was placed on the city payroll in Los Angeles to act as a public health nurse. Nurses were being hired in a similar capacity all over the country. In 1903, Reba Thelin was hired by Johns Hopkins Hospital to work in the homes of people infected with tuberculosis. Her job was to make sure that clients received fresh air, rest, and regular meals, and that the danger of transmitting the disease was kept to a minimum.[1]

Public health nursing affirmed its political identity by establishing its own organization, which would set standards of practice and guide the further expansion of the specialty. The resultant National Organization for Public Health Nursing (NOPHN) was chartered in 1912 and was the first nursing organization to admit non-nurse members.[2] Even in those formative years, there was much discussion about titles, position requirements, and protocols. For instance, while Wald endorsed the title "public health nurse," others advised the use of "visiting nurse," "district nurse," or even "instructive visiting nurse."[15] By 1912, visiting nurses had, for the most part, become known as public health nurses, and they numbered more than 3000 nationwide.[12]

As early as 1901, there was concern about the salaries of public health nurses on the one hand and their cost-effectiveness on the other. At the turn of the century, public health nurses were working from 8 to 10 hours a day and were being paid $45 to $60 a month. The typical working day was summed up as follows by a visiting nurse from Brooklyn, New York:

> It is a hand-to-hand struggle against disease, poverty, and dirt, and against the most pitiful ignorance and inherited prejudice. . . . going from house to house, mounting flight after flight of stairs—for it is a curious but true fact that tenement house patients always live on the top floor of a very tall house—here making beds, preparing nourishment, giving sponge-baths, there bandaging a leg or applying a dressing, but in all cases carrying out the doctor's orders, being certain the medicine will be properly administered. . . . In short, doing everything in her power for her patient's comfort.[15]

Despite the various difficulties, the aspect of the job that caused the most anxiety and required the most time and skill was keeping the various written records in good order.[15]

By 1910, overall death rates, especially those attributed to infectious diseases, were declining, and general sanitation had improved. Public health nurses were managing case loads, and the majority of large urban visiting nurse associations had initiated preventive programs for school children, mothers, and clients with tuberculosis. Under the nurse's care, clients could go for months without seeing a physician.[16]

Many issues that confront contemporary community health nurses are issues that arose in earlier times. For example, as soon as the role of the public health nurse became fairly well known, controversy arose over what constituted the role functions of the nurse as opposed to the role of the social worker, the physician, and even layworkers in some charitable organizations. In 1911, a self-appointed but fairly eloquent spokesperson for nursing, C. E. A. Winslow, summarized the three areas of responsibility of most concern to public health nursing practice: (1) promoting school health, (2) decreasing morbidity and mortality associated with tuberculosis and other communicable phenomena, and (3) reducing the nation's high infant mortality rate. In addition to these concerns, Winslow pointed out that public health nurses of the day were viewed as capable of inspecting factories, schools, and homes with respect to the adequacy of the physical environment and atmospheric conditions (such as lighting and sanitation) and of assessing these areas to determine if appropriate mechanisms were in place that would contribute to worker or family safety and well-being.[17]

Another recurring issue revolved around what constituted appropriate educational preparation for a public health nurse. Winslow felt that the principles of physiology and bacteriology should be mastered, as well as the fundamental laws of hygiene and sanitation. He felt that an intellectual mastery of these principles was not enough.

The public health nurse also must be able to apply and teach these principles in actual community settings.

One of the earliest definitive attempts to provide the additional education required for public health nursing practice was at Teacher's College in New York under the direction of a registered nurse, Adelaide Nutting. The program began in 1899 with two students and had an enrollment of over 1000 by 1933. Nurses who had completed both high school and a hospital-based nursing program were admitted to the program. The 1-year course of studies was designed to prepare "teacher nurses" for school health care, home health care, and prevention and control of communicable diseases.

Not everyone agreed that nurses needed more education. In fact, some people—especially physicians—argued that nurses were already being overeducated for the realities of practice. However, Dr. William Welch, an epidemiologist and a friend of nursing, said the following at a commencement exercise:

> Now I think nothing is more absurd than to talk even of the possibility of the overeducation of the trained nurse. That it is possible for a nurse to know too much, to be too highly qualified on the practical, scientific and intellectual side of her profession seems to be highly absurd.[18]

Early public health nurses were employed either by an official agency, such as a city or county health department, or by an unofficial or voluntary agency, such as a visiting nurse association. Originally created to deal with the health problems of large immigrant populations, the voluntary agencies found that there was less need for their services as the number of immigrants decreased. In contrast, public health nursing in official agencies experienced a steady expansion. By 1924, 54% of all public health nurses were employed by official or governmental agencies, and that number would continue to grow for the next four or five decades.[16]

Public health nursing as a discipline was beginning to have a noticeable effect on the health and well-being of Americans. Welch said on May 24, 1916 that: "The public health nurse has become one of the very greatest agents in the advancement of health, both individual and public, in this country."[18]

Nursing, in general, received further positive recognition as a result of nurses caring for soldiers and civilians alike during World War I. The two nursing specialities that grew the most as a result of wartime activities were military nursing and occupational health nursing. When World War I began in 1917, there were 403 nurses on active duty, and that number increased to 12,186 1 year later. Several nurses were wounded, but none died as a result of enemy action, although 200 died from the swine flu epidemic. As a result of their service during the war, three Army nurses were awarded the Distinguished Service Cross and another 23 received the Distinguished Service Medal.[19]

Occupational health nurses fared well because it soon became apparent that their efforts resulted in decreased absenteeism among workers that were producing vital wartime equipment and supplies.[2]

During the Great Depression, public health services suffered from decreased funding, salary cutbacks, personnel reduction, and curtailment of most basic services, including public health nursing. Thousands of hospital nurses were unemployed. However, through New Deal employment programs, 10,000 nurses were assigned to jobs at official health agencies. Although these jobs gave thousands of nurses exposure to public health nursing, the nurses' general lack of preparation in public health science and their lack of field experience served to minimize their impact.[20]

■ *Public Health Legislation*

Physicians and nurses held very different opinions on how midwives should be supervised and trained. In essence, organized medicine felt that midwifery should be abolished and the whole field of obstetrics turned over to physicians. The Sheppard–Towner Act of 1921 stipulated that public health nurses should be used to instruct local lay midwives on the principles of safe delivery of newborns.

While the Sheppard–Towner Act was aimed essentially at improving maternal and child health, it indirectly stimulated the organization of state health departments. The Public Health Title VI of the Social Security Act of 1935 went even further. Through grants to state health organizations, it stimulated the growth of local health services, provided funds for the recruitment, training, and supervision of public health personnel, and promoted the expansion of services in research, prevention, and treatment of major health problems.[20] One of the public health nursing leaders who helped draft the legislation associated with the Social Security Act of 1935 was Pearl McIver. McIver believed nurses could improve the health of individuals, families, and entire communities. She worked toward appointing a well-prepared nursing director in every state health department, since she believed the scope and quality of local public health nursing services depended heavily on wise leadership at the state level.[20]

Although the 1930s was a decade marked by growth in public health nursing on state and local levels, there were still 1077 counties (over one-third of the total) and 26 cities with a population of 10,000 or more with no local public health nursing services.[20] By 1940, all 48 states, as well as the territories of Alaska, Hawaii, and the District of Columbia, had established public health nursing programs.

Even though the National Organization for Public Health Nursing had taken responsibility for promoting educational standards since its inception in 1912, by 1940 only 26 approved postgraduate courses in public health nursing existed. Funds generated through the Social Security Act enabled about 1000 nurses to complete their educational programs in public health by 1936. Although progress was being made, the National Health Survey of 1938 revealed

> . . . grossly insufficient preventive services, alarming malnutrition, one-third of the population with little or no medical care, excessive disease and death rates in low-income groups, and while threats of communicable diseases were diminishing, the chronic diseases—syphilis, tuberculosis, heart disease, cancer and stroke—had become the leading causes of death.[20]

World War II

In response to the demands created by World War II, attention was refocused on guarding the health of military personnel, families in containment areas, and workers in essential industries. With nurses and physicians actively involved with the needs created by the war, people who normally would have been hospitalized were treated at home instead. Since family members had to cope with the care of acutely ill members at home, they needed instruction, support, and assistance. These family caretakers looked to public health nurses to provide that assistance. With the help of agencies such as the American Red Cross, which organized courses in home nursing and training programs for nurse's aides, public health nursing mobilized to meet the home health care needs.

While many nurses had been unemployed just a few years before, at the height of the war effort, nursing shortages became apparent. United States Representative Frances P. Bolton had funds appropriated to support basic, postgraduate, and graduate education for nurses. As a result, 4200 nurses were able to complete their graduate studies, half of them completing studies in public health. Another stimulus to nursing education was the United States Cadet Nurse Corps program, which successfully enlisted and trained 95,000 nurses.

Although the initial intent of these two pieces of legislation was aimed at increasing the numbers of trained nurses, they ultimately acted to change nursing education dramatically. Not only were traditional programs being critically and systematically evaluated, but basic baccalaureate programs were increasing markedly. Notably, junior colleges began to provide experimental programs in nursing.[20]

Post World War II

Experiences in military health care during the war served to increase the public's expectations of the peacetime health care delivery system. Health problems related to peacetime readjustment included an increase in emotional problems, accidents, and alcoholism. Simultaneously, many scientific breakthroughs made traditional patterns of medical practice obsolete. Antibiotics became available for the treatment and prevention of numerous infectious diseases, such as rheumatic fever, and some sexually transmitted diseases, such as syphilis and gonorrhea. X-ray techniques, such as the photofluorogram, were perceived as mechanisms that would greatly facilitate mass screening for tuberculosis.

Instead of federal monies for state services being withdrawn after World War II, as they were after World War I, funds were funneled into categorical programs such as tuberculosis, sexually transmitted diseases, cancer, and mental health problems. There was renewed and aggressive emphasis on early diagnosis of diseases such as tuberculosis and the provision of preventive services in the care of individuals, families, and high-risk groups. The G.I. Bill enabled many nurses to return to school. A good number of those who returned specialized in public health.[20]

A survey published in 1945 by a subcommittee of the American Public Health Association revealed that some segments of the United States population were assigned to local health units whose staffing was so sparse that even the most basic services, such as communicable disease control and health education of the general public, could not be provided. The survey's recommendation that more public health nurses were needed had a substantial impact on the growth of local health departments, as well as on job opportunities for public health nurses. In fact, from the post-World War II years through the 1950s, state and federal health departments, through funding and philosophical endorsement, became increasingly active in promoting the establishment of local health departments. By 1950, 56% of the 3070 counties in the continental United States were covered by full-time local health services. By 1955, this figure had increased to 72%.[20]

The Hill-Burton Hospital Construction and Survey Act of 1946 provided matching money for construction of public health and hospital facilities. While the use of these funds by some inpatient institutions became controversial in that excess beds were created, health departments were able to move nursing offices and clinics into safer and more modern settings. Also in 1946, the constitution of the World Health Organization was drafted with input from such people as American Surgeon General Thomas Perran and the Executive Secretary of the National Nursing Council, Elmora Wickenden. From the start, the World Health Organization identified public health nursing as a district unit. Although it has undergone structural and programmatic changes since that time, public health nursing continues to play an important role in the World Health Organization.[20]

In 1952, three smaller national organizations (the National Organization of Public Health Nurses, the National League for Nursing Education, and the Association of Collegiate Schools of Nursing) were dissolved and their functions redistributed between the National

League for Nursing (NLN) and the American Nurses' Association (ANA). From that point on, the professional development of public health nursing was to be directed primarily by the NLN with the support and collaboration of the Public Health Nursing sections of the American Public Health Association (APHA) and the ANA. One of the first ideas pushed by the newly formed NLN and inspired by Esther Lucille Brown's 1948 Study of Nursing Education, was that all basic collegiate nursing programs should be required to integrate social and public health concepts throughout the curricula in order to prepare the students for beginning positions in public health. In addition, the NLN publicly supported the notion of providing education and training on the master's level for public health nursing specialists. This last idea of basic education for entry level and master's preparation for public health specialists essentially has endured up to the present day.

In the NLN's zeal to upgrade public health nursing practice by strengthening educational preparation, new requirements were sometimes implemented without a thorough look at resources for effecting the change. For instance, there was nothing wrong with suggesting that public health didactic and clinical content be made a part of undergraduate program curricula, but a problem that went unseen was that there was not a sufficient number of public or community health faculty prepared to teach the content and supervise clinical experiences. Because most faculty members lacked the necessary background, public health nursing became erroneously synonymous with "out-of-hospital nursing" and the real "contextual fiber of public health," i.e., the concept of the group and the larger community, was lost.[20]

Even though it was required that public health concepts be visible in curricula for accreditation before an adequate number of faculty could be made available to identify and teach the content, for the first time there was recognition (if not consensus) that public health nursing was a legitimate specialty within nursing that required specialized content and clinical practice. Despite the fact that increasing numbers of nurses were being educationally prepared in public health in the 1950s, nursing service directors of public health agencies complained that new graduates were unable to function clinically in public health agencies without long and intensive staff development training. The unfortunate truth is that the same complaint is still heard today.

▮ *1960 to the Present*

America in the 1960s experienced population growth, a stable economy, and space explorations, as well as rising racial tensions, increasing environmental pollution, and inequities in health care. The Economic Opportunity Act of 1964 provided funds for neighborhood health centers, Head Start, maternal and child health programs, men-

tal health and mental retardation programs, and regional medical programs for heart disease, cancer, and stroke. Chronic diseases had become the major killers of Americans, and federal funds were targeted
at their prevention and control.

After years of heated debate and in an attempt to provide health
services to the people least protected by health insurance, Congress
amended the Social Security Act in 1965 to include benefits such as
hospital and home nursing care for the elderly (Medicare), and more
types of services to the indigent (Medicaid). Although nursing organizations had pleaded that their preventive services and home health
care be included among the benefits, the bill that became law did not
allow for health promotion or preventive care as a part of home care.
Reimbursement for home care was limited to those interventions prescribed by physicians.

Much has been written about the effects of Medicare and Medicaid, but their effect on home health care was notable for several reasons. First, home health agencies that survived implementation of
Medicare and Medicaid benefited from acquisition of new skills such
as modern fiscal management, revised and standardized care procedures, and expanded nursing programs that included physical therapy, occupational therapy, specialized nutrition programs, and social
services. Additionally, in an environment of financial reimbursement
for prescribed home health care services, official agencies offering
home nursing care grew from 250 agencies in 1960 to 1328 in 1968.
Medicare reimbursement also prompted the very rapid growth of the
proprietary home health agency that was financed by entrepreneurial
groups with no interest or even particular expertise in home health
care.[20]

This unprecedented expansion of home health care agencies
combined to create considerable competition for clients. In addition,
there were perceived inequities relating to continued care for indigent
clients. In some instances, an agency would provide nursing services
as long as Medicare would provide reimbursement, but would then
drop the client or refer him to official agencies like county health departments when Medicare or Medicaid no longer covered needed visi-
tations and the client in question was unable to pay. Some of these
agencies ended up with a disproportionate number of indigent clients, partly because home health clients were referred to official or
tax-supported agencies when there was not a visible means of reimbursement. Not only did this situation create negative feelings between members of competing agencies, but it ultimately acted to frag-
ment nursing care. Finally, when a particular agency was carrying a
large load of indigent home health clients, it needed a much larger
operating budget to pay salaries and operating costs because the rate
of client reimbursement was lower.

By 1965, federal regulations made it necessary for states to submit written plans for reducing major health problems. Thus the era of

systematic evaluation of the effectiveness of public health programs formally was born. In order to prepare these plans, research and extensive documentation were needed, and those efforts continued into the 1970s and 1980s. Peer review, outcome measures, accountability, and quality assurance are now familiar processes.

By the 1970s, the notion of disease prevention had regained wide acceptance. Human behavior was recognized as a contributing factor to illness, and the birthrate was dropping sharply as safe contraceptive methods gave American women family-planning options. Public health professionals continued to develop new roles to meet the changing health care needs. One of these new roles, that of infection control nurse, began in England in 1959 and became established in the United States in 1963. Essentially, these nurses combined nursing and public health science to monitor, prevent, and control nosocomial or hospital-acquired infections. By the late 1970s, accreditation agencies required that every hospital have an active infection-control program, and the cornerstone of these programs was the infection control nurse. By the early 1980s, there were over 5000 infection control nurses nationwide, and their practice was beginning to include long-term facilities like nursing homes and home health care agencies.

In the late 1960s and 1970s, many clinical nurses moved outside the hospital as part of programs that frequently were financed by federal money. These programs were directed at early diagnosis and treatment of major health problems like caridovascular disease and diabetes. The nurses practiced in a variety of nontraditional health settings such as ambulatory clinics and health departments. Although these nurses worked in community-type settings, they lacked the specialized academic preparation and clinical experience necessary for public health practice. Because they lacked public health preparation, they focused on their clients on a one-to-one basis instead of focusing on the individual as a part of a family and a member of numerous peer groups, including a community. By 1979, there were over 64,000 registered nurses employed by state and local health agencies or boards of education. Sadly, almost half of these (49.6%) had no public health preparation.[20]

It comes as no surprise then that there was much confusion throughout the 1970s and 1980s about what actually constituted public health nursing. Not only was there confusion about the parameters of the role and what constituted appropriate preparation for that role, but a new title emerged at this time. The term "community health nurse" came into general use when the ANA sought to create an organizational entity to which nurses working in scattered community settings could belong. These nurses would come from settings such as doctors' offices, schools, and similar community sites where nurses practiced.[21]

Although several organizations, including the APHA have attempted to address the problems and clarify the issues surrounding the community health nurses such as who they are, what they should be called, and exactly what constitutes their practice base, confusion over titles and practice parameters still continues. As illustrated by the preceding historical overview, educational preparation has been an issue since the late 19th century, but by the mid-1980s, most people were agreeing that the bachelor's degree constituted adequate preparation for beginning practice, whereas specialized practice required a master's degree. Large factions in the nursing education field and in nursing practice adopted the term "community health nurse" as a replacement for the term "public health nurse." In fact, the division over titles is illustrated later in the text when the various national organizations present a definition of the role: the APHA refers to "public health nursing," whereas the NLN and ANA refer to the "community health nurse."

In September, 1984, the Division of Nursing, Bureau of Health Professions of the Health Resources and Services Administration sponsored a national invitational conference in Washington, D.C. to identify critical issues confronting community health nursing. Other goals of the conference were to examine the kind of educational preparation needed to practice in the field, and to develop some degree of consensus on the collective goals of public health nursing in the future. While the meeting was coordinated by the APHA, the major national organizations, including the ANA and the NLN, were represented. The members of that conference made the following statements:

1. At the basic level, a public health nurse is one who holds a baccalaureate degree in nursing that includes some content and clinical experience in public health nursing; this nurse may or may not practice in an official health agency, but has the initial qualifications to do so.
2. A public health nurse specialist receives preparation at the graduate level with a focus in the public health sciences. This person holds a master's or doctoral degree and may or may not practice in an official public health agency, but is educationally qualified to do so.
3. Community is a setting for practice. Just as some nurses practice in a hospital or other institutional setting, others practice in the community.
4. A "community health nurse specialist" is a nurse with at least a master's degree in any area of nursing who is practicing in the community. So the term "community health nurse" is simply an umbrella term used for all nurses who work in the community.[21]

The participants of this conference essentially agreed that the term "public health nurse" should be used to describe a person who has received specific educational preparation and supervised practice in public health nursing. Yet, the fact remains that the term "community health nurse" is used extensively by both educators and administrators. Eventually this issue of title will most likely be resolved. In the meantime, it may not be as important to focus on what we call ourselves as it is to base our practice on a synthesis of nursing and public health sciences.

Summary

*A*lthough the federal government in Colonial America left the provision of health services to the individual states and communities, federal involvement has escalated over the years. By the mid-1980s, some form of government paid for 42% of all health care expenditures compared to only 10.8% in 1965 at the dawn of Medicare/Medicaid legislation.[22] Slowed economic growth and persistent inflation during the 1980s brought curtailment in the federal funding of health services as well as limitations in other programs such as nutritional supplements for school children and food stamps for the marginally poor. With the enactment of the Gramm-Rudman Act in 1986, which was targeted at balancing the federal budget, cuts in virtually all federal programs were made.

At the end of the 1980s, population and social changes are producing new health care needs that were unthought of at the beginning of the 20th century. Human evolution and multiple technical developments are affecting and continuously reshaping the health care delivery system of which community health nursing is a part. Community health, as a nursing specialty, evolved from early efforts to promote health of human populations in factories, schools, and homes. The visiting nurse aspect of community health nursing is barely 100 years old. The concept of public health and even public health science is much older than organized nursing or nursing science, yet modern precepts from both constitute a viable basis for community health nursing practice in contemporary times. Many issues in community health nursing, such as educational preparation, title, and role functions, have been raised and addressed over the last 100 years. They have not been resolved. Resolution of these issues now lies in the hands of a new generation of nurses who have chosen to practice in the developing and innovative specialty of community health nursing.

References

1. Spradley BW: Community Health Nursing: Concepts and Practice, 2nd ed. Boston, Little, Brown & Co, 1985

2. Bullough VL, Bullough B: The Emergence of Modern Nursing, 2nd ed. Toronto, Collier–Macmillan Co. 1969

3. Hanlon JJ, Pickett GE: Public Health, Administration and Practice, 8th ed. St Louis, Times Mirror/Mosby College Pub, 1984

4. Zinsser H: Rats, Lice and History. Boston, Little, Brown & Co, 1935

5. Monteiro LA: Public health then and now: Florence Nightingale on public health nursing. Am J Public Health 75(2):181–186, 1985

6. Seymer L: Selected Writing of Florence Nightingale, p 362. New York, Macmillan, 1954

7. Kramer HO: The beginnings of the public health movement in the United States. Bull Hist Med 21:352–276, 1947

8. Tinkham CW, Voorhies EF, McCarthy NC: Community Health Nursing: Evolution and Process in the Family and the Community, 3rd ed. Norwalk, CT, Appleton-Century-Crofts, 1984

9. Bureau of the Census: A Century of Population Growth: 1790–1900. Washington, DC, Government Printing Office, 1909

10. Dulles FR: The United States Since 1865, p 91. Ann Arbor, University of Michigan Press, 1959

11. Hill HW: The New Public Health, p 30. New York, Macmillan, 1916

12. Shyrock H: The History of Nursing, pp 297–300. Philadelphia, WB Saunders, 1959

13. Jacques M: District Nursing, pp 411–425. New York, Macmillan, 1911

14. Wald LD: Windows on Henry Street. Boston, Little, Brown & Co, 1934

15. Fulmer H: History of Visiting Nurse Work in America. Am J Nurs 2(6):411–425, 1902

16. Buhler-Wilderson K: Public health nursing: In sickness or in health? Am J Public Health 75(10):1155–1161, 1985

17. Winslow CEA: The role of the visiting nurse in the campaign for public health. Am J Nurs 11(11):909–921, 1911

18. Welch WH: Papers and Addresses, vol III, p 165. Baltimore, Johns Hopkins Press, 1920

19. Shield EA: Highlights in the History of the Army Nurse Corps. Washington, DC, US Army Center of Military History, 1981

20. Roberts DE, Heinrich J: Public health nursing comes of age. Am J Public Health 75(10):1162–1172, 1985

21. United States Dept of Health and Human Services, Public Health Services, Human Resources and Services Administration, Bureau of Health Professions, Division of Nursing: Consensus Conferences on the Essentials of Public Health Nursing Practice and Education. Report of the Conference. Rockville, MD, September 5–7, 1984

22. Myers BA: Social policy and the organization of health care. In Last JM (ed): Maxcy-Rosenau Public Health and Preventive Medicine, 12th ed, chap 55, p 1656. Norwalk, CT, Appleton-Century-Crofts, 1986

Epidemiology: A Community Health Science

LEARNING OBJECTIVES

After reading and understanding the contents of this chapter, the student will be able to:

1. *Identify the seven major applications or uses of epidemiology in community health nursing practice.*

2. *Describe the process of case finding in relationship to the community health nursing role.*

3. *Outline the steps in the epidemiologic method.*

4. *Explain the relationship between the epidemiologic method and the nursing process.*

5. *List the mandated services of public health.*

6. *Define the scope of public health practice.*

Introduction

*E*pidemiology is a community or public health science. This definition is based on the innate nature of epidemiology as a scientific process applied to solve problems in the community. The nursing process also is a scientific process using observations to assess and evaluate nursing intervention in patient care. Nursing and epidemiology are both process-oriented sciences applied in practice to various and widely different situations. Looking at what nurses do for different patients in different settings leads to an understanding of nursing as a professional entity. Similarly, a discussion of epidemiologic approaches to nursing is easier to understand by examining the uses of epidemiology for addressing community problems.

■ Uses of Epidemiology

In 1975, Morris published his interpretation of the seven major uses of epidemiology as a public health science.[1] These seven areas describe general purposes for applying epidemiology to community situations.

The Uses of Epidemiology

1. To study the effects of disease states in populations over time and predict future health needs.
2. To diagnose the health of the community.
3. To evaluate health services.
4. To estimate individual risk from group experience.
5. To identify syndromes.
6. To complete the clinical picture so that prevention can be accomplished before disease is irreversible.
7. To search for cause.

Each use of epidemiology will be discussed and related to nursing in the community.

1. To Study the Effects of Disease States in Populations Over Time and Predict Future Health Needs

Morris stated that epidemiology is used in a historical context to study events over time. By looking at a population over several years or several centuries, reasonable predictions can be made about the future health of the group. This method can be used to forecast a person's average lifespan. For example, the mortality rate for a community over a series of years will indicate how long someone born in the community can be expected, on the average, to live. Epidemiology can be used to monitor changes in community characteristics over time. For example, a community that has been served by a nursing agency or institution for 50 years can be assessed for occurrences of diseases and the ongoing health status of that community. If this information has been collected continuously and responsibly, then changes in the needs for nursing services over time can be categorized. If shifts in the average age of the population, housing needs, and socioeconomic status of the population can be calculated, then the need for nursing services over time can be estimated. Predictions for future nursing care needs can be made from historical studies of the population receiving services.

2. To Diagnose the Health of the Community

Another use of epidemiology identified by Morris is community diagnosis and the identification of community health hazards. Epidemiology is used to identify outbreaks of communicable and chronic diseases wherever they may occur. The areas studied as communities may include geographic areas, such as counties or states, or they may include schools, hospitals, or industrial areas—in fact, anywhere a group exists with common interests or needs. Special epidemiologic research designs, methods, and tools have been developed to make accurate community diagnoses when a surge of similar health complaints are received. The parameters of the problem and the boundaries of the community at risk are measured using epidemiologic techniques to accomplish a complete, valid community diagnosis. In a literal sense, the area, group, or community is the subject of analysis to diagnose the state of health.

A problem in identifying an epidemic is distinguishing between an unexpected but naturally occurring chance cluster of events and indicators of hazards which are preventable or controllable. It is a challenge to the ability of the nurse to distinguish between a chance occurrence and a real threat to a group, large or small. For example, an unusual number of deaths occurred recently in an intensive care unit (ICU) in a hospital in the Midwest.[2] It was crucial to obtain facts to support the postulation that a real environmental hazard was causing this high death rate. It was logical to ask about the quality of nursing care or medical care, faulty equipment, or unusual infections that may have been associated with these deaths. The deaths had to be regarded as something other than just a selection of unusually sick patients admitted to the ICU. It was determined that the increase in the number of deaths occurred after the instigation of the Diagnostic Related Groups (DRGs). (Most hospitals experience a decrease in length of stay and a concomitant rise in seriously sick patients after the change to prospective payment systems.) In the circumstances being described, competing reasons for the unexpected rise in mortality

were not considered. Unfortunately, the deaths were said to be associated with the practices of a nurse in the unit. This charge could not
be substantiated, even after a thorough investigation in a court of
law. The nurse and, indeed, the hospital as a whole—as a community—experienced a great deal of unnecessary anxiety. Subsequently,
an epidemiologic investigation appeared to substantiate that an unusual group of sick patients had been admitted into the ICU and the
deaths were a random event. No other reason was evident. This example of the need to employ epidemiological methods in an ICU
shows that an "epidemic" investigation may be large or small. Epidemics may be concerned with death, infection, disease, accident,
precursors to disease, or threat of disaster. In all cases, epidemiology
is used to collect scientific evidence to separate chance occurrence
from the real hazards that occur to aggregates of people wherever
they may be.

Another diagnostic technique for the community is an assessment of need. Community assessment is a method of defining the
burden of disease already prevailing in a community. When this information is obtained, nursing care can be organized to meet the
needs identified during the assessment to maintain the health of the
group. The epidemiologic methods developed for diagnosing the
health of the community are consistent with public health principles
and assist the delivery of nursing services in the community.

3. To Evaluate Health Services

Epidemiology is used to estimate the utilization of health services and to investigate the reasons the services are chosen by clients
in the community. Closely associated with utilization of services is the
quality of care delivered to clients. Patient/client satisfaction is a relevant concern affecting utilization rates. Utilization, therefore, is not
only an assessment of how often services are used, it can also be an
indication of community satisfaction with nursing services received.
Knowing how often a nursing service is used contributes to the evaluation of the effectiveness of the nursing care. It is important to know
the utilization of nursing services in order to organize delivery systems that will meet the needs of the community. Access to nursing
care is, of course, an important variable in assessing utilization, and is
influenced in part by costs, transportation, and public awareness of
what is available. Nursing and medical diagnoses, including the men-
tation or mobility status of clients, must be considered as possible de-
terrents to the use of nursing services.

Mietinnen called epidemiology the "study of confounding."[3]
This means that factors ascribed to influencing an event, such as utilization of services, must be separated from factors that confound or
interfere with the true reason for choice of services. Ignoring the confounding factors may lead to erroneous conclusions called spurious
associations. If an evaluation of clinical nursing services in a commu-

nity shows that attendance at the clinic is low because the clients are too poor to afford available and necessary transportation, access to care is influencing utilization rather than dissatisfaction with the quality of nursing services. Thus poverty is confounding the choice of using nursing clinics through the clients' lack of money for transportation.

The measurement, surveillance, and utilization of services affects the organization and structure of all public health services. Data substantiating quality and impact of many kinds of care, including nursing services, affect the legislative and regulatory decisions at the political level. Information on health services, their utilization and evaluation indicates the demands and needs a community has for health care. Political action groups use these data to substantiate claims for changes in the delivery of services. Often in response to these demands, the health care system seeks new methods of delivering services. Health and social maintenance organizations (prepaid care) and preferred provider organizations (health care at a discount delivered by groups of physicians and nurses) are examples of voluntary entrepreneurial efforts to respond to societal demands concerning rising cost of care.[4]

The scientific observation and assessment of the many factors involved in delivering high quality health services is essential information, especially in times of limited financial resources. Epidemiology is the public health method of choice to provide the information necessary to make decisions on health care delivery to communities. Providers of care, such as public health nurses, use information on evaluation of services to substantiate the need for funds to make changes in delivery of services to the public.

4. *To Estimate Individual Risk from Group Experience*

Morris says that estimating individual risks from group experience is a salient use of epidemiology. The ability to identify patient/client individual risk in any hazardous event is based on the collection of information from ongoing observations of similar occurrences. This may be accomplished through epidemiologic research studies or through surveillance systems requiring registration for specific problems. Surveillance through registration is most likely to be applied when the cause of the problem event is either unknown or unsubstantiated, or when intervention for protection of the public is ineffective. Many of these problems require a distinction between inherited and environmental variables and often involve chronic diseases. To establish the individual, average risk of an event requires accurate surveillance and recording systems. In many parts of the country there are now registers for cystic fibrosis, cancer, and sudden infant death syndrome (SIDS).[5] Most of the surveillance systems for these diseases are still on a voluntary basis but provide excellent information for estimating the average risk to a family.

Community health nurses are often responsible for maintaining accurate records in surveillance systems and for educating the public on registration and recording systems. The knowledge gained from an epidemiological approach to community problems makes the consequences of poor reporting systems all too clear. The scientific principles of validity and reliability are indispensable and integral to epidemiologic methods to ensure the effective surveillance of the community. It is through these scientific principles of accuracy and consistency that epidemiology provides guidance to nurses as they collect relevant facts concerning community problems.

Community health nurses use their special education and expertise when caring for the sick and their families and for promoting healthy lifestyles. Nursing theory and nursing skills enable them to elicit information from families under the most difficult and stressful circumstances. For example, surveillance of SIDS occurs in grief-stricken families. Community health nurses may provide care and support for the bereaved. In addition, information often is gathered in circumstances associated with unlawful behaviors, such as child and elderly abuse. Also, surveillance data must be gathered on diseases that lack general societal sanction, such as acquired immune deficiency syndrome (AIDS). The balance between epidemiologic necessities and professional nursing care in such sensitive situations is a hallmark of effective community health nursing.

Many instances of individual risk have already been established through epidemiologic research and are used for the education and guidance of clients in community health nursing. For example, epidemiology showed that there is a greater risk of trisomy 21 (Down's) syndrome in pregnancies occurring in women 35 years of age or older.[6] With diagnostic methods now available for early recognition of this condition, clients can be advised of the choices available in this situation. By examining worker experience over time, epidemiological research has identified the individual risk for asbestosis or byssinosis among workers in industries that use asbestos or process cotton.[7,8] Community health nurses provide assistance and solace to individuals at risk after exposure in working situations. Surveillances in industry as well as hospitals record the history of exposure to hazards and case occurrence. Epidemiologic approaches and methods of measurement increase the ability of the community health nurse to ensure effective monitoring and recording of observation occurring within the environment to define risk from exposure to multiple hazards.

5. To Identify Syndromes

Identification of syndromes is another use of epidemiology. Through epidemiology, diseases and syndromes (a collection of signs and symptoms thought to be similar) can be identified. Syndromes or cases are differentiated by identifying a difference in epidemiologic patterns. For instance, gonorrhea and syphilis long ago were thought to be the same disease. Their epidemiologic characteristics, such as the incubation period (the time from exposure to signs of illness) were the facts that assisted in identifying two different diseases caused by two different organisms. Another example of case identification occurred in herpetic infections caused by Herpes hominis I (herpes simplex virus) and Herpes hominis II. The different epidemiologic characteristics produced by infections from these two viruses were distinguished in the 1970s by observing the different distributions or patterns of the characteristics associated with the two infections. Herpes hominis I infection occurs at an earlier age in crowded family circumstances and in lower socioeconomic groups. In contrast, Herpes hominis II infection occurs with the onset of sexual activity.[9] These distinctions are important in directing community health nursing interventions for prevention and control. Identifying new syndromes is also the purview of epidemiology. Toxic shock syndrome, a staphylococcal infection causing severe illness and sometimes death, is an example of a new syndrome of the 1980s that threatened the community.[10]

In nursing, epidemiology can be applied to case finding and/or syndrome identification during the delivery of care. The community health nurse has access to homes, schools, and agencies in the community. In these (and other) settings, clients take advantage of the proximity of the nurse to share concerns and physical complaints that may be obscure enough to be called a syndrome but are not severe enough to promote self-diagnosis or care-seeking behavior. Nurses must make judgments concerning the referral of clients to other disciplines, the giving of emergency nursing care, and the education and counseling of clients according to their needs. It is diverse settings that provide the community health nurse with the opportunity to identify syndromes and cases of disease, and it is the knowledge of nursing care for the sick that establishes the credibility of the community health nurse as a trustworthy resource to solve health problems in the community. During delivery of care to the sick, the nurse has the opportunity to identify the needs, syndromes, and illnesses of the group or family members who have no overt complaints.

Case finding and the identification of persons requiring medical and nursing care and syndrome identification is a responsibility of the community health nurse (CHN). In the context of the epidemiologic approach, case finding must be grouped and classified for similarities and commonalities. The activity of syndrome/case identification should be placed in the context of groups of cases in order to be the most effective guide for nursing services. The community health nurse is in a singular position to identify and accumulate similar complaints within a given community. Observation of frequent and similar occurrences may identify a wider community threat. The perspective of placing observed events and associating them as a group occurrence is an epidemiologic approach enabling the nurse to unite events in a logical way in order to intervene for the well-being of the whole community.

> 6. *To Complete the Clinical Picture of Disease so that Prevention can be Accomplished Before the Disease is Irreversible*

The sixth use of epidemiology identified by Morris is completing the clinical picture before the disease is irreversible. This involves identifying the precursors of diseases so that groups at high risk can be identified. This use of epidemiology can be interpreted as identifying intermediate steps in a cycle of events so that the evolution of a disease can be elucidated, or it can refer to physiologic changes predicting a state of illness, such as high blood pressure. Historically, malaria (literally "bad air") was thought to be spread through the miasma associated with water in low-lying marshes. Today it is known that the mosquito of the genus *Anopheles* carries a protozoan parasite of the genus *Plasmodium*, which breeds in shallow, still water. The protozoan is injected into humans through the salivary glands of the female mosquito and reproduces asexually in the human liver. The clinical picture typically is recurrent chills and fever, depending on the time required to develop a new generation of parasites that periodically invade the bloodstream. Thus, the clinical picture for malaria was incomplete until the discovery of the route of transmission through the vector in the life cycle of the protozoan. Thus the clinical picture of disease was completed, and the occasion for intervening for prevention was clarified.

Another example of the sixth use of epidemiology is in the treatment of cardiovascular disease. Advances in cardiovascular disease have identified certain physiologic conditions that exist before this disease is diagnosed. High cholesterol and lipid levels in the blood indicate a greater chance of developing heart disease. High blood pressure levels indicate a greater chance of a cerebrovascular accident. Disease indicators, such as high levels of blood cholesterol, high lipid levels, and high blood pressure readings are called precursors to disease. By controlling these precursors, the mortality rate for cardiovascular disease can be reduced. This, in fact, has been accomplished through public health efforts that screen populations for precursors, identify high-risk groups, and deliver services to control not the disease but the precursors of the disease. Community health nursing has played an important role in organizing and executing these multidisciplinary efforts aimed at disease prevention.

Much work still needs to be done to complete the clinical picture of disease. For instance, community health nurses play an important and indispensable role in the care of patients with diabetes mellitus—a disease in which the development of complications is still obscure. Early death occurs in some diabetics from complications, and the reason remains obscure. It has been postulated that there is a special group of diabetics at high risk for rapid onset of complications. As yet, there are few indicators or precursors to disease that would identify this high-risk group. Completing the clinical picture by identifying precursors to the complications of diabetes will provide a method of identifying high-risk groups. Nursing intervention then will be more effective because it will be directed to the antecedents of this disease.[11] It is a community health nurse's responsibility not only to intervene in the disease process but also to participate in gathering observations to identify precursors that will complete the clinical picture.

7. To Search for Cause

The final use of epidemiology identified by Morris is to search for cause. When the cause of a disease is known, prevention, control, and treatment can focus on the most precise and effective methods of intervention. However, it is not necessary to know the cause before initiating protective procedures. It has already been noted that in the control of smallpox, vaccinations took place without the causative agent being known. Even when the agent is known, it does not always indicate curative care. In AIDS, the agent(s) causing the problem have been identified; however, we still do not know how to promote effective treatment for this deadly disease. The search for a cause may be interpreted in a slightly different context for nursing care. Nursing is interested not only in the cause of a disease but also in the reasons for the delay in rehabilitation, the cause of recidivism in health behaviors and the cause of lack of client/patient compliance. These other "causes" suggest nursing interventions that can be focused with more precision and directed to meet the needs of the community.

▪ Epidemiologic Method and the Nursing Process

The uses of epidemiology illustrate the scope of the science as it is used for public health and for nursing care in communities. Epidemiology has developed methods and measuring tools designed to enhance the effectiveness of applied epidemiology to solve community problems. The methods of epidemiology are inductive, that is, they are scientific methods adapted for researching community needs. Induction is a method of collecting facts from which generalizations are derived. The formulation of hypotheses, statements of expected relationships between cause and effect, is part of the method. Testing of the hypothesis, repeatedly if necessary, leads to conclusions for prevention and control of hazards to groups. The epidemiologic method is a process, a series of steps inductive in nature, designed to solve problems in communities requiring immediate attention and clinical intervention.[12] The steps of the method are outlined in Figure 2-1.

The model is traditional because it is a method identified as the

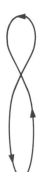

1. Establish the existence of an epidemic or community problem
2. Verify the diagnosis of the cases causing the problem
3. Make a quick survey of known cases and the community situation
4. Formulate tentative hypothesis concerning the possible cause of the problem
5. Plan a detailed epidemiologic investigation
6. Conduct the investigation
7. Analyze data collected during the investigation
8. Test the hypothesis
9. Formulate conclusions
10. Put control measures into operation
11. Make report

F I G U R E   2 - 1
Outline of the traditional epidemiologic method.

process used to solve acute communicable disease problems in the past. It is still used today to solve acute problems. During the application of the epidemiologic process, the hypothesis may be rejected. In this case, reformulation of other hypotheses is necessary, and the process must be repeated until solutions implied in the hypotheses can be verified. Thus, the epidemiologic process can be called a linear model, which is iterative and dynamic.

The nursing process can also be called a linear model, one concept leading to another, as illustrated in Figure 2-2.

Reapplication of the nursing process also creates an iterative and dynamic process for patient care. The epidemiologic method and

A Comparison of Nursing Process and the Epidemiologic Model

NURSING PROCESS	EPIDEMIOLOGIC METHOD
• Assess	• Establish the existence of an epidemic
	Verify the diagnosis of the cases
	Make a quick survey of known cases and the community situation
• Formulate a nursing diagnosis	• Formulate a tentative hypothesis
• Plan and intervene	• Plan and conduct the investigation
• Evaluate	• Analyze, test, and formulate conclusions

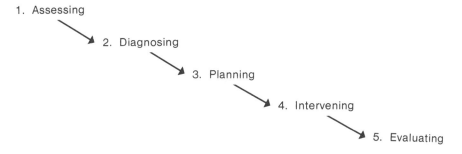

F I G U R E   2 - 2
The nursing process as a linear model. (Adapted from Stanton M, Paul C, Reeves JS:
An overview of the nursing process. In George JB [ed]: Nursing Theories: The Base for
Professional Nursing Practice, 2nd ed, pp 14–33, Englewood Cliffs, NJ,
Prentice-Hall, 1985)

nursing process are analogous: establishing the existence of an epidemic, verifying the diagnosis of the cases, and making a quick survey of known cases and the community situation is similar to making
a nursing assessment. Formulating a tentative hypothesis is equivalent to making a nursing diagnosis. Planning and conducting the
investigation is like planning nursing intervention. Evaluation of the
results of the nursing plan is similar to analyzing and testing epidemiologic data, and formulating conclusions. Besides these obvious procedural parallels, both processes are based on the use of observations
to make judgments. In the application of the epidemiologic method
and the nursing method, there is a constant, dynamic interaction so
that assessment, evaluation, diagnosis, and planning intervention are
recurring events. In the epidemiologic process, the testing of the hypothesis may result in rejecting a hypothesized causal relationship.
This requires reexamination of the situation and formulating another
hypothesis on which to plan the investigation of the community problem. The difference between the nursing process and epidemiologic
method is that the epidemiologic process is applied *only* to groups;
the nursing process is individualistic and applies to groups only when
the concept of community is clearly understood to be the focus of the
nurse. Both processes are inductive, both are based on observations,
and both are based on scientific evaluation. Although the nursing
process can be used to assess community problems directly, it is the
epidemiologic process and its methods of quantification that augment
the nursing process. Together they provide an effective program of
assessment, diagnosis, and intervention in the community. The difference between the two processes is that epidemiologic method extends
the nursing process to include a well-defined hypothesis rather than a
diagnosis for nursing care. The hypothesis relates to community problems requiring a postulated cause. In the nursing process, the diagno-

sis is more circumscribed and based on known facts rather than unknown relationships.

Cholera and the Broad Street Pump—A Classic Epidemiologic Investigation

An example of the application of the epidemiologic method and the role of the hypothesis in the inductive process is the classic investigation of cholera made by Dr. John Snow in London in 1856. This investigation of a cholera epidemic that was caused by contaminated water from the Broad Street pump in the Soho district heralded the era of modern epidemiology. The Broad Street pump has become a symbol of prevention and control of disease in communities.

Cholera is no longer a dreaded disease except in third world nations. In the middle of the 19th century, however, cholera ravaged urban and rural populations, leaving death and chaos in its wake. Dr. Snow's investigation took place before sanitation changed the environment of cities. A discussion of the epidemic requires some understanding of what life was like in London, England, where Snow lived and worked. In 1856, London was the largest city in the world. Chadwick and other social reformers inspected the districts in London by going on what were called "walking tours," making observations as they strolled along the streets and squares of the community.[13] Their written observations are difficult to comprehend by today's standards, for they reported conditions of the utmost filth that were inexcusable, even in those days. Common privies were available, but frequently overflowed. As a result, most people avoided the privies and stored fecal matter in their homes. Disease and poverty were commonplace, and the stench of the streets was often unendurable. Chadwick commented that even in comparatively "healthy" districts, or parishes as they were called, heaps of rubbish lay decaying. It was under these community conditions that the cholera epidemic broke out in the 1850s.

Dr. Snow had been working in several parts of the city and came upon Broad Street in the Soho district on September 1, 1856. He observed a water pump situated in the middle of a square formed at the intersection of Broad Street and another thoroughfare. There was a percussion cap factory on the street and a church in the vicinity, but the area was mainly residential. During Snow's preliminary survey of the community situation, he discovered that 500 deaths from cholera had occurred in a 14-week period. The signs and symptoms of cholera were too familiar to doubt the diagnosis: an epidemic existed in the area, and it was pervasive and spreading rapidly. The pump was the only supply of drinking water for the area. Snow investigated 89 fatal cases of cholera and found that 68 people who died drank water from the Broad Street pump. He formulated a hypothesis that was extraordinary for his time: he said that something unseen was contaminating the water and spreading the disease! On September 7th, he took the handle off the pump to keep people from drinking the water in an effort to prevent and control the epidemic. Then he made his report and published it, mainly, as he said, to allay the fears of the people by demonstrating how he had controlled the spread of the disease.

According to Chave, the General Board of Health of the parish rejected outright Snow's hypothesis of spread of cholera by a contaminant in the drinking water.[14] The Board preferred the alternate hypothesis that cholera was spread by a widely diffuse agent that was not infectious and therefore not passed from person to person. The Board held a meeting and appointed a committee to investigate Snow's hypothesis. The committee, composed of several church wardens and physicians, was chaired by Dr. Earl Lancaster. Lancaster's committee appealed for monetary support from the Board of Guardians of the Poor, but the Board was reluctant to release funds to continue the study because trade was depressed; besides, they said, the hypothesis of contaminated water was absurd. A motion was made in committee to discontinue the investigative work, but it failed by one vote. Lancaster then requested that information about the cases of cholera around Broad Street be made available to the committee by the Boards of the Parishes. This request also was refused because it was thought that the investigation of the epidemic should be independent of local government. After becoming informed of this decision, the committee decided to circulate a questionnaire to all households with cases of cholera in an effort to collect their own information. They found that a questionnaire was a most unsuccessful way to collect data because most people in the parish around Broad Street could not read. At this point, the committee decided to conduct personal interviews and invited Dr. Snow and Henry Whitehead, the vicar of the church near Broad Street, to conduct the investigation. Dr. Snow gave a copy of his preliminary findings to Whitehead and left to investigate a cholera outbreak in another part of London. After reading Snow's report, Whitehead disagreed with the "Snovian" hypothesis and set out to establish that it was wrong. He formulated yet another (alternate) hypothesis, which said that the reason for the spread of cholera was miasma, or stench around drains, in the streets (shades of malaria!).

At this point in the investigation, the following three hypotheses existed: (1) the epidemic of cholera was caused by something contaminating the water in the well (Snow's postulation); (2) the epidemic of cholera was caused by a diffuse agent in the atmosphere; and (3) the epidemic was associated with stench or "effluvia" from drains in the streets. To test these hypotheses, Whitehead planned to interview every resident on Broad Street, including those who stayed well. Some had moved away from this district, but he was undeterred and followed them to their new homes. As a pastor, he was known and trusted by the local people, and they welcomed him as he went to see them repeatedly to make inquiries about the epidemic and confirm his information. He found out fairly quickly that the number of cholera cases was not greater among people close to drains; whereupon he started to collect information to test Snow's hypothesis. Whitehead was a cautious epidemiologist who documented as much information as possible, including the age, sex, and household position of the people occupying the houses of the deceased or ill. He categorized the sanitary arrangements and collected information on the sources of drinking water. He knew the number of persons occupying each residence and the hour of onset of illness. He verified that the two private water companies in the town did not supply the Broad Street pump. He became interested in the cases that drank the water but did *not* become ill, for he admitted that he himself had taken a little water from the pump to dilute the brandy which he occasionally imbibed. All in all, he contacted 497 people on whom he had taken extensive notes.

In addition, he used a clinical case history, a method used in epidemiology, to provide an illustrative example of group experience. A widow and her two sons who lived a distance from Broad Street on the edge of Whitehead's parish died from cholera. When he went to visit their home, he discovered that she was the owner of the percussion cap factory located near the Broad Street pump and that her two sons had managed the factory. Each evening when they came home, they filled bottles with water from the pump to carry to their mother; subsequently all the family perished from cholera.

After collecting his information, Whitehead organized the data to test the hypothesis. In analyzing 84 deaths, he found that of 56 who were residents of the Broad Street area, only two did not drink water from the pump. He counted 28 nonresident deaths, of which 24 people worked in a factory near the pump on Broad Street and had access to the pump. These findings are shown in Figure 2-3.

Snow noted that the aged and infirm did not get cholera as much as the healthy young population. He assumed that, since the aged and infirm had no children to fetch water from the pump, they drank sparingly and avoided large doses of the contaminated water. Snow found that at the peak of the epidemic, on August 31st, 35 of the cholera victims had consumed pump water after August 30th and 34 had an onset of symptoms on September 2nd. When Whitehead investigated people who had not been ill, he found that 43 of 279 people drank the water. He also noted that there had been a decline in cholera cases after September 2nd and there were no cases after September 6th until the time the pump handle was reconnected. As Whitehead continued, he discovered that of 50 recovered cases, 35 consumed water from the pump after the handle had been replaced, which was about a month after Snow removed it. After analyzing all

Deaths from cholera, London, 1865

	Pump water used	Pump water not used	
Residents	54	2	56
Nonresidents	24	4	28
	78	6	84

F I G U R E   2 - 3
Relationship of deaths of residents and nonresidents in Broad Street areas to using water from the Broad Street pump. (Chave SPW: Henry Whitehead and Cholera in Broad Street. Baltimore, Johns Hopkins, 1946)

the evidence, Whitehead concluded that Snow's hypothesis was correct and formulated a further hypothesis of intermittent contamination of the pump water in view of the fact that too many people drank water from the pump and survived. However, he still could not understand how contamination occurred. After extensive review of his records, Whitehead decided he had to make his report to the committee and present the findings without knowing the source of the contamination. On the way to the meeting, he recalled that a baby who lived close to the Broad Street pump died. Instead of continuing on to the meeting, he went back to review the mortality records at the church and reinterviewed the baby's mother. She confirmed that when the baby became ill, she threw the soiled water from washing the diapers down a drain conveniently situated on the corner of the square near the pump. Armed with this information, Whitehead hurried to keep his appointment with the committee and persuaded them to examine that drain. They ultimately found that the wall had crumbled between the drain and the pump and, indeed, the soiled water was contaminating the pump water. With the baby's death on September 2nd, the known source of gross contamination ceased, and subsequently the number of cholera cases also started to decline. Thus, Whitehead confirmed that cholera was spread through water and that contamination of the water was intermittent, through the waste water from the laundering of diapers.

A review of these facts raises a question concerning the effectiveness of taking the handle off the pump as a measure of prevention. If the death of the baby prevented any further gross contamination of the drain with soiled water after September 2nd, it is reasonable to expect that after the date of the baby's death, the epidemic would begin to subside. Whitehead was able to document the decrease in cholera cases after that date. Did Snow's famous preventive measure of disconnecting the handle really control the epidemic, or would the epidemic have waned even if the pump had remained intact? It is worthy to note that the baby's father became ill on September 8th and died on the 12th. If the wife continued to contaminate the drain from the father's excretions, just as she had with the baby's diaper water, then the absence of the handle probably prevented further illness and death, for the handle was restored at least three weeks later. The question of evaluating the preventive action must remain as an example of trying to establish what might have happened if there had been no intervention to control disease.

This historic epidemiologic study demonstrates the importance of hypothesis formulation in the application of epidemiologic method and the quantification of data. It also describes the dynamic quality of the process of reevaluation, the collection of details, and the testing of hypotheses through the application of scientific logic. The nursing process uses a similar approach in cases where nursing diagnoses are important guides to intervention and reevaluation based on observations. The union of nursing process and epidemiologic method is a powerful alliance for assessing, diagnosing, planning, intervening, and evaluating problems in public health.

■ *A Model For Clinical Practice of Community Health Nursing*

The epidemiologic method has been presented as a linear model. The nursing process, according to Stanton and colleagues, is also a linear model that can be arranged in a circular pattern to indicate iteration of the decision-making process[15] (Fig. 2-4).

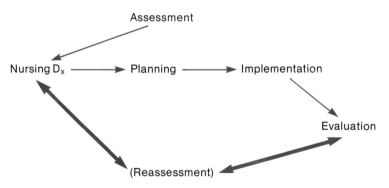

F I G U R E 2 - 4
Nursing process as a "forward movement" model. (Stanton M, Paul C, Reeves JS: An overview of the nursing process. In George JB [ed]: Nursing Theories: The Base for Professional Nursing Practice, 2nd ed, pp 14–33. Englewood Cliffs, NJ, Prentice-Hall, 1985)

Models are defined as diagrammatic or mathematical displays of logical constructs used to develop hypotheses and to guide practice by forming a "blueprint" or template of conceptualizations on which practice is based. According to Fitzpatrick and Whall, conceptual models or frameworks contribute to understanding the nature of nursing by demonstrating the general relationships of nursing practice.[16] Eventually, theories can be developed from nursing models composed of many levels of abstractions. In community health nursing, not only is it necessary to identify a model conceptualizing the nature of nursing, but it is also necessary to identify models contributing to the nature of the field of public health. The epidemiologic process is consistent with the philosophy or concepts of public health because epidemiology was designed to fulfill public health principles of prevention and control of disease. The identity of community health in nursing care in the community is a critical factor in defining the roles and responsibilities of the community health nurse as an epidemiologic function. As Banta says, "unless we have a common definition of what we are seeking, it will be impossible to articulate goals and objectives that can be translated into action."[17]

Archer and Fleshman have developed an approach for defining the uniqueness of any nursing specialty area.[18] They suggest that a field of specialization in nursing has two main components: the art and science of nursing and the art and science of the area of specialization. The area of overlap of the two areas indicates the unique blend of nursing and the field of the critical discipline (Fig. 2-5).

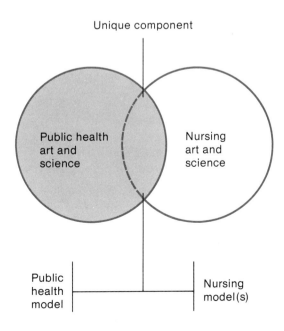

FIGURE 2-5
Archer and Fleshman model for identifying nursing specialty areas. (Archer SE, Fleshman RP: Community Health Nursing: Education and Practice. NY, NLN, 1980)

There are many models for nursing, such as Roy's adaptation model, Orem's self-care model, Orlando's collaborative model, Johnson's behavioral system, Fitzpatrick's rhythm model, and Rogers' humanistic model, to name a few. White's value model is designed for community health nursing and Betty Neumann's health model is also applicable to community health nursing.[19,20] Both models attempt to combine nursing and public health principles or constructs.

Henderson and Nightingale formulated definitions of nursing from which models can be derived. Abstracting principles from a definition constitutes deductive reasoning because a definition is a canon from which constructs and concepts are taken to form a framework to guide practice. To simplify the present discussion of the unique properties of public health from a generalistic point of view, the nursing component is stipulated as nursing process—a process that is intrinsic to all nursing models so that the need to justify a particular nursing model for public health is obviated. We will use a deductive approach similar to the models that have been derived from definitions of nursing. The public health clinical model will be abstracted from a definition of public health.

To begin the deductive process, a definition of public health will be chosen from which constructs and concepts for a public health clinical model will be derived. C. E. A. Winslow's definition is the one most often quoted in the field of public health. It was published in 1945, but it is as relevant today as it was then.[21] Moreover, Dr. Winslow was a proponent of community health nursing and appreciated the singular contribution of the community health nurse to community health. The complete definition by Winslow is quite long and includes a direct reference to nursing services and medical care, as well as a list of the public health services required by law.[22] Because of the legal mandate to deliver these services, they are called the basic activities of public health departments. The mandated services of public health are

1. To collect vital statistics
2. To control sanitary conditions
3. To control communicable diseases
4. To provide laboratory services
5. To protect the health of mothers and infants
6. To educate the public for promotion of health

The definition of public health by Winslow is paraphrased to form the basis of a clinical model for public health practices. In brief, the definition says that "public health is the art and science of prolonging life, promoting health and preventing disease through organized community efforts." The definition then is completed by summarizing the basic activities of public health. It seems reasonable to abstract the first construct for applied public health as the delivery of professional services. Bixler described a profession as a body of persons employed in an autonomous calling requiring higher education and research, exalting service above personal gain, and ensuring freedom of action for its members.[23] The nursing profession exemplifies these criteria, and so do many other providers of public health services in the community.

■ *Concepts of Multidisciplinary Care and the Community*

Public health services are distinguished by their multidisciplinary nature as well as their professional character. The mandated services are diverse and complex and require the participation of several professions. In public health, services are often delivered by many professionals acting together and involve many professional groups, of which nursing is an indispensable and separate discipline. Alternately, the other professions act as resources for the nursing profession to ensure that all the needs of the community receive appropriate care. The multidisciplinary nature of professional services in public health is pervasive. It is the secondary concept characterizing public health and is intrinsic in the definition. It is a natural step in logic to deduce that professional services emphasizing a multidisciplinary approach must have a special focus to distinguish these services from individualized patient care. The community orientation of public health supplies this focus. Community is a multifaceted concept; it may be defined geographically, as a state or a county; it may be defined as the target population for nursing services; or it may be defined by demographics such as sex, race, and age, or by need, such as the sudden infant death syndrome (SIDS) community. A definition of community consistent with Winslow's public health definition is that a community is any group that has common needs and common demands, and seeks solutions through cooperative efforts. The construct of community is basic to public health and is included in the model for clinical practice.

The Family as a Concept within the Community

It is reasonable to question how small a group can be in order to meet the definition of a community. In nursing, this depends on the need of the population concerned. Communities may be intramural (literally "within walls," such as the hospital, a school, or an industry), or they may be extramural (defined by space, by culture, or by neighborhood). What is important is that the community, the aggregate or group, assumes a totality of its own when group needs are addressed—this being the most effective way to protect the individual family. Within a community, the smallest groups are called "units of concern," and it is these units that are related to the whole community during nursing assessment. In public health nursing, the unit of concern, according to Freeman, is the family.[24] Family is a concept subsumed within the construct of community and may be defined as a commune, a group with genes in common, or an extended family including those related by marriage. A definition useful for organizing nursing care is that a family is the support system around any individual. This enables individuals living alone to be perceived, conceptually, as a family unit. It also enables the family support system to assume a place in relationship to the broader community. In caring for this unit of concern, this family, the needs of the outer community are served. Family is, therefore, an important concept as the smallest unit in the aggregate and an indispensable conceptualization in the delivery of professional community nursing services.

■ *Levels of Prevention*

Up to this point, we have identified the constructs of delivery of professional services and of community from which we have derived the concepts of multidisciplinary care and the family. In public health, all services, including nursing care, are delivered for a specific purpose so important that it forms another major construct for the public health model. The fundamental reason for public health practice is the prevention of disease and disability in the community and the control of unpreventable diseases. Prevention and control has been defined by Leavell and Clark as a three-tiered concept consisting of primary (1°), secondary (2°), and tertiary (3°) levels. Primary prevention occurs before the disease is present in the community. Examples of primary prevention are health education of groups, the maintenance of nutritional status by support of food programs for high-risk populations, legislation for safety belt use, anti-smoking campaigns, and environmental programs for sanitation and safety. Secondary prevention is the early diagnosis of health problems in the population. Typical of these services are community assessment, screening groups for case/syndrome identification, early recognition of nosocomial infection in hospitals and nursing homes, and the early documentation of exposure to toxins and noxious agents in the community. Within the family and community, early findings of previously undiagnosed conditions is a secondary level of prevention. The third level of prevention is rehabilitation of chronic disabilities and diseases. The principle of prevention is applied by reducing the effects of disabilities and promoting the self-reliance and independence of the chronically ill. Rehabilitation includes nursing care to promote a return to work in the community for people with mental and social problems, as well as assisting disabled groups in maintaining self-sufficiency and productivity so that the burden on the community is lightened and the health of the general population is enhanced.

■ *Surveillance and Provider Outreach*

Public health has two other concepts that influence the philosophy of delivering care to the community and contribute to the identity of public health as a specialized orientation. These two concepts are constant surveillance and provider outreach. Both principles are fundamental to the basic nature of public health through their ability to effect methods of prevention and control. Surveillance is defined as a method of monitoring emerging hazards in the community. Surveillance is operationalized through the epidemiologic method, or, to put it another way, it is through surveillance that epidemics are identified and the health of the community is diagnosed. The threat to community well-being may manifest as immediate dangers or gradually emerging problems evolving over time. It is a professional nursing responsibility to apply surveillance activities in order to find new cases within family units and relate this activity to the community as a whole. Locating and identifying individuals with problems as early as possible requires constant monitoring to relieve the burden of illness in the total community as efficiently and effectively as possible.

Closely allied to the concept of surveillance is the concept of provider outreach. It is through provider outreach that services are provided for problems identified by monitoring systems; however, the concept of provider outreach requires a more detailed explanation. Provider outreach ensures intervention in the community, preferably before the target population is aware of its own needs. Typically, provider outreach is an intermittent activity even though it may be provided for long periods of time. This principle is exemplified by setting up clinics in the community for preventive services such as immunizations, well-baby care, family planning, and community screening in search of specific health problems. Provider outreach epitomizes the principle of prevention and control. It prescribes the ultimate practice to ensure maximum safety for the health of the community. The definition of provider outreach is summarized as the delivery of services in the client/patient's own environment, such as the school, home, place of employment, or neighborhood, that require intermittent client contact over time to meet a need defined previously by the provider(s) of care.[25]

Three constructs and four concepts are derived from C. E. A. Winslow's definition of public health. These seven principles encompass and identify the nature of all services delivered in the community. When activated by the nursing process, they provide a clinical model for community health nursing. The seven principles are

1. *The delivery of professional services*
2. The concept of *community*
3. The *prevention and control* of disease to promote the health of populations

4. The use of *multidisciplinary* resources for service delivery
5. The *constant surveillance* of the community to monitor hazards to the health of the public
6. The concept of *provider outreach* or providing intermittent services to groups to meet previously defined needs
7. The *family* as the unit of concern within the population

The conceptual framework is interrelated and is applied simultaneously to form a "blueprint" for public health practice. These interrelationships are shown as overlapping circles in Figure 2-6.

The nursing process of assessing, diagnosing, planning, intervening, and evaluating operates in the context of these interdependent principles and brings a dynamic quality to the public health model. This model, when viewed as interrelated and inseparable components, identifies the unique activities of public health nursing and distinguishes this specialty area from any other area of nursing care. It has been used effectively to research clinical situations requiring the identification of community health nursing activities during delivery of care.[26] The model does not include the principles of management of nursing services; it is a model for clinical nursing practices in public health and is confined to practice occurring during day-to-day interaction with clients, with families, and in communities by providing

FIGURE
2 - 6
A public health model for practice. (Reprinted with permission from Chavigny KH, Kroske M: Public health nursing in crisis. Nurs Outlook 31[6]:312–316; © 1983, American Journal of Nursing Company)

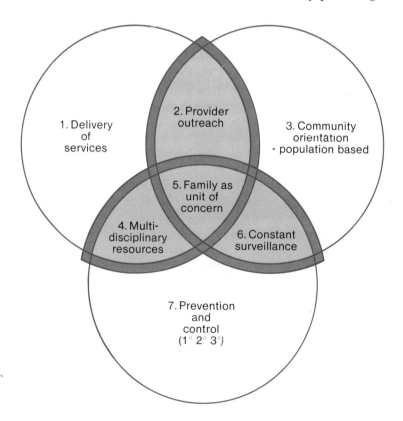

1. Delivery of services
2. Provider outreach
3. Community orientation - population based
4. Multi-disciplinary resources
5. Family as unit of concern
6. Constant surveillance
7. Prevention and control (1° 2° 3°)

hands-on, applied services. The application of this model reflects the role of the community health nurse as a generalist rather than a specialist, such as a nurse executive, or a nurse researcher; however, the model also may form a basis for practice for the clinical community health nurse specialist at the graduate level through the use of an advanced nursing model.

Summary

*A*ccording to Morris, there are seven main applications of epidemiology in nursing care. Epidemiology is used to describe the changes over time in community characteristics and to predict future nursing care needs. Community health nurses have developed unique skills from many areas for nursing the sick and well. When these skills are combined with epidemiologic methods, community health nurses can diagnose the presence of hazards to groups in many settings. The utilization of health services in the context of an epidemiologic approach provides facts to promote a logical basis for political and legislative changes that will benefit the community. Epidemiologic approaches ensure that optimum surveillance and collection of information will take place and that reliable data banks will be provided for future investigation. Identification of syndromes and new facts contributing to disease, when analyzed for commonalities or clusters within community settings, assist in identifying high-risk groups and in organizing effective nursing interventions. Finally, epidemiology is used to identify cause. It is effective in identifying not only the cause of a disease but also the causes influencing the effectiveness of nursing actions in the delivery of health care to populations.

Epidemiology enhances the nursing process by expanding the inductive approach of nursing so that it can be effective in planning and evaluating nursing intervention in groups. Also, epidemiology is a public health science designed to accomplish the major objectives of public health initiatives. The nature of public health for clinical practice is explored through a clinical model consisting of seven interrelated conceptualizations of community, delivery of professional services, multidisciplinary resources, family, constant surveillance, provider outreach, and prevention and control of diseases. These principles provide a framework for clinical practice in community health nursing that is consistent with an epidemiologic approach.

References

1. Morris JN: Uses of Epidemiology, 3rd ed. New York, Churchill Livingstone, 1975
2. American Medical News: Does profit overpower quality of nursing home care? June 7, 1985, p 2
3. Miettinen OS: Theoretical Epidemiology: Principles of Occurrence Research in Medicine. New York, John Wiley & Sons, 1985
4. Lefton D: Hospital Chains Open National PPOs, HMOs. American Medical News 28(34):1;11–14, September 13, 1985
5. SIDS Surveillance System Oregon State Department of Health and Human Resources, 1986, personal communication
6. Hook EB, Lindsjo A: Down syndrome in live births by single year maternal age internal in a Swedish strictly comparison with results from a New York State study. Am J Hum Genet 30(1):19–27, 1978
7. Selikoff IJ, Hammond EC, Churg J: Asbestos exposure, smoking, and neoplasia. JAMA 204(2):106–112, 1968
8. Schilling RSF, Hughes JPW, Dingwall I et al: An epidemiologic study of byssinosis among Lancashire Colter Workers. Br J Ind Hygiene 12:217–227, 1955
9. Engelburg A, Piacigelli G, Petersen M et al: Medical and industrial hygiene characterization of the cotton waste utilization industry. Am J Ind Med 7:93–108, 1985
10. Rawls WE, Gardner HL, Flanders RW et al: Genital herpes in two social groups. Am J Obstet Gynecol 110:682–689, 1971
11. Centers for Disease Control: Toxic-Shock Syndrome—United States. MMWR 29(20):229–230, 1980
12. Chavigny KH: Epidemiology and Outbreak Investigation. In Gurevich I, Tafuro P, Cunha BA (eds): The Theory and Practice of Infection Control, pp. 28–46. New York, Praeger, 1984
13. Flinn MW: Report on the Sanitary Conditions of the Labouring Population in Great Britain 1842. Edinburgh, University of Edinburgh Press, 1965
14. Chave SPW: Cholera and the Broad Street Pump. Baltimore, Johns Hopkins, 1946
15. Stanton M, Paul C, Reeves JS: An overview of the nursing process. In George JB (ed): Nursing Theories: The Base for Professional Nursing Practice, 2nd ed, pp. 14–33. Englewood Cliffs, NJ, Prentice-Hall, 1985
16. Fitzpatrick JJ, Whall AL: Conceptual Models of Nursing: Analysis and Application. Bowie, MD, Robert J Brady, 1983
17. Banta JE: Definition of community health. In National League for Nursing, Southern Regional Assembly of Constituent Leagues for Nursing: Community Health: Today and Tomorrow (Pub No 52-1768), pp 5–13. New York, The League, 1979
18. Archer SE, Fleshman RP: Perspectives of community health nursing education. In National League for Nursing: Community Health Nursing: Education and Practice (Pub No 52-1834), pp 13–41. New York, The League, 1980
19. White MS: Constructs for public health nursing. Nurs Outlook 30(9):527–530, 1982
20. Neuman M: Theoretical Models. Norwalk, CT, Appleton-Century-Crofts, 1986

21. Winslow CEA: The evolution of public health and its objectives. In Simmons JE (ed): Public Health in the World Today, pp 23–24. Cambridge, Harvard University Press, 1949

22. Hanlon JJ, Pickett GE: Public Health: Administration and Practice, 8th ed, p 4. St Louis, Times Mirror/Mosby College Pub, 1984

23. Bixler G, Bixler RW: The professional status of nursing. Am J Nurs 59(8):1142–1147, 1959

24. Freeman RB, Heinrich J: Community Health Nursing Practice, 2nd ed. Philadelphia, WB Saunders, 1981

25. Chavigny KH, Kroske M: Public Health Nursing in Crisis. Nurs Outlook 31(6):312–316, 1983

26. Chavigny KH, Kroske M: A Method of Identifying Nursing Specialty Areas. Abstracts of the International Conference on Nursing Research, Edmonton, Alberta, May, 1986

The Natural History of Disease—A Preventive Model for Community Health Nursing Practice

LEARNING OBJECTIVES

After reading and understanding the contents of this chapter, the student will be able to:

1. Name the three components that influence the onset of any disease process or health phenomenon.

2. Describe the relationship between the levels of prevention and the natural history model.

3. Explain the concept of multiple causation.

4. Define each of the levels of prevention and give examples of each related to community health nursing practice.

5. Identify each of the stages of the natural history of disease.

Introduction

The natural history of disease schema was first described formally by Leavell and Clark in the early 1950s. It was designed to guide public health personnel in their endeavor to promote optimum health, to prevent departures from health, and to prevent disabling illness after the onset of disease. Epidemiologists used the term "natural history" as far back as 1860 in the United States as an analogy for the clinical course of disease. However, the term remained largely undefined and unassociated with specific preventive strategies prior to 1953.[1]

By using the components of this model and consulting contemporary literature to ascertain the level of current knowledge, community health nurses are able to clearly identify priorities for preventive activity for any health problem in virtually any population segment. Although the model was once primarily associated with infectious diseases, it can be used quite effectively to explore preventive modalities for chronic, accidental or mental health phenomena.

■ *Definition*

Originally designed by two public health physicians, the model of the natural history of disease contains many epidemiologic concepts and has enjoyed wide applicability to other disciplines, such as nursing. The natural history model may be defined as follows:

> A narrative and schematic representation which portrays a chronological sequencing of departures from health. The sequence begins with the factors that promote health, but the model also addresses the very first forces that inaugurate pathological departures. An innate function of this model is to describe various approaches to prevent and control pathological processes, and this function is known collectively as the levels of prevention.[2]

These are the same levels of prevention incorporated into the public health model described in Chapter 2. The schema in Figure 3-1 fuses the natural history of disease with primary, secondary, and tertiary prevention activities. Figure 3-2 includes the interaction between the agent, the human host and environmental factors that are essential components influencing the onset of any disease process. This trio of elements interacts to challenge the state of health progressing along the continuum of pathogenesis and, without intervention, may culminate in death of the host. This is a famous conceptual action called the epidemiologic model of disease causation and is included in Figure 3-2.

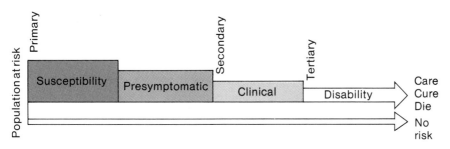

FIGURE 3-1
Natural history models with levels of prevention.

▋ *Assumptions*

Before exploring the model, it is necessary to make some preliminary statements about the assumptions upon which the model is based. Understanding these assumptions will help focus on vital aspects of epidemiologic and public health science and philosophy and provide an understanding of the intent of the model.

- *Assumption One: Health is a Relative State*

  The assumption made by referring to health as "relative" is that everyone possesses some degree or level of health, and that health may be affected by living and nonliving disease agents, by the inherent or acquired characteristics of people, and by the many factors that are a part of the environment in which people live. The authors of the nat-

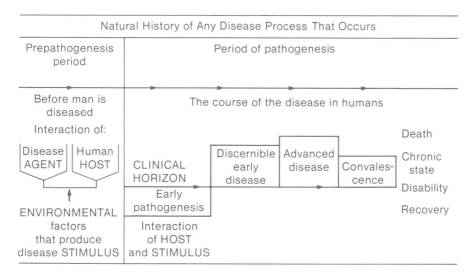

FIGURE 3-2
Prepathogenesis and pathogenesis periods of natural history. (Leavell, Clark: 1953, 1979)

ural history of disease model subscribe to the World Health Organization's definition that "health is a state of complete physical, mental and social well-being, not merely the absence of disease or infirmity."

• *Assumption Two: Disease is a Process*

The disease process in humans depends on the nature and characteristics of disease agents, individual and group characteristics, as well as a person's response to disease-producing stimuli. The disease-producing stimuli may arise from the enviroment or from within the individual. Neither health nor disease is stationary or static; both are processes that actually begin before the individual is affected. In other words, the conditions that promote either health or illness are present in the biological, physical, emotional, and social environments as well as in the organism itself.

• *Assumption Three: Multiple Causation*

The condition of health (as well as any number of deviations from health) is the result of constantly interacting forces. Likewise, the actual occurrence of disease is contingent on a triad of factors. This triad refers to an epidemiologic triangle composed of the host, the agent and the environment (H–A–E). The *host* refers to the individual or population affected. The *agent* is an element, a substance or a force, either animate or inanimate, whose contact with a susceptible host under proper environmental conditions, serves as a stimulus to initiate or perpetuate a disease process. Agents are generally biological, chemical or radiological in nature. For example, the agent in drug abuse is usually chemical in nature, whereas the biologic agent in acquired immune deficiency syndrome (AIDS) is a retrovirus. *Environment* is the aggregate of all the external conditions and influences affecting the life and development of the host or the agent. This epidemiologic model of disease causation is shown in Figure 3-3.

F I G U R E
3 - 3
The epidemiologic model.

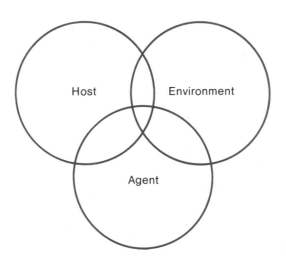

All three components of the epidemiologic triad (host, agent and environment) form what has been called "the Web of Causation" or multi-causation since the occurrence of disease never depends on a single component, but develops as a result of favorable interaction among the elements of host, agent and environment. Since no single force causes disease to occur; there must be (1) a susceptible host; (2) a causative agent or factor even if the exact nature of the agent is not known; and (3) an environment which is conducive to the interaction of the host and the agent. The precise mechanism whereby disease is produced by one interaction and is not produced by another interaction is not fully known.

As an example of multiple causation, consider the situation where several health professionals come into direct contact with a client who has active tuberculosis, and they administer cardiopulmonary resuscitation. Even though the members of the health care team have come into contact with an infectious agent through their experience, the probability is that none of the workers will become infected. Some may convert to a positive skin test, but others will retain their negative skin test for the tuberculosis antigen. Why? Because exposure to causative agents is necessary, but not sufficient to cause disease. Host and environmental factors must be considered along with how much exposure the workers actually had to the mycobacterium. Another example of exposure to an infectious agent without subsequent infection is illustrated by occupational exposure to the AIDS virus, HIV (human immunodeficiency virus). Although thousands of health care workers have had documented accidental exposure to this virus, less than 1% have become antibody positive unless they belonged to another risk category for the disease.

■ *Overview of the Natural History Model*

Leavell and Clark's work[1,2,4,5] visualized the natural history of any given health anomaly as occurring in two stages: the stage of prepathogenesis and the stage of pathogenesis. Prepathogenesis, or the predisease stage, is identified as that varying period of time that begins with the initial confrontation among the host, the agent, and the environment, including the intricate changes produced by the interaction, and ending just short of the point when the disease can be objectively or subjectively detected (Fig. 3-4).

The disease or pathogenic period begins at the point where the anomaly can be clinically detected. This stage lasts until the host recovers, is disabled, or dies.[6] Prepathogenesis may then be associated with a prodromal or incubation period, and pathogenesis represents that time period when the disease or other anomaly manifests itself and causes some kind of host response.

Intervention strategies, called the levels of prevention, are then sequenced to coincide with predictable events within the stages of prepathogenesis and pathogenesis, as shown in Figure 3-5. Applying the levels of prevention requires anticipatory action based on a knowledge of the natural history of a given disease. In other words, one cannot apply preventive strategies when none are known or they are unavailable. For example, the necessary technology is available to prevent tetanus by active or passive immunization. However, a specific vaccine for some infectious diseases is not available, nor is the sufficient technology available to protect people from contracting most chronic disease phenomena.

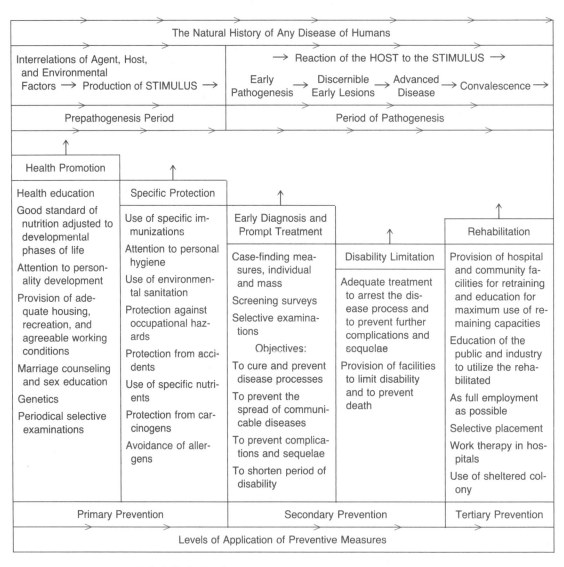

F I G U R E   3 - 4
Levels of application of preventive measures in the natural history of disease.

■ *The Levels of Prevention*

There are three major phases to prevention strategies associated with the natural history model. They are primary, secondary and tertiary prevention. Within these three phases of prevention, there are five distinct levels at which preventive practices may be applied—again depending upon the level of knowledge about the history of the disease. All levels of prevention are applied to human populations in a holistic fashion in that people are visualized as possessing emotional and psychosocial domains as well as physical ones.

Primary Prevention

Primary prevention strategies are aimed at preventing the initial interaction between the H–A–E. If there is complete success with primary prevention, the disease will not occur because the components of the H–A–E will not interact. There are two types of primary prevention: general health promotion and specific protection measures.

General Health Promotion

In general health promotion, nursing intervention strategies may not be directed at any particular disorder, but may serve to promote a general well-being. For example, provision of conditions at home, work, school, and play that favor good health, such as health education, are based on general health promotion as a part of primary prevention. In the instance of general health promotion, the focus is on promoting individual and group well-being since a healthy host or population is one that is generally less susceptible to illness.

Specific Protection

Specific protection consists of measures applied to a particular disease entity or group of diseases in order to literally intercept the known causes of disease before they affect people. Examples include immunization, environmental sanitation, protection against accidents and occupational or environmental hazards, genetic counseling, improvement of nutritional intake, stimulation of proper personal hygiene and control of disease vectors like mosquitoes, and even the use of suppressive drugs.

The whole idea behind primary prevention strategies is to alter the host, the agent or the environment in such a way that disease is averted. Certainly not all primary prevention strategies fall directly within the realm of nursing practice, but awareness of prevention modalities will enable the community health nurse to counsel clients intelligently. For instance, the community health nurse should know where in the community clients should be referred to receive immunizations for family members and pets.

Secondary Prevention: Early Diagnosis, Treatment, and Disability Limitation

Secondary prevention strategies are used to diagnose disease at an early stage, to slow the disease process, and to prevent complications. Because knowledge is limited about the cause of some diseases, primary prevention strategies may not be known, and therefore efforts at controlling many of the chronic diseases may center primarily around secondary prevention. For example, because a specific agent for diabetes or high blood pressure is unknown, primary prevention strategies for these two diseases are minimal. The emphasis is on secondary prevention strategies instead.

Another point to consider is that in some instances, it may be possible to simultaneously use primary and secondary prevention strategies in different populations. For instance, early treatment of persons with sexually transmitted diseases on the community level is an example of secondary prevention. But because treatment of infected persons may serve to protect potential contacts from acquiring the infection, primary prevention strategies are employed also.[7] The two types of secondary prevention are early diagnosis and treatment, and disability limitation. Both are aimed at slowing or halting the disease process, but they are slightly different in nature.

Early Diagnosis and Treatment

As the words imply, the objectives of early diagnosis and treatment are to prevent spread to others when the disease is communicable, to cure or arrest the disease process in order to prevent complications or disease sequelae, and to prevent prolonged disability. One of the assumptions here is that case finding in the early stages of a disease is advantageous because the subsequent treatment may be more effective in minimizing the effects of the illness in question. For example, it is well known that *in situ* carcinoma has a very favorable prognosis if diagnosed and treated very early in the disease process.

Disability Limitations

The objective in disability limitation is to prevent or delay the consequences of clinically advanced diseases. Nursing measures such as back care and passive range-of-motion exercises for an immobile client are examples of disability limitation strategies. Individualized health teaching for the insulin-dependent diabetic is another example. In this pathogenic stage of the natural history of the disease, the H–A–E have interacted to produce a clinically apparent disease, so one concentrates on how to minimize the potential effects of that disease process.

Tertiary Prevention

In tertiary prevention, the emphasis is on rehabilitation or restorative nursing interventions. At this point in the natural history, primary and secondary preventive strategies are either ineffective or unknown. Tertiary prevention occurs late in the pathogenic stage of a disease, and irreversible changes have occurred as the result of the disease process. Tertiary prevention is not so much an effort to slow the disease process as it is an attempt to prevent complete or unnecessary disability after anatomic and physiologic changes have more or less stabilized. Rehabilitative strategies are used to maximize the potential for health that remains. For example, when the residual damage from the disease process is blindness, paralysis, or some other type of irreversible pathology, the client nonetheless retains some potential for realization of maximum health potential.

At this point in the discussion, it is important to note that not all health anomalies result in irreversible change, and that secondary prevention strategies are often quite effective in deterring the progression of the disease process. When the client or group recovers without irreversible changes, there is no need to consider tertiary prevention strategies since secondary prevention interventions produced full recovery.

This same sort of mutually exclusive relationship exists among all the levels of prevention, because if primary prevention is totally effective, the H–A–E would not interact and no health deviation would be seen. Thus, when primary prevention techniques are totally effective, there is no need to consider secondary prevention; likewise, when secondary prevention techniques are totally effective, tertiary prevention is unnecessary.

■ Host, Environmental Risk Factors, and Agent

Host Risk Factors

One example of a host risk factor associated with an increased rate of some diseases is genetic make-up. For instance, people with type A blood have an increased risk of gastric cancer, while those with type O blood are more likely to develop a duodenal ulcer.[7] Another example of a host risk factor is past history of exposure. Exposures can range from exposure to infectious diseases to smoke in the environment, or to exposure to various occupational hazards. Personality is another host risk factor which may influence response to illness, or even the tendency to seek health care or to comply with health advice. Other host risk factors, besides genetic make-up, history of exposure, and personality, are listed below.

- Emotional make-up
- Health-seeking behaviors (such as safe sexual practices, adequate nutritional intake, weight control, and adequate rest and exercise)
- Social class membership
- Level of health knowledge (also considered an environmental factor)
- Habits, customs and attitudes (mental risk factors)

Environmental Risk Factors

Environmental risk factors may be classified as biologic, economic, social, or physical. By definition, environment is the "aggregate of all the external conditions and influences affecting the life and development of an organism."[8] The environments associated with an increased risk of disease are listed below and were adapted with permission from Mausner and Kramer.[7]

- Biologic environment—includes presence of infectious disease agents, environmental reservoirs of infection, vectors that transmit disease (for example, flies and mosquitoes), and plants and animals that are hazardous to people.
- Social environment—includes the overall socioeconomic and political organization of any given community that affects the technical level of medical care, as well as the mechanisms through which care is delivered. The social environment includes the adequacy and severity of codes and laws that control health-related environmental hazards (pollution, fire, accidents, housing standards, occupational safety). Various social customs such as types of food eaten and degree of cooking also may be considered environmental risk factors as may the degree to which individuals are integrated into or isolated from their respective societies.
- Physical environment—includes such things as heat, light, air circulation, water, radiation, gravity, atmospheric pressure, and a variety of chemical agents. In addition, adequate shelter, water purification, sewage treatment, air, noise, water, and other types of pollution affect human health.

Agent Factors

The final consideration of risk factors that may favor the development of disease is the agent portion of the epidemiologic triad. A disease agent is defined as "an element, a substance, or a force, either animate or inanimate, the presence or absence of which may, following effective contact with a susceptible human host under proper environmental conditions, serve as a stimulus to initiate or perpetuate a disease process.'' The agent that initiates or perpetuates a disease (with the simultaneous interaction of the host and environment) may be classified as biologic, chemical, nutrient, physical, and mechanical. Examples of agents in each category are shown below.

Before concluding the discussion on (H–A–E) risk factors, it is important to make three points. First of all, risk factors may or may not be susceptible to change or manipulation through employing the levels of prevention. For example, host risk factors, such as age, sex, and race, are often associated with a high risk of some diseases, but these factors cannot be altered. Manipulation of risk factors is also limited to what is reasonable and prudent. For example, one might be able to prevent alcoholism by removing all the alcoholic beverages from the markets; however, Prohibition showed that such drastic action had little impact on the availability of alcohol.

The second point is that even when there is a strong statistical relationship between a risk factor and a disease, one cannot automatically conclude that all individuals with the risk factor will develop the disease nor that the absence of the risk factor will ensure subsequent absence of the disease. For instance, not all smokers contract lung cancer, and some who have never smoked develop the disease.

The third point is that there is frequently some overlapping of risk factors that raises a question as to whether they are host, agent or environmental factors. As an example, is smoking tobacco a host risk factor because the individual chooses to smoke, or is smoking an environmental risk factor because some environments are more conducive or permissive to smoking plus the fact that exhaled smoke is found in the environment? Is smoking an agent-related risk factor be-

---

- Biologic agents—those disease-producing organisms such as the arthropods and helminths (worms), protozoa, fungi, bacteria, rickettsiae, and viruses.
- Chemical agents—include useful substances (such as iodide and fluoride) or detrimental substances (such as noxious gases, volatilized drugs, airborne solid particles), or those substances taken as medicine.
- Nutrient agents—include fats, carbohydrates, proteins, vitamins, minerals and water.
- Physical agents—includes abnormalities in atmospheric pressure, temperature, and humidity; unusual intensity of sound; abnormalities of radiation and mechanical forces that add unexpected stresses to body mechanics. These agents are usually associated with certain occupational exposures.
- Mechanical agents—include mechanical forces that result in crushing, tearing or penetrating wounds, and other accidental injuries.

cause smoking is statistically associated with the occurrence of several diseases? The answer is that smoking might have ramifications for the host, the agent, and the environment, depending upon one's perception.

■ *Chronology of the Natural History Model*

Now that the various risk factors associated with the occurrence of disease have been discussed and the various components of the levels of prevention have been explored, let us next examine the structure and timing of events in the natural history of disease. Instead of using the two phases of prepathogenesis and pathogenesis, a newer modification of the natural history model will be examined. This model is divided into four clear-cut stages: the stage of susceptibility, the stage of presymptomatic disease, the stage of clinical disease, and the stage of disability. Dividing the natural history into four stages allows a clearer visualization of both the period of time when the disease is present but not detectable, and the period of time when disability may occur as a result of the disease process. Additionally, separating the natural history into four stages helps in understanding exactly where the levels of prevention must be applied (Fig. 3-5).

As depicted in Figure 3-5, it is possible to generally categorize any given population into one which is at high, low, or no risk for a given disease. For example, in assessing a population's risk for AIDS, the groups at high risk would be intravenous drug abusers and people who engage in anonymous sex on a frequent basis. A group at low risk might be health professionals who care for clients with AIDS or an AIDS-related syndrome, but use appropriate precautions when exposed to body secretions and excretions. The group that might be considered at lowest risk (arbitrarily, "no risk") would be people who are not sexually active and do not use intravenous drugs.

The stage of susceptibility and the stage of presymptomatic disease in the Mausner and Kramer model correspond to Leavell and Clark's stage of prepathogenesis. (Compare Figure 3-4 to Figure 3-5.)

Stage of Susceptibility

In the stage of susceptibility, host, agent and environmental risk factors of various intensity are present but not yet interacting to cause disease. As seen in the outline of the Mausner and Kramer model, in this stage the risk factors specific to the disease or health anomaly in question are identified. When a thorough epidemiologic study is completed, it is possible to address the associated risk factors in detail. However, when relatively little is known about the anomaly, especially the specific agent involved (as in Creutzfeldt–Jakob disease or Kawasaki disease), it is difficult to elaborate on the risk factors.

Stage of Presymptomatic Disease

The stage of susceptibility ends and the stage of presymptomatic disease begins when the H–A–E interact at the cellular level. Actually, the stage of presymptomatic disease correlates with that period of time called the incubation period in communicable disease. In chronic processes, the presymptomatic stage is that period of time that stretches from the interaction of the H–A–E to just before signs and symptoms are present.

As an example of how difficult it is to detect activities in the presymptomatic stage, suppose a 42-year-old male died of accidental drowning. An autopsy determined that the cause of death was drowning, but the beginning evidence of oat cell carcinoma of the lung was found. This man was then in the stage of presymptomatic disease for cancer even though he died of drowning. So even though the presymptomatic stage of illness cannot be diagnosed, it is known to exist because there is a variable period of time between interaction of the H–A–E and onset of clinical illness.

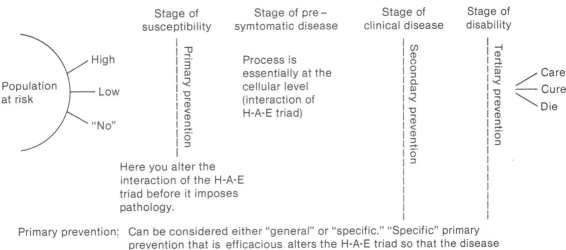

Primary prevention: Can be considered either "general" or "specific." "Specific" primary prevention that is efficacious alters the H-A-E triad so that the disease does not occur. Example: Immunizations for tezanos, typhoid, etc. General primary prevention is aimed at promoting well-being by altering susceptibility or reducing exposure to risk factors for susceptible hosts.

Secondary prevention: Focuses on early diagnosis and treatment. Measures are instigated that are directed at slowing the progression of the disease process or its handicapping disabilities.

Tertiary prevention: Deals with rehabilitation activities for clients in an effort to return the client to a maximum level of wellness/productivity/self-care.

FIGURE 3-5
Levels of prevention as viewed through the natural history of disease. (Natural History format adopted from Mausner, Bahn: Introduction to Epidemiology)

Logically, the length of the presymptomatic stage in the natural history of a disease varies greatly. It can be instantaneously short, as in accidental injuries; it can be a few hours to a few months long, as in infectious diseases; and it can be many years long, as in chronic diseases like heart disease and diabetes. Because the presymptomatic stage is not detectable under normal circumstances, there is no corresponding preventive strategy. For purposes of the natural history model, as soon as a diagnosis is possible, the client or group has entered the next stage, the clinical stage of illness.

Stage of Clinical Disease

As stated, the presymptomatic stage, regardless of duration, ends when signs or symptoms make a diagnosis possible. At that point, the disease is in the clinical stage of development. Nursing management in the clinical stage is centered around secondary intervention strategies. Early diagnosis and treatment play a very significant role in those diseases for which there is a very effective treatment for the early stages of disease. For example, it is quite advantageous to diagnose and treat cervical or breast cancer in the early stages. However, for other diseases such as Alzheimer's, early diagnosis and treatment make a questionable impact on the outcome, given present knowledge of the disease. There are other reasons why early diagnoses are required for some social services that may be vital to the well-being of some clients.

Disability limitation strategies in the clinical stage of disease are aimed at prevention of disabling sequelae that would cause further morbidity or even permanent disability in some instances. Disability limitation strategies may be as simple as providing various measures to soothe itching in the client with chickenpox to avoid infection or permanent scars. Strategies for disability limitation may be very complex, involving several body systems including the psyche. Although the following has already been mentioned, it merits repetition: all preventive strategies visualize the client as a holistic entity who is a member of a family and of larger communities, and all care should reflect consideration of these two variables.

Stage of Disability

The stage of disability begins when secondary preventive strategies used by the entire health care team have been ineffective in preventing irreversible pathology. It is in the stage of disability that tertiary prevention modalities are used to restore the client to the fullest possible potential for health and well-being.

As mentioned in the discussion on tertiary prevention modalities, some health anomalies are self-limiting, or respond to primary or secondary prevention interventions. When the disease or illness is such that it responds to secondary prevention strategies, the stage of disability is usually not entered. A point to remember is that the stage of disability is entered only when there is some kind of irreversible pathology as the result of the disease process.

*W*e have expended considerable effort discussing the notion of the natural history model. When used correctly, the natural history model is a tool that allows identification and even prioritization of prevention-based health care. The model can be applied to individuals or to entire populations. Clients are visualized holistically and as members of families and larger communities. Health anomalies are viewed as resulting from multiple causes from within and without the person affected. Further, the model synthesizes public health, preventive nursing, and epidemiologic concepts into an understandable and highly useful tool for practice.

Summary

References

1. Leavell HR, Clark EG: Preventive Medicine for the Doctor in His Community. New York, McGraw-Hill, 1953
2. Leavell and Clark: Preventive Medicine for the Doctor in His Community, An Epidemiologic Approach, 3rd ed. Huntington, NY, RE Dreges, 1979
3. MacMahon B, Pubh TF: Principles and Methods of Epidemiology. Boston, Little, Brown & Co, 1970
4. Leavell and Clark, 1958
5. Leavell and Clark, 1965
6. Leavell and Clark, p 21, 1979
7. Mausner JS, Kramer S: Epidemiology—An Introductory Text. Philadelphia, WB Saunders, 1985
8. Leavell and Clark, p 19, 1979
9. Leavell and Clark, p 50, 1979

The Community— The Nursing of Aggregate Groups

SECTION

II

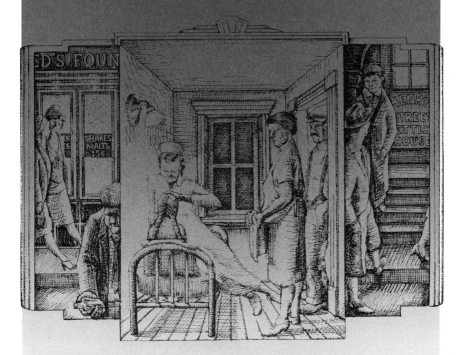

Wald called herself and the other Henry Street Settlement nurses "public health nurses." The basic idea behind their enterprise was that the nurse's peculiar introduction to the patient and her organic relationship with the neighborhood constituted the starting point for universal services to the area.

Epidemiology and Community Health Nursing

LEARNING OBJECTIVES

After reading and understanding the contents of this chapter, the student will be able to:

1. Describe the use of epidemiology in relation to public health science and community health nursing.

2. Discuss the terms "community health nursing" versus "public health nursing."

3. Explain how epidemiology parallels the nursing process.

4. Construct a situation in which a secondary attack rate would be useful.

5. Identify the importance of epidemiologic markers and give examples.

6. Define an epidemiologic rate, ratio, and proportion and give examples of each.

7. Differentiate between incidence rates and prevalence rates, and demonstrate the use of each in community health nursing practice.

8. List the basic differences between crude or summary rates, specific rates, and adjusted rates.

Introduction

*T*he unique components of public or community health nursing have been identified in the public health model in Chapter 2. The concepts of public health and the nursing process are used to guide the curriculum in schools of nursing, to assist nurse executives in the hiring of staff with special preparation to meet the needs of the community, and to define the scope of practice of community health nursing. Knowledge of the conceptual framework guiding all public health workers is a necessary prerequisite to ensure the incorporation of special perspectives for delivery of care to aggregates. This is especially true when the complex needs of the community are met through a team of multidisciplinary providers requiring the coordination of group actions to deliver optimum care. Epidemiology, a public health science, has evolved in order to quantify and measure the needs of the community and evaluate public health services. Knowing the basic concepts of public health initiatives and their purpose in the community facilitates the incorporation of epidemiologic approaches to enhance nursing services.

▌ *Public and Community Health Nursing*

Historically, as we have seen, the term "public health nursing" was used and promoted by Lillian Wald. During the last 20 years, most nursing agencies in public health and nursing educational programs have changed the term "public" health nursing to "community" health nursing. Many reasons were given for the change. The most frequent justifications for the change to community health nursing will be reviewed here. It was claimed that "public" is a word often associated with public funding or government subsidy. To label nursing care delivered in the community a public service would irrevocably associate nursing services with government and federally supported programs. Another reason for the change from "public" to "community" was that nursing services would become associated with public welfare systems and the stigma of receiving care directed to indigent populations would affect their utilization. On the other hand, the word "community" was all-encompassing, and the use of this term would avoid the connotations ascribed to the word "public." These arguments (and others) were convincing enough to be accepted by the majority of nurses across the country. The title "community health nursing" was adopted in an effort to broaden the view of nursing services delivered to aggregates and to avoid the association attached to recipients of the public welfare referred to in Chapter 2.

The change from "public" health to "community" health does not appear to have affected the perceptions of clients, patients, and non-nursing health care providers. There is little evidence to support a change in perceptions of the public in general or the view of other health care professionals; other disciplines in the field still refer to public health nursing programs, perhaps because schools of public health have never relinquished the traditional title.[1] There are indications that baccalaureate programs in community health nursing have been integrated into undergraduate curricula in schools of nursing. Unfortunately, integration has become synonymous with anonymity. A transfer of scope of practice to a broader community base may have compromised the identity of public health nursing as a specialty area.[2]

A definition of public is "related to government," but it also means "being in service to the community" or "relating to or affecting all people or areas of nations or states."[3] Another appropriate definition of public is "relating to community as opposed to private affairs." Definitions of community are equally diverse. Community is defined as "a state or commonwealth." As such, it includes the public or government domain. It is defined also as "geographic areas with common concerns" and "a body of persons with a common history, or political interests." As Banta says, there is so little difference between the two words that little is gained by using "community" instead of "public."[4] This is especially true when a change in title has failed to affect perceptions thought to be deleterious to the utilization of nursing services. The reasons for using "public" or "community" are unresolved and unsubstantiated.[5] The terms are used interchangeably in this text.

▌ *Epidemiology*

Epidemiology is a public health science. As such, it is applied in a multidisciplinary context to evaluate professional services and to prevent and control diseases in the community through scientific methods. The language, methods, and quantification of epidemiology are used by all workers in the field of public health. Although it goes back to the days of Hippocrates, epidemiology was first identified as a unique process during the epidemics that devastated the world from the 13th to the 17th centuries. Epidemiology and public health developed side by side. Today, the modern methods of epidemiology are used to solve contemporary health problems, for large and small units of people.

In order to approach community health nursing from an epidemiologic point of view, the principles of public health have been identified. Epidemiology accomplishes the purpose of public health through special characteristics and contributes to nursing care through these same properties. Epidemiology is a method of conducting inquiries concerning aggregates or groups, and is an inductive process of thinking from which conclusions are drawn to enhance nursing care. More than this, however, epidemiology parallels the nursing process as a method of assessing, diagnosing, planning, intervening, and evaluating. As a scientific approach, it is similar to the nursing process, yet epidemiology provides its own special techniques for measuring and observing groups rather than individuals. It differs from the nursing process because its focus and only concern is the health or threats to health in communities. Epidemiology differs from the nursing process by providing methods of hypothesizing new relationships. The language of epidemiologic methods and research are held in common by all public health workers who may be unfamiliar with nursing process. Epidemiology contributes to community health nursing by providing a scientific language that is common to all public health workers concerned with the common good. Thus, it creates an avenue for communication between public health nursing and the other providers of community care. Epidemiology generates a knowledge of factors that can modify or prevent disease occurrences. It defines the burden of disease that is present in the community, and it identifies individuals at high risk for catastrophic events. Epidemiology also reflects the philosophy of public health and is consistent with a public health model or conceptual framework of concepts that guide clinical nursing practice in the community.

Public health nursing is the nursing of aggregates; applied nursing care is generalistic in nature encompassing all practices learned at the bedside. The nursing of aggregates, however, requires skills, tools, and special methods, many of which are provided by an epidemiologic approach. The methods or processes of epidemiology assist in the decisions made for delivery of nursing services, the assessment of community needs, and evaluation of the programs of nursing care. The contribution of epidemiology to nursing can be explored through discussion of the characteristics which delineate epidemiology as a public health science.

Distinguishing Characteristics of Epidemiology

1. An observational science for public health
2. Delineated by methods and tools used to quantify observations, including:
   - Statistics
   - Laboratory tests
   - Comparisons of quantifications
3. Clients are served as populations (as communities)
4. Outcome event of concern is illness and health

■ *The Characteristics of Epidemiology for Community Health Nursing*

Epidemiology has certain defining characteristics or features that make epidemiology different from the other public health sciences, such as the environmental sciences and the behavioral sciences. The first characteristic of epidemiology states that it employs standardized, meaningful tests of known accuracy which are as quantified as possible. There are many examples of these kinds of tests known as the tools of epidemiology. These tools, or markers, are applied to accomplish measurement and quantification. Many tools are laboratory-based tests. It is important to review some of the laboratory tests most frequently used to guide and direct nursing intervention.

Tools is a comprehensive term used in the text to denote all methods of measurement in epidemiology. It includes statistics, screening tests, and epidemiologic markers or tags. The latter are used to assure the epidemiologist that cases are caused by the same organism (virus, fungus, or bacterium). Epidemiology and the era of sanitation and bacteriology evolved side by side the last two centuries. Methods of disease prevention, such as vaccination, antibiotics, and pure water supplies, have improved the health of the public dramatically and indelibly. As science produced accurate methods of testing for bacteria, toxins, and pollutants in the environment, these laboratory tests, or tools, proved to be invaluable in documenting the effects of sanitary measures. Blood tests measured the response to vaccinations, and laboratory methods and *in vivo* observations monitored the effectiveness of antibiotics. Tests became invaluable in epidemics as markers or tags for communicable and chronic diseases. These epidemiologic tools assist community health nurses in contributing meaningfully to investigations of epidemics and in counseling and consoling families. Such knowledge helps in the prevention of infection and in allaying the fears of the spread of infectious disease to family members. Tools are a way of assessing environmental exposure to families and groups and providing evidence to ensure compensation for work-related exposures for nurses and others.

Before going further, it is necessary to review some basic principles of microbiology and molecular genetics; but first an example of the use of epidemiologic tools and markers will show their relevance to nursing practice. Imagine a mother with several small children at home. Her youngest child, about 6 months old, is seriously ill with pneumonia. The organism identified from a laboratory culture is *Hemophilus influenzae*. The mother fears that her friend's new baby has been exposed to her own child and may also contract the disease. She is concerned also that other members of her young family are at risk for the same disease. What should the young mother be told to allay her fears and educate her in prevention and control? The nurse's response would be based on the nurse's understanding of epidemiologic quantifications from laboratory-based information. Such data is seen in Figure 4-1 which shows the rates by age groups for *H. influenzae* infections. These age-specific rates are rates of infection predicated on being in a certain age group; they are known as secondary attack rates. Secondary attack rates simply mean the rates occurring in a family *after* the index, or first member, has fallen ill. These rates quantify the risk of infecting other family members. With this knowledge, the nurse can counsel the mother, confident that scientific facts substantiate the accuracy of nursing care. Figure 4-1 shows that the risk of being infected secondary to another family member is probably nonexistent after 6 years of age. The younger children (under 6 years) should not be exposed to the sick baby. The friend's baby, who is younger than the sick child (or the index case) is at greatest risk because younger infants are more susceptible. Perhaps the friend's baby indeed becomes ill from the same disease. If a different strain of *Hemophilus influenzae* is the cause of the infection in her friend's baby, the mother of the index case can gain comfort, for in all probability, the sickness in the neighbor's child was *not* caused by cross-infection between the two infants. This assurance can be given only if epidemiologic markers from laboratory tests have established that the strain of bacteria is different for each *H. influenzae* infection. Pathogens can be of the same genus and species, but before they can be labelled as being from the same strain of virus or bacteria, epidemiologic markers or tools must be applied. Without these facts, assurance of lack of cross-contamination or, in the worst scenario, the likelihood of cross-infection may not be given to the mother by the nurse. Laboratory tests are used in many ways. These epidemiologic tools are applied during the screening of small and large groups for phenylketonuria (PKU). They are used to examine the blood of populations to find out the proportion of people who are susceptible to the virus of hepatitis B or those who have been infected with the human immune virus (HIV) of AIDS. Sometimes laboratory tests are used to verify nursing assessments of families in the community. For instance, the nursing assessment of the rise in lead poisoning of children in low-income

Age-group	Risk of disease
Under 2 years	3.8%
2–3 years	1.5%
4–5 years	0.1%
6 and over	0%

F I G U R E   4 - 1
Risk of hemophilus influenzae disease among household contacts of cases, during 1 month after onset of disease in the index case. (Adapted from CDC: MMWR 24[38]:329, 1975)

housing varies significantly, from tests for blood lead levels taken by undergraduate nursing students in community health according to Parson's article in 1981. When accurate laboratory tests are applied to groups of people, populations can be studied for the levels of protective antibodies to infectious diseases. These are called sero surveys that help predict the degree of hazard existing in a community from a specific infection and help to plan immunization programs. It is important that the nurse is able to interpret these tests for families and groups so that meaningful intervention can be planned and executed. For instance, in the care of patients with AIDS, a frequent question is whether the virus has always been in the community or whether it is new. Examination of banks of sera (collections of blood samples from several populations stored frozen in laboratories all over the world) have been examined for antibodies to the HIV. No antibodies to this virus have been found in any sera banks before 1972. It appears that the virus may be a new mutation. Using DNA probes, sophisticated methods of marking strains of viruses, it seems clear that more than one virus is responsible for the disease. These DNA probes are called epidemiologic markers. The enzyme-linked immunosorbent assay (ELISA) test, a serological test for antibody presence that identifies congenital transmission of AIDS to neonates and identifies high-risk groups, is also an example of using laboratory tests as a tool to guide the nurse in providing intervention, counseling, and support to stricken families.

Epidemiology applies tools as markers to identify cases in epidemics and individuals at high risk of problem events. There are several markers, such as phage typing,[6] biocin typing,[7] and antibiograms[8–10]—a series of measurement of sensitivity reactions of a microorganism to several antibiotics. These markers reveal many things about the aggregate of concern. For example, they denote invasion of populations by the same organism; multiple typing confirms that groups of cases have the same diagnostic pathogen. These tests also can distinguish between newly infected cases and old cases, that is, those infected in the past. At this point in the discussion, and indepth review of the use of these epidemiologic markers in quantifications will illustrate their wide application to community health nursing. For example, reports of the level of antibody to an infection or toxins are usually annotated as ratios, such as 1:8, 1:16, and 1:32. These ratios are the results of a common laboratory strategy known as serial dilution. In serial dilution tests, the sera of clients/patients are compared with a measured aliquot of known antigen or test substance diluting the test sample if necessary to a level denoted by a standard observation such as precipitation or flocculation. The higher the dilution required to meet this standard, the greater the degree of reaction and the higher the level of antibody. To show how ratios are generated and interpreted from serial dilution tests, the following example is used to assess antibiotic susceptibility.

When the community health nurse is called on to provide public health services to a hospital or an industrial group, early identification of series of infections by the same organism can be indispensable in guiding the nurse's actions. A series of susceptibility patterns to several antibiotics are called antibiograms. Antibiograms mark two or more cases infected by the same organism. Traditionally they are used to assist in choosing the most appropriate antibiotics for patient care and are easily available for epidemiologic use. Not only do antibiograms assist in identifying a break in aseptic nursing techniques to control cross-infection, but they identify the invasion of a hospital community by a highly resistant organism detrimental to patient care. The use of epidemiologic markers are essential in identifying cases caused by the same strain of virus in bacteria. When a bacterium is retrieved from blood specimens collected in a community and sent to a laboratory, it is usual to submit the identified pathogens to a battery of antibiotics to test for susceptibility or resistance to a series of antimicrobials. By arranging the results of several tests in a linear fashion, a pattern of susceptibility can be seen. This pattern of susceptibility or lack of susceptibility (resistance) of a pathogen to a series of antibiotics is called the antibiogram. The antibiogram is used to mark or identify cases of infection defined as similar when the antibiogram patterns match. A serial dilution test will now be described for one antibiotic.

An antimicrobial is serially diluted in a broth to which the test organism, usually species of bacteria, has been added. A broth or culture medium (0.5 ml) is placed in each of 11 test tubes, ten of which are seeded with an inoculum of bacteria. For example, 100 μg of the selected antibiotic is diluted in 0.5 ml of broth in the first tube that contains no bacterial inoculum, and left as a control. Half the contents of this tube is added to the second tube containing the organisms. Half the contents of the second tube are transferred to the third, and half of the third is transferred to the fourth, and so on. The last test tube receives no antibiotic solution and acts as the second control for bacterial growth. After 18 hours of incubation at 35°C (both may vary with the organism, of course), the tubes are examined for the visible growth of bacteria. The tube that shows no visible growth prior to the bacterial growth is called the minimum inhibitory concentration (MIC) level. *In vivo* test results, already known from clinical observations, indicate the dilution level of MIC that is sensitive (S) or resistant (R) to treatment from the antibiotic. In this example, the 100 μg of antibiotic has been diluted to 50 μg ml in the second tube to 25 μg ml in the third, and so on. The less antibiotic required to inhibit bacterial growth the greater the sensitivity of the pathogen to the antibiotic. The usual denotation of this dilution as a ratio is 1:1, 1:2, 1:4, 1:8, 1:16, 1:32, which shows the progressive dilution of the antimicrobial in successive test tubes. Either the dilution level (the ratio), the S and

R to a series of antibiotics can be entered into an array to form a marker for epidemiologic purposes.

Serologic tests act on the same principle as the serial dilution test but are much more complex with endless variations in application occurring. In general, according to Boyd and Hoerl, three major serological testing techniques exist.[11] In the first, antigens are separated through diffusion, osmosis, and electrical charges. In the second, soluble antigens or antibodies are attached to cells, such as red blood corpuscles or latex particles, in order to view analysis or agglutination reactions. In the third technique, marker labels are conjugated to antibodies or antigens to identify their presence. These markers include fluorescent dyes, electron-dense materials viewed through electron microscopes, and radioactive substances. ELISA, the test used to detect antibodies in AIDS, is a good example of a laboratory test used for population screening. In the ELISA, the chemical color change is proportional to the concentration of antibodies in the patient's serum. This test has also been used to identify antibodies to viral hepatitis B infection and infection by rotaviruses. As previously mentioned, ELISA is proving to be a valuable test in identifying groups at high risk for AIDS.

Serologic tests are a salient example of the use of meaningful quantifications in epidemiology. Their value to individual patient care is obvious. They identify etiologic agents of diseases, confirm diagnoses, and assist in following the course or severity of illnesses. In epidemiology, serologic tests are important: they determine pathogenic serotypes—the antigenic differences in pathogen identification required for epidemiologic studies. They also can be used to establish the levels of protection against certain diseases that exist in communities. The knowledge of the genus and species of bacteria and viruses is not enough to identify a group of cases in a suspected epidemic. Antibiograms, biocin typing, and phage typing establish that all cases in a group are probably caused by the same pathogen. This knowledge in nursing is used as a guide to management decisions relating to staffing and other resources. It also affects clinical interventions such as the planning of immunization clinics by nursing agencies and the implementation of prevention and control measures to inhibit epidemics in hospitals as well as extramural communities.

Epidemiologic markers just discussed are examples of "standardized meaningful tests." Although the standardized tests help nurses define the risk of disease for an individual family, their significance lies in their application to groups, particularly in estimating the level of resistance or susceptibility to disease. However, quantification is not limited to laboratory tests. Mathematical quantifications also are used to measure observations in communities. Some of these include biostatistics and the comparison of quantified phenomena. The most important computation or basic measurement of the health of the public is the rate. There are many rates—rates of disease occurrence, rates of birth, rates of death, rates of utilization of services, and many more. Rates are designed to quantify events or occurrences in communities and are used as indices of community health and well-being. Rates are so important for the practice of community health nursing that they will be detailed a little later in this chapter. For the present, it should be emphasized that rates are the basic components of risk ratios, which quantify the effects of exposure. Exposure is not always a threatening experience. Exposure may include care, such as immunization clinics or specialized services (for example, nursing). When the exposure is a hazard, it is usally a toxic agent such as lead, asbestos, or an infectious organism or other noxious event.

The measure of risk from exposure is so important that epidemiology has been called the study of risk. It is now possible to quantify the risk of life style choices, of exposure to infectious organisms and toxic waste, or even the risk associated with the lack of nursing care. Special mathematical measures have been developed to quantify risk that are relatively simple to calculate. The measures are called risk ratios (RR). The RRs are computed by comparing two rates with one another. The rate of disease in the group exposed to a hazard such as smoking is compared with the rate of disease occurring in the group not exposed to a hazard. The nurse can then say that scientific evidence shows that risk of disease or death is doubled, or more, by certain choices made by clients.

A brief overview of quantification in epidemiology would not be complete without reference to biostatistics. This tool of epidemiology has many applications, not the least of which is quantifying the probability of an event arising by chance—an event such as a rise in infections, an increase in illness in a school, or a geographic grouping of cases of disease such as multiple sclerosis. It is important to measure the chance that the occurrences are accidental and have no etiology beyond a random or chance event. This is a function of biostatistics in public health.[12]

Epidemiology, as a public health science, bases investigations on populations or communities. There are some differences among epidemiologists on the size of the population to be investigated. Some epidemiologists confine their studies to large geographic areas, such as states and countries. Other prefer to define smaller groups as target populations or high risk aggregates. This latter approach is particularly appropriate for public health nursing, as many nursing agencies divide their catchment areas into census tracts or neighborhoods. Special nursing programs are directed also to small groups with special needs, such as migrant workers or ethnic minorities. The immediate concern of the public health nurse is to deliver care to the neighborhood or tract and serve the needs of the smaller community.

Epidemiology is distinguished by its ability to provide methods of surveillance of communities, large and small, and its ability to quantify important observations. Epidemiology has one thing in common with all inductive approaches: it is mainly an observational science. In contrast to the basic sciences, the observations of epidemiology are restricted to people in groups. Epidemiologists concentrate on serving human beings within communities. As such, epidemiologists cannot conduct standard experiments or organize observations in a way that is destructive, manipulative, or confusing to human life and liberty. In order to conduct research and solve problems threatening people, epidemiology has developed and refined special methods of observation and comparison. Field studies in epidemiology observe naturally occurring phenomena as they happen in order to measure the effects on populations. The eruption of Mount St. Helen's in Washington State is a case in point. Immediately after the eruption, surveillance of the population for the long-term effects of exposure to volcanic ash was initiated. Another example of a field study of an occurring phenomenon involved the catastrophe at the Chernobyl nuclear plant in the Soviet Union—an event which facilitated the observation of the effects of exposure to different degrees of radioactivity. Even in unavoidable catastrophes, epidemiologic methods are applied to learn as much as possible from the event. Observations are collected and analyzed using comparisons as well as statistical and laboratory tools to glean information that will be used to promote safety and health in present and future generations.

The final characteristic of epidemiology to be considered is the outcome event, which is the focal point of epidemiology. This event is the *raison d'etre* of this public health science. Illness and health are outcome events of concern in epidemiology. They are polar concepts, that is, they are at opposite ends of a continuum with one concept negating the other. Breslow has made a good argument for the epidemiologic study of health rather than disease as the outcome of interest; however, it is difficult to measure health.[13] Parsons says that health is "the state of optimum capacity of an indiviual for the effective performance of the roles and tasks for which he has been socialized."[14] Thus, health is defined with reference to the individual's role in the social system. Others believe a healthy person is one who has been inadequately studied! In the World Health Organization's definition of health, it is said that the condition of health is "not merely the absence of disease but is the state of complete physical, mental and social well-being."[15] An ecological definition of health would include the degree to which an individual can operate with effectiveness within the limits of heritable, physical and cultural environments. Epidemiology quantifies phenomena and constantly refines its approaches to measurement; but health is inadequately defined and uses many subjective terminologies that are difficult to measure. This problem has compelled most epidemiologists to define health in terms of disease since it is the more tangible and observable outcome event. Special symbols have been assigned to label a case of disease and its

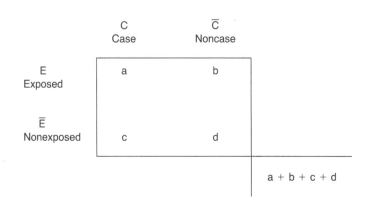

FIGURE 4 - 2
Outline of the Classical 2 × 2 table used in epidemiology. (Adapted From Susser MW, Watson W: Sociology in Medicine, 2nd ed. London, Oxford Univ. Press, 1971)

absence. C and $\overline{C}$ denote a case and a non-case, respectively. A variation of this scheme is D and $\overline{D}$, which denote disease and non-disease, respectively. These denotations form the basis of the classical two-by-two table that shows the relationship between exposure to disease and disease and non-disease occurrence (Fig. 4-2). This table is used to measure effects or calculate risk ratios.[1]

It is of the utmost importance that the definition of "case" is viewed creatively for optimum utilization of epidemiology for nursing. Modern epidemiology provides the opportunity to define cases or outcome events as those that are specifically nursing concerns rather than the concerns of other disciplines. From this perspective, "case" may be defined as cases of recidivism, lack of ability to perform the daily activities of living, lack of attendance at nursing clinics, as well as cases of mental confusion, cases of nosocomial infection, cases of contamination, and cases of illness. According to Jacox, morbidity is a relevant nursing concern as well as health. Nurses (and physicians) have a special understanding of the care of those who are ill. Knowledge of the effects of disease and the required treatment assures a unique appreciation of the role of promoting health. Similarly, quantifying the absence or decrease of illness produces an appreciation of disease as an estimate of community health. Moreover, the education of families to acquire healthy lifestyles is most effective when presented by a nurse **during the delivery of nursing care to the sick and disabled.** The outcome of epidemiology is the case and non-case, C and $\overline{C}$, but also can be defined as events relating to nursing services for the ill and the well. Public health nursing is unique among the disciplines in its ability to meet the needs of the sick and the healthy in the community.

■ *Rates: The Basic Statistics of Public Health*

The outcome in epidemiology is measured by rates. Rates indicate the severity of physiologic and psychosocial problems in groups. They also indicate the effectiveness of public health services. The infant mortality rate is used as a measure of the health of society. Rates of communicable diseases such as poliomyelitis and smallpox are cited to show the effectiveness of immunization programs. Rates of visits to a clinic show the usefulness of or need for community nursing services. Most of all, rates are observations of people—people who are ill and well, people who are anxious and confused, and people who have benefited from efforts to meet their needs. No matter how dull or impersonal rates appear to be, the public health nurse knows that they measure the problems of a group as well as the successes of all health workers in meeting the needs of society.

It is important that the community health nurse reads rates accurately and knows how they relate to the illnesses and health of aggregates. The numerator is a count of an outcome event such as illness, birth, death, and behavior. The denominator is the population or group at risk for illness, birth, death, behaviors, and so forth. This population at risk is summarized as p.a.r. (usually not capitalized except out of habit). The p.a.r.'s alternate title is target population, which is the community that suffers or benefits from the event in the numerator. The rate is meaningless for nursing without knowledge of the group from which the rate is derived.

How the numerator and denominator are counted or how they are defined is critical for understanding rates. Every rate and ratio relates to a time period—for example, 1 day, 1 month, 1 year, or 10 years. The longer the time spent counting the event in the numerator, the greater the numbers will be. But what is a rate, what does it reveal, and how is this basic statistic of public health used?

A rate is a probability statement concerning the risk of occurrence of an event. Fleiss explains that the rate is a measure of the likelihood that a special event or characteristic occurs to or is possessed by a "typical" member of the population.[18] Clearly, there is no typical member of a community. In fact, in nursing it is important to maintain the integrity and singularity of each client and patient. The challenge of public health nursing is to interpret rates meaningfully for families receiving care. Knowledge of group parameters and measures of health such as rates increase the nurse's awareness of the needs of small groups in relation to the larger community. Rates used with knowledge and perspective can improve nursing care of aggregates and can be used to justify change in nursing services. There are many kinds of rates. They should be interpreted with a knowledge of how rates are defined, collected, and compiled; most important, the interpretation should be tempered with practical clinical observations. Rates, when used as guides to nursing practice, must be used with judgments that are based on nursing care; clinical judgment must always supercede mathematical computation when there is an inconsistency.

Rates are not the only statistics used to quantify community events. Proportions and ratios may also be applied as indices of health. There are differences among ratios, proportions, and rates. A ratio divides one quantity by another, but the two quantities relate to different items or events. A ratio compares or relates two different things—one in the numerator and one in the denominator (for example, men to women, professional nurses to technical nurses, oranges to apples). In a ratio, the numerator is *not* included in the denominator. In contrast, a proportion is a fraction where the numerator is included in the denominator. It may be expressed as a percentage of the whole by multiplying the fraction by 100 ($X/X+Y \times 10^2$). A rate is defined for the physical sciences as the rate of change in one variable, X, per unit change in another variable, Y, on which Y depends. In epidemiology, the rate is defined as the proportion of disease (or other event) occurring in a specified time period per unit of population, such as 10,000 (10^4), or 100,000 (10^5).[19] In a true rate, the denominator must represent the entire population at risk for the event occurring in the numerator. The time period must always be specified, not only for all rates, but also for ratios and proportions. The rates used in public health give an approximation of the probability of events, which is most useful for epidemiologic purposes. The rate may be defined as an approximate measure of the risk of occurrence of an event or state. This risk is expressed as the proportion of people experiencing the event per unit of population during or at a specified time period.

For discussion, rates will be defined (1) by time; (2) by cases in the numerator; and (3) by the p.a.r., that is, the target population or denominator. This trichotomy is artificial: in reality rates include all these variables—time, numerators, and denominators, as described above. However, it is a useful strategy to discuss the rates for public health nursing under these three headings.

(1) Rates Defined by Time

The rates defined by time are called incidence rates and prevalence rates. Incidence rates are collected over a continuous period of time, and new cases occurring during this period accumulate in the numerator. The formula for an incidence rate is the number of new cases divided by the p.a.r. consisting of (new) cases and non-cases, times 10 raised to an exponent. Incidence rates are composed of cases observed on a continuum in time, or longitudinally. More accurately they are called cumulative incidence rates because they are counted and accumulated over a specified period, such as a month, a year, 5 years, or even 10 years, when case occurrence is small. Cumulative incidence rates are represented diagrammatically in Figure 4-3.

Prevalence rates are different. Prevalence rates are also defined by time but the cases are collected as though they occurred at one point in time. The numerator refers to all cases of a disease, whether they are new or old, and the denominator contains new and old cases

New case ↓	New case ↓		New case ↓

T_0 _____ T_1

where T_0T_1 represents a defined time period

Formula:

$$\frac{\text{New cases}}{\text{New cases and noncases}} \times 10^a \text{ for a time period } T_0T_1$$

$$\text{or } \frac{C}{C + \overline{C}} \times 10^a \text{ for } T_0T_1$$

FIGURE 4 - 3
Cumulative incidence rates.

and non-cases of the disease event under scrutiny. The formula for a prevalence rate, using disease as the event of concern, is shown in Figure 4-4.

For a prevalence rate, a day may be specified on which all cases, both new and old in a community, were counted. For instance, a rate of disease on June 1, 1987, will include all cases prevailing in the community on that date relative to the total number of people in the community. The prevalence rate is influenced greatly by the duration of the disease; for instance, if the disease is a chronic condition not causing death, then old cases will accumulate in the community. Compared to the new cases, the occurrence of old cases will be much greater when the disease is chronic. Thus, prevalence approximates incidence when the duration of the disease is known, or $P = I \times D$ (P is Prevalence Rate, I is Incidence Rate, and D = the Duration of Disease). This formula works best when the duration of the disease is predictable and stable. Although the prevalence rate is defined as a rate occurring at one point in time, it is obvious that it is impossible to gather information so quickly. It takes time to complete a survey of all cases in a community. The collection period is confined to as short a timespan as possible, and the date quoted in connection with prevalence usually indicates the final day of completion of the survey done to measure prevalence of disease.

Formula:

$$\frac{\text{New cases + old cases}}{\text{New cases + old cases + noncases}} \times 10^a \text{ for } T_1$$

or

$$\frac{C}{C + \overline{C}} \times 10^a \text{ for } T_1$$

where C includes new cases and previously diagnosed (old) cases of disease and *a* equals any exponent of 10

FIGURE 4 - 4
Prevalence rate.

■ *Application to Nursing Practice*

Of what use are incidence and prevalence rates to nursing? Incidence rates indicate the risk of a new disease in the community. This information helps the nurse's efforts in the community to reduce the risk of specific diseases through education, early detection through case finding, and clinical intervention such as rehabilitation. The best indicator of the impact of nursing care is the incidence rate, which helps compute the effect of nursing services. An incidence rate, because it is collected over time, is also more likely to identify precursors to disease or disability. When precursors are identified, nursing interventions will be of greatest effect in preventing the occurrence or perhaps the recurrence of disease. Prevalence, on the other hand, is the rate used when making an assessment of the need for nursing services in a population. By specifying the prevalence of disease in the community, nursing resources can be deployed to meet the current needs of the sick and the well. Many times a description of the burden of disease, old and new, which is present in a community, is of vital concern to enable the optimal use of scarce resources.

Rates Defined by Numerator

A rate has a numerator shown above the line and a denominator shown below the line in the fraction. When we define a rate using the numerator as the basis for the definition, we use the type of case referred to in the numerator. When we define a rate as a morbidity rate, we mean illness rate, because the numerator refers to illness. When the illness is specified, then the rate is a cause-specific morbidity rate such as cardiac disease, hepatic disease, or mental confusion. When the numerator relates to recidivism or activities of daily living, it is also defined by the content or event observed in the numerator. It is necessary for the nurse to determine whether the numerator refers to a single person, a case, or an episode. When the numerator indicates episodes, it is important to remember that a few patients may experience many recurrences or episodes of a disease such as arthritis or schizophrenia. In hospital infection control, the episodes in the numerator may apply to only ten patients, each sharing several episodes of nosocomial disease. The use of episodes as numerator data may be useful in tracking down epidemics of nosocomial infection and in distinguishing autoinfection (self-infection) from exogenous spread through person-to-person contact. Recurrent episodes of chronic diseases are important parameters for nursing care; however, they should be used cautiously. For example, the nurse must consider that a new episode of the same disease is not counted as a new case but as a recurrence of an old case. A rate with episodes in the numerator can be interpreted as the risk of a total population for a disease rather than an average risk to an individual. Compare this to a rate with cases in the numerator, which is interpreted as the average or overall risk for a person having a disease. Rates defined by numerator data specifying a diagnosis are referred to as cause-specific rates and are not to be confused with specific rates where the numerator *and* denominator are restricted to a specific population.

(2) Rates Defined by the Denominator

Rates defined by the denominator are called specific rates and are, by definition, a conditional probability where the condition affects the population, or p.a.r., as well as the cases in the numerator. Specific rates define the probability of a condition given that a certain characteristic exists in the p.a.r. This is stated statistically as P(D)lC, the probability of disease given that the condition exists. The characteristics most often specified as the condition are demographic variables. Demographic variables are those characteristics that are shared by all human beings and are used to describe the group. Age, race, sex, and ethnic background are the most frequently used demographic variables in public health. Age-specific rates apply to a particular age group or age stratum; sex-specific rates are confined to one specified sex; race-specific rates define a case in one ethnic group. The p.a.r. of a specific rate includes only people with the demographic characteristic. What is important is that the numerator event occurs only to the population specified by the denominator. Specific rates are confined or curtailed in both numerator and denominator in exactly the same way so that the cases of illness apply only to an age group or other defined demographic group. Specific rates are extremely useful for comparing populations. If two nursing agencies wish to compare disease occurrence in each of their communities, it would be useful to make this comparison by specific age groups so that the comparisons would be valid. Disease occurrence increases with age. By comparing age groups, the effects of age distribution in each population will be taken into account. Although the discussion has examined rates by time, by numerator, and by conditions restricting the denominator (and numerator) to a population with specific characteristics, it is essential to recall that the trichotomy is artificial. Incidence or prevalence can also include morbidity rates and specific rates at the same time.

Given these simple principles, rates can be structured with special meaning for nursing care. For instance, if one wanted to know the number of first visits to a nursing clinic of the over-65 age group, the specific rate would be composed of the number of first visits divided by a total of the first visits and non-first visits made by clients over 65 years old and occurring in a particular time period. The rate can also be the number of patients not returning for follow-up, divided by a total of patients not returning for follow-up and those returning for follow-up in another clinic. These are just one or two examples of how rates can be specially structured so that they can be useful for evaluating populations receiving nursing services.

In public health, the term summary rate is used. There are two important summary rates: a crude cause-specific mortality or morbidity rate and an adjusted rate. A summary rate is just that—an overall rate that summarizes the occurrence of an event in a community. The overall mortality rate for the United States is a summary rate. It is not a specific or conditional rate nor does it apply to only part of the country. A summary rate is a crude quantification of a health-related event in a community.

Adjusted rates are used often in public health and occur constantly in the literature. The most frequent use of adjusted rates in nursing is probably for nursing management. They will be mentioned here briefly so that the staff nurse in community health nursing can recognize and appreciate the use and interpretation of the adjusted rate. Before discussing the general principles of using an adjusted rate, an example of a situation where adjusted rates are useful will illustrate the point. It is most likely that the use of adjusted rates for delivery of nursing services will be used when comparing the costs of two nursing agencies or the costs of two nursing services for different groups. In the present system of delivery of community services, hospital cooperations may wish to compare the rates of disease and costs of administration for home health nursing agencies or their ambulatory care clinics. It would be unfair to compare costs of services and rates of disease between an agency serving a group of elderly and another agency serving adolescents! The clinics populations are different—the elderly population require many services and have increased frequency of disabilities and diagnoses compared to the adolescents. Therefore, an adjustment for the difference in age groups must be made before the rates and costs can be compared. On a more global basis, a comparison between countries can be made only if life expectancy in both countries is about the same and the proportions of older people to younger people are similar in the two countries (Fig. 4-5). It can be postulated that Chileans do not live as long as people in the United States, where heart disease is a more frequent cause of death. The difference in the adjusted rates of the two countries is considerably narrowed by using the rates adjusted so that the differences in the ages of the two groups being compared has been eliminated. By adjusting the rates for age differences, a more valid comparison can be made. Other factors besides age are influencing death from heart disease in the United States according to this comparison.

Adjusted rates are summary rates; that is, they summarize a rate for a total population. Adjusted rates have a special advantage. They are used for comparisons between two or more populations, and they are used to compare two or more subpopulations within the same group. It has already been noted that the best way to draw comparisons between rates occurring in groups is to compare similar levels of

	Crude rates	Age-adjusted rates
Chile	67.4	58.2
United States	316.3	136.4

Crude and age-adjusted death rates from heart disease for Chile and the United States for 1967. (Mausner, Baum, 1972)

specific rates—rates that are stratified on a variable such as age. By comparing age-specific rates, the effects of differences in age composition of the populations will not compromise comparisons between different groups. Another way of expressing this is to say that age-specific rates control for the distributional differences in a confounding variable (like age) when comparing rates between the groups. Age is the variable most likely to confound the outcome of disease or death because illnesses and deaths increase as the community becomes older. If age is not homogeneous in both groups, the rates will reflect the age difference between groups rather than a true difference in rates of disease. Suppose that a comparison is being made of summary rates of abortion between two communities served by two nursing agencies. In order to compare risk of abortion between the groups, one would have to adjust the rates for the confounding variable of age. It seems reasonable to expect different risks of abortion if one group has more older, postmenopausal women than the other group; thus, the rates for each group will be influenced by the different distributions of age in the two populations. Methods of adjusting rates have been developed so that valid comparisons can be made. How is an adjusted rate interpreted? One can safely say the risk is greater in one group than another only after knowing that an adjustment has been made to take away the error that would occur if the comparison were between a young population and an old population. When the rates have been adjusted, these differential distributions will have no effect and one can compare adjusted rates for directional differences between the two groups. An adjustment can be made for any variable that confounds the outcome event. To compare a risk of sickle cell anemia, a genetic-linked illness, an adjustment would be needed to compare the risk between two populations in which the distribution of blacks may be different.

A word about identifying the correct denominator is in order. The denominator for an incidence rate can be calculated as the middle point in a time period that is stable and reasonably reliable. Most cities and large geographic areas have large populations. People come and go but usually the numbers do not significantly alter or compromise the character of the p.a.r. or the size of the denominator. An assumption is made that those who leave the area are replaced by those entering the area. If there is no evidence to challenge this assumption, such as a sudden influx of immigrants to a city, or the closing of a large army base near a town, the p.a.r. may be assumed to be fairly constant over a short time span. If the observations of the public health nurse confirm that the area is relatively stable, the cumulative incidence rate with a denominator obtained from census information can be used with confidence.

Prevalence rates usually have a denominator that is well identified as the total group under observation. The problem with the prevalence rate is that it involves new and old cases in the numerator and denominator. As an expression of risk, the prevalence rate is less useful than incidence rate because nursing interventions to decrease risk of contracting a new disease are different from interventions for an old episode of disease. The probability of being an old or previously identified case of disease has little merit for clients or patients who already know they are stricken with illness. But preventions of further disability is an important nursing responsibility. Prevalence rates, though they denote the probability of being an old or a new case at one point in time in a community, are seldom used to denote risk and never used to denote casual association. Prevalence rates are used for management of nursing care in the community, for community assessment, and to generate rates as an index of the health of the community.

Summary

*T*he distinguishing characteristics of epidemiology are as follows: (1) epidemiology is (mainly) an observational science for public health; (2) epidemiology is delineated by methods and tools used to quantify observations and include the use of statistics, laboratory tests, and comparison of quantifications; (3) clients/patients are studied as populations, or communities; and (4) the outcome of illness or health is the dependent variable and is the outcome of interest for epidemiology. In general, the dependent variable of epidemiology may be viewed as a responsibility of the public health nurse. Epidemiology is a method of calibrating the effects of public health services through quantifying disease, quantifying risk, and measuring interventions. Are these characteristics solely the domain of epidemiology? Other social sciences have similar features. Anthropology is intermittently involved with communities and groups, as are sociology, demography, political science, and other disciplines. But the outcome event of the social sciences are different and therefore their focus is different. Anthropology's focus of study is the cultural mores in groups and the observations of behaviors that result from the influences of culture. Sociology studies the interactions of groups in the community and how value systems affect behavior. In demography, population trends for marketing are predicted; and in political science, observed group behavior is used to determine the influence of group interactions on political organizations and the use of power. All these sciences are interested in the community. They use statistics, perhaps not to the degree that epidemiology does, but certainly quantifications are an important part of their purview. The real difference between epidemiology and other group sciences is that epidemiology concentrates on the outcome of disease and health. It is this concern that distinguishes epidemiology in its approach to defining community problems. This science is of great importance to nursing, for it has the same outcome of concern as public health nursing—improving the health of communities by diminishing disease occurrences. Quantifications in epidemiology are accomplished by markers or tools from laboratory tests and by the use of statistics to identify change occurrences. Risk of disease is measured by special quantifications (rates); risk of exposure is measured by a comparison of two rates (risk ratios).

The basic statistic of public health is the rate. Rates are defined by time, such as incidence and prevalence; by numerator, such as cases of disease or episodes of cases; and by restricting the target population by applying a condition such as specific rates. Nursing prerogatives and priorities can be influenced by these statistics. Rates are used to show new problems requiring nursing services. They indicate the need for hiring new staff or staff with specialized nursing skills. They denote hazards in schools, hospitals and industry—in fact, in any setting where nursing surveillance is group-oriented. It is of the greatest importance that rates are understood by the public health nurse and nurse executives so that applications for nursing care in the community are made with increased scientific rigor. Rates also influence health policy and often summarize the evidence that provides a logical basis for change in health regulations and standards.[20]

References

1. School of Public Health, University of North Carolina at Chapel Hill, School of Public Health, University of Minnesota
2. Chavigny KH, Kroske MF: Public health nursing in crisis. Nurs Outlook 31:312–316, 1984
3. Webster's New Collegiate Dictionary. Spring Hill, MA, G & C Merriam, 1980
4. Stenger FE, Banta JE, Morris MH: Community Health—Today and Tomorrow. New York, NLN Publication No. 521768:1–130, 1979
5. Anderson E, Meyer AT: Report of the Conference. Consensus Conference on the Essentials of Public Health Nursing Practice and Education. Rockville, MD, U.S. Department of Health and Human Services, 1985
6. Snider, DE, Jones WD, Good RD: The usefulness of phage typing mycobacterium tuberculosis isolates. Am Rev Respir Dis 130 (6):1095–1099, 1984

7. Bauernfeind A, Petermuller C, Schneider R: Bacteriocins as tools of analysis of nosocomial *Klebsiella pneumoniae* infections. J Clin Microbiol 14(1):15–19, 1981

8. Grimwood R, Chavigny KH: A statistical test for classification of pathogens according to antibiotic sensitivity patterns. Biometrics 37:753–761, 1982

9. Chavigny KH: The antibiogram as an epidemiologic tool. J Urol Care and Infection Control (Part IV) 2:15, 17–21, 1977

10. Ashenafi M, Gedebou M: Salmonella and Shigella in adult diarrhea in Addis Ababa—prevalence and antibiograms. J Res Trop Med 79(5): 719–721, 1985

11. Boyd RF, Hoerl BG: Basic Medical Microbiology, 2nd ed. Boston, Little, Brown & Co, 1981

12. Remington RD, Schork MA: Statistics with Applications to the Biological and Health Sciences. Englewood Cliffs, NJ, Prentice–Hall, 1970

13. Breslow L, Hoagin L, Rasmussen G, Abrams HK: Occupations and cigarette smoking as factors in lung cancer. Am J Public Health 44:171–181, 1954

14. Parsons T: Definition of Health. Essays in Sociological Theory, rev ed. New York, Free Press, 1964

15. World Health Organization: The First Ten Years of the World Health Organization. New York, WHO, 1958

16. Susser MW, Watson W: Causal Thinking in the Health Sciences. New York, Oxford University Press, 1973

17. Mausner JS, Baum AK: Basic Medical Statistics. New York, Grune & Stratton, 1982

18. Fleiss JL: Statistical Methods for Rates and Proportions. New York, John Wiley & Sons, 1973

19. Elandt-Johnson RC: Defintions of rates: some remarks on their use and measure. Am J Epidemiol 102:4:267–271, 1975

20. Ibrahim MA: Epidemiology and Health Policy. Germantown, MD, Aspen Systems Corporation, 1985

Family as Client

LEARNING OBJECTIVES

After reading and understanding the contents of this chapter, the student will be able to:

1. *Adapt or create a definition of family that is consistent with the student's practice philosophy.*

2. *Differentiate the characteristics and functions typical of most family units.*

3. *Demonstrate the relationship between overall social class variables and population morbidity and mortality.*

4. *Identify the cultural background of any given family and relate how culture affects its health beliefs and behaviors. (You may also wish to refer to the discussion in Chapter 7.)*

5. *Review the ten traits or characteristics associated with healthy families.*

6. *Explain how nursing care of the family provides opportunities for case finding.*

7. *Describe how individual health is affected by the family, and how family health is affected by the well-being of each of its members.*

8. *State the basic components and rationale for family assessment.*

9. *List predominant demographic characteristics or trends among American families.*

Introduction

*F*amily" is a concept familiar to each of us, yet it can be a very complex and sometimes difficult one to grasp. There exists an extraordinary number of volumes and a variety of literature on the various facets and functions of the family unit. This literature has been generated over the years by scholars in disciplines such as anthropology, sociology, psych-mental health, marriage and family counseling, and nursing. As an entry-level nurse in community health, you will be dealing with the family as a unit, and thus it is important to understand the related body of knowledge that has evolved to the present day. The single, most important lesson to be learned is that the family is the basic unit of society, and it is a unit of service rather than merely a collection of individuals. In other words, the family is more than the sum of its parts.

The family structure, composition, heritage, lifestyle, communication patterns, and health beliefs have definite, if not always predictable, effects on the relative well-being of each family member. For this reason the community health nurse's concern is with the whole family unit. Whether the purpose of the nursing episode is preventive, curative, or restorative in nature, the nursing process and the resultant care plan should include the whole family instead of focusing unilaterally or exclusively on the one member whose health status may be compromised.

▋ *Family Defined*

If you were to ask ten people how they would define family, you'd very likely get ten different definitions. That same variety of definitions is present in the literature. Each person's definition reflects his own understanding and life experiences as well as his own value system. Likewise, there is a wide variety of opinions among scholars on the best definition of family, and those differences are reflected in the following sampling.

List of Definitions of Family
1. A group of two or more people who are emotionally involved with each other and choose to identify themselves as a family.[1]
2. The family involves people who are related in a traditional or non-traditional sense by marriage, blood, adoption or friendship.[2]
3. Primary group of people living in a household in consistent proximity and intimate relationships.[3]

4. A nuclear family is a small group consisting of parents and their non-adult children living in a single household. A family may also be defined as a "cluster of people whose relationship is stipulated by law in terms of marriage and descent, and whose precise membership varies according to circumstances."[4]

5. The family is a social group characterized by common residence, economic cooperation and reproduction. It includes adults of both sexes, at least two of whom maintain a socially approved sexual relationship, and one or more children. . . ."[5]

6. The coexistence of more than one human being involving continuous presumably permanent sharing of living facilities, a perception of reciprocal obligations, a sense of common-ness, and sharing of certain obligations toward others.[6]

7. As a rule of thumb, a family may be considered to be people related by blood and marriage, whether or not they reside in the same household, and immediate family to be those people related by blood or marriage who reside in the same household.[7]

8. A group of two or more persons related by birth, marriage or adoption and residing together in a household.[8]

9. Family is composed of people (two or more) who are emotionally involved with each other and live in close geographic proximity. Emotional involvement means that there is a perception of reciprocal obligations, a sense of common-ness, and a sharing of certain obligations, coupled with a caring and commitment to each other."[9] The author goes on to say that this definition is purposely broad so that it will include relationships such as are represented by two members of the same sex linked through homosexual attachment or two friends living together for a sustained period.

10. Family is defined as a human group with significant emotional bonds, usually living together in the same household. Significant emotional bonds are those of emotional gratification, affection, and caring, and those of interdependence, responsibility, loyalty, accountability, and commitment."[10]

11. Family is a "relationship community of two or more persons" in which individuals may come from the same or different kinship groups.[11]

Some of the listed definitions are quite traditional in nature whereas others include nontraditional concepts of families, such as two members of the same or opposite sex who are not related by marriage or blood. Other definitions in the list differentiate nuclear families from extended families in that nuclear families live together and are usually related, whereas extended members live outside the primary residence. In essence, the way one chooses to define family is based on one's experience with family and one's individual philosophy and value set. For example, from a public health science viewpoint, family is defined in terms of social support systems, as seen in Chapter 2. None of these definitions is right or wrong. Some are just broad or restrictive as to what can actually be called a family.

■ *Characteristics of Family*

Regardless of how one defines the family, it is important to realize that the prevalence of nontraditional family units is growing in contemporary America. A person in a nontraditional family, like one in a traditional family comprising a mother, father and child, affects the health and well-being of all family members. Therefore, it is important to view members of both traditional and nontraditional families as a unit in each phase of the nursing process.

Reviewing the various definitions of family illustrates the differences in family structure and composition, but there are also universal characteristics that may be considered applicable to nearly all family units regardless of their makeup. Spradley has identified five of these universal characteristics which are as follows:

Five Universal Characteristics of Family

1. Every family is a small social system.
2. Every family has its own cultural values and rules.
3. Every family has its own structure.
4. Every family performs certain basic functions.
5. Every family moves through stages of the life cycle.

As a social system, families interact with the greater community as well as with their own nuclear and extended members. Further, families interact with the animate and inanimate environment or surroundings and, in turn, are affected by the community in which they live, play, go to school, and work. For example, if a given community lacks needed recreational or educational facilities, family units will suffer the consequences or go outside the immediate community. On the other hand, when resources or facilities exist but are not used or supported by families, the community is, in turn, adversely affected. As will be seen in subsequent chapters, a healthy community is one that provides the conditions and resources that promote a healthy family life. In turn, the relative health of any given neighborhood or community is at least partially dependent on its larger community such as the state, the nation, the world, and even the solar system. Thus, family and individual health would suffer if conditions in the larger system were not supportive of basic human needs such as safety, access to food and water, adequate sanitation, clean air, and adequate shelter.

Another variable that impacts on family life and, therefore, individual development and well-being, is social class. Educational level, occupation, and income are factors that help to determine social class, but family background is also a consideration—especially for members of the upper class. It is important to consider social class because the identification of socioeconomic factors can better help the community health nurse to anticipate family resources, potential health stressors, and even individual family structure and function in some cases.[9]

The relationship between social class and subsequent morbidity and mortality has been observed for centuries, and evidence has shown consistently that members of the lower classes have a greater incidence and prevalence of illness, a higher rate of disability, and an overall decreased life expectancy. The most frequent explanations associated with this phenomenon include poor housing, crowding, low income, poor education, unemployment, nonavailability or nonutilization of health care resources, and increased exposure to noxious agents.[13]

To further illustrate the relationship between social class variables such as education and mortality, one study found that white males with low educational levels had age-adjusted mortality rates 64% higher than men with higher educational levels. For white women, those in the lower educated groups had an age-adjusted mortality rate 105% higher than those in the higher educated groups.[14]

As will be discussed in Chapter 7, every family is characterized by varying cultural values and rules. In the most basic sense, it is membership in a family that instills individuals with not only specific cultural beliefs and practices, but also with a knowledge of how these practices are recognized and celebrated. Clearly there are cultural differences between families of the Jewish and Christian faiths, for example, but even more differences may be noted among individual families within each faith. For instance, although Christians philosophically believe in holidays such as Christmas and Easter, each family may vary in the way and extent to which these holidays are celebrated. Some families place a high value on attending religious ceremonies that mark these holidays, whereas other families place more importance on the family's celebration within the home.

The community health nurse's cultural value set is often quite different from the families being served, but the important points to be learned by the nurse are the following. First, it is important to ascertain what the family's cultural values and rules are so that plans for care will not conflict or negate these rules and values. Cultural beliefs may have a profound effect on health behaviors, and thus they may be ascertained during the assessment phase. Second, as is true of all care settings, it is imperative that the nurse be accepting and insightful of cultural backgrounds, and that personal values not be imposed on the client caseload.

▮ *Every Family Has Its Own Structure*

As reflected in the various definitions of family, families vary in their structural makeup. While traditional families may be composed of mother, father and offspring, there are also many single-parent families as well as childless, married couples. Nontraditional families may be composed of several adults who may or may not have children, as seen in communal groups whose members share a single dwelling. In some instances, three or more generations of the same family may cohabit, or persons of the same gender may reside together with or without children. There has even been some argument that single individuals may be conceptualized as family units under some conditions.

Every family member has various roles to play, and the stability of the family unit is at least partially dependent on the successful enactment of those roles. Individual roles are allocated and defined by the family and are related to the things the family must accomplish to remain functional. Examples of family roles are nurturer, disciplinarian, wage earner and meal planner. Multiple roles may be played by given family members, and there is usually some flexibility in the assigning and acting out of these roles. When role responsibilities change abruptly or role expectations vary, confusion develops and the relative wellness of the family unit may be compromised. In essence, when roles are not performed, the family may fail to accomplish the things necessary for maintenance or even survival of the family. For example, suppose a female head of a household becomes an alcoholic. Time may be lost from work, resulting in decreased monies available for food purchases and other household expenses. Further, the inebriated member may subject either herself or other family members to various safety hazards, and her allocation of time to the family as a whole may be seriously compromised. In situations where there is an alcoholic spouse or parent, it is frequently necessary for other family members to assume additional roles to keep the family functioning in any fashion. When other members of the family are forced to assume role behaviors previously assigned to another, considerable stress is generated and the result may manifest itself in unstable family functioning.

Just as every family allocates roles to help conduct overall family living, each family has an operative power system. Although the nature and allocation of power may vary from family to family, power in the form of decision-making must necessarily exist. Sometimes the power for decision-making may rest primarily with one individual; other times, decisions are formed in a more democratic or egalitarian fashion. When the decision-making capacity of the family is compromised, equilibrium is disrupted and overt emotional or physical illness may follow.

Every family performs certain basic functions, such as meeting individual needs for affection, security, identity, affiliation, socialization, and controls.[12] It is important to note that family functions, like the structure and composition of families, change over time. Historically a family was viewed as having five major functions.[15] Examples of family functions are found in the following list.

Family Functions

- To achieve economic survival
- To provide physical protection to individual members
- To pass on the religious faith
- To educate its young
- To confer status

For nearly 100 years, if a family met those five criteria, they were considered a healthy or "a good family." But in recent years, these five traditional functions of family have changed and largely disappeared in response to societal needs. For example, large families with multiple offspring were thought to ensure economic survival in the past because children were expected to participate in family wage-earning and to care for aging parents. But now children are no longer economic assets, but costly luxuries. For instance, a couple with the national average of 1.8 children face a $124,000 responsibility dispersed over a minimum of 18 years for a middle-class lifestyle.[15]

A more contemporary approach to family is to examine what goes on inside the family, such as whether there is effective communication and provision for needed emotional support. Fifteen traits can be identified in the healthy family, including communication skills and emotional support. These traits, along with a brief description, are listed below.

*Fifteen Traits of a Healthy Family**
1. The family communicates and listens. This trait or strength is based on the notion that the major function of a family is relational rather than physical. Instead of dominating family members, healthy spouses complement one another.

*With permission, from Curran D: Traits of a Healthy Family. Minneapolis, Winston Press, 1983

2. The family members affirm and support one another. The family realizes that support doesn't mean pressure, so the members help to develop realistic goals and control expectations of self and others. Additionally, the family's basic mood is positive.
3. The family teaches respect for individual members and others. The family respects individual differences in family members and accords respect for a variety of outside groups.
4. The family develops a sense of trust between and among its own members.
5. The family has a sense of humor and play. The family recognizes its need to play, but doesn't necessarily equate play with spending money.
6. The family exhibits a sense of shared responsibility. In this instance, responsibility is geared to individual capability, and responsibility is paired with recognition.
7. The family teaches a sense of right and wrong, and parents or adults share a consensus on important values.
8. There is a strong sense of family in which rituals and traditions abound, and there is often an identifiable locus (either person or place) for family activity.
9. The family has a shared religious core and respects religious differences.
10. The family members respect the privacy of one another.
11. The family values service to others within and outside the family unit.
12. The family fosters family table time and conversation, and encourages expression of individual feelings and independent thinking.
13. The family shares leisure time and values opportunities to spend time together.
14. The family has a balance of interaction among its members. Family members listen and respond, and they recognize verbal and nonverbal messages among members. The family members interrupt one another, but equally, and there is an intensity and spontaneity of exchange.
15. The family admits and seeks help with problems that cannot be solved among its membership.

Curran's 15 traits of a healthy family have important ramifications for nursing assessment of family, for when a family possesses some or all of these strengths, it may be able to withstand physical, social or emotional disability and remain a relatively healthy family unit. In fact, when families possess these skills, crisis situations may result in growth of the family unit and acquisition of new coping skills.

Conversely, families who possess few of these traits may have trouble dealing with daily living activities and may be devastated by disability or illness in one member. There are many situations where families are able to ensure serious health threats or even the death of a member. But when families have serious deficits in communication skills or a power imbalance, they are at a much greater risk of becoming permanently fragmented or even dissolved when crisis does occur.

■ *The Nursing Process Applied to Family*

Different practice settings provide the nurse with a variety of experiences in family health care. In acute care settings, it is often mandatory that the individual client be the focus of nursing attention, especially when physiologic or emotional crises occur. In such instances, the family may necessarily be peripheral, although it should become more central to the nurse's concern as the intensity of the episode lessens.

Exchanges with family members may be limited to keeping them informed and taking moments to listen to family concerns when there is a nursing or medical emergency. However, when the individual client's status becomes less acute, the family should once again be the unit of concern. For example, in critical care settings, family visitation and involvement with client care is contingent on a number of factors, including the relative severity/stability of the client's condition. When the client improves, the family can be incorporated into the nursing plan of care. As discharge nears, nursing emphasis should be focused firmly on the entire family unit.

The amount of attention given the family unit is partially contingent on individual nursing philosophy and is sometimes limited by structural or functional care settings. Some nursing specialities emphasize the individual client as the unit of immediate concern, but the traditional and ongoing unit of care for public health nurses has been the family as well as the family's physical, social, and emotional environment. Just as with individuals, the nursing process provides the basic framework for nursing practice with families.[16]

The reason that the family unit is the unit of care for the community health nurse is because the more we know about family, the more we realize that the individual's potential for wellness is influenced, in incalculable ways, by the family unit. In essence, if the family (however it is defined) does not value and understand a plan of care, or does not have the necessary resources to carry out the plan of care, the prescribed regimen for the individual family members will most likely not be carried out effectively.

Another reason that identifying the family as the unit of care is essential to community health nursing is because such an approach provides rich case-finding opportunities that suggest any of the levels of prevention. For example, many home health nurses gain access to the family because of a referral identifying some nursing deficit in one given family member. Even though the initial reason for the home visit may revolve around the individual client's health problem, the community health nurse incorporates and involves the family in the client's care as soon as possible. Thus, the database for effective community health practice includes data on specific family members, as well as data on the psychosocial and physical environment of the family. Inclusion of the family into the plan of care helps to enhance the changes that the plan of care will be carried out. Collection of data on all family members also allows rich opportunities for case finding.

As an example of case finding, assume that a given home visit was originally conducted to help an obese, insulin-dependent diabetic to self-administer insulin. As the nurse gathers rudimentary family data, it is learned that the 13-year-old daughter is also obese and frequently misses school due to recurrent headaches. Thus the community health nurse started out teaching the diabetic client how to self-administer insulin; however, knowing that obesity makes diabetic control very difficult and that diabetes is familial, the nurse enlarges the plan of care to include both the initial client and the daughter. Additionally, the nurse makes a note to further assess the remaining family members, and to perform a physical assessment on the mother and daughter on a return visit. Through epidemiologic case finding, the nurse has identified the 13-year-old girl as an individual who is at high risk for diabetes. By using primary prevention strategies (general health promotion) such as weight control, the daughter may be able to avoid becoming clinically diabetic; through secondary prevention strategies (early diagnosis and treatment), the daughter may be diagnosed ultimately as diabetic. In the latter instance, treatment/management modalities may be instituted to limit the disability associated with diabetes.

One of the reasons that the family is the unit of concern in community health nursing is that an individual's relative potential for wellness is frequently and deeply affected by the family unit's structure, composition, heritage, lifestyle, communication patterns, level of education, and health beliefs. Additionally, by focusing on the family unit, valuable opportunities exist for epidemiologic case finding and intervention based on the levels of prevention. Finally, a full understanding of a family cannot be developed by dealing only with some of the family members. As illustrated in the following material, the substance and sequencing of the nursing process does not change; rather, the unit of concern is modified from individual to family.

Assessment

In some instances, the database collected on the family will be dictated either by an instructor or a clinical agency where clients are selected. It is sufficient to say that there are numerous ways to approach family assessment, just as there are many variations in individual client assessments. It is also true that complex family assessments constructed from specific conceptual or theoretic frameworks are probably best left to the nurse with a master's degree or a doctorate. The fact that several texts exist that center on different kinds of family assessment is testimony to the variations in approaches to the process.

Family assessment is typically an ongoing process since single nurse–client encounters are rarely lengthy or concentrated enough to gather a complete database. Methods of data collection in the assessment phase include interviewing, observing the physical environment, subjectively appraising the family by interacting with the family to note communication patterns, task allocation and nonverbal behaviors. Another valuable source of assessment data consists of written or verbal communication with other health care team members.[9]

The following family assessment is adapted from Burgess and consists of several different categories of health-related information.[17]

- Basic information about each member
- Resources available to the family
- Environmental considerations
- Health status of each family member
- Family health practices
- Family lifestyle
- Summary of assessment data and formulation of nursing diagnosis

Basic Information About Each Family Member

Names, addresses, and telephone numbers, as well as information relating to the location of the home are collected and recorded. The initial date of service should be noted as should the referral source and the reason for the referral. Other useful information includes age, sex, family position, occupation(s), educational level, and language spoken and understood by each member. The nurse must be sensitive to the implications of data such as unemployment, inability to speak English, or different surnames. Also, it is necessary to obtain further information if significant members are not currently living in the home. The nurse must be aware that family pets often play a significant role in family life: their names, types and presence should be noted. As mentioned earlier, because a family's religion and/or ethnic or cultural background bear on the family's health beliefs and behaviors, this information should also be obtained.[17]

Resources Available to the Family

Family resources include a multiplicity of factors that might conceivably be mobilized to help the family meet physical and/or emotional health care needs. For example, does the family have an adequate income, savings and/or substantial health and life insurance coverage? What health care delivery mechanisms and personnel are currently being used to meet health maintenance needs? Are these agencies and personnel able to meet continuing health care needs of the family in question? If the nuclear family unit is unable to meet specific health needs, are there extended family members who could be mobilized? What kind of access does the family have to health care providers and agencies? What is the nature and extent of the family's involvement in social networking; that is, do family members belong to religious or paternal organizations in the community? Which family members work which hours, and how flexible is the work schedule?

Obtaining answers to the above questions allows the community health nurse to help the family plan for present and future health care needs, as well as to make appropriate referrals to community resources when indicated. Some of the data required, especially that pertaining to income and savings, is usually a sensitive issue. It is probably better to obtain this sort of information using skillful interview techniques after some degree of therapeutic relationship is established.

Environmental Considerations

Systematic observation of both the intramural and extramural family environments should be made. The intramural (within walls) or home environment should be assessed to ascertain if the physical structure provides for hygiene, safety and the special needs of the family. It is important for the nurse to record specific information on the state of the physical structure as well as the number of rooms in relation to the number of inhabitants since the amount of living space required depends on numerous factors, including socioeconomic and cultural considerations. For example, some Spanish–American homes may appear too small to the nurse, whereas the family's perception may be quite different.

Aside from notations on the size of the home, the general state of repair, both inside and outside, should be noted. Are there obvious safety hazards, such as open wall sockets, in the presence of toddlers? Is there sufficient light, ventilation, cooling, and heating (depending on climatic conditions)? Are kitchen, bath, and laundry facilities functional and adequate for the family's need? Are disease vectors such as flies, roaches, or rodents a problem in the home? Most of these environmental considerations can be assessed as the opportunity arises, and complete assessment of the home may necessitate several visits since "inspection tours" are obtrusive.

The experienced community health nurse uses every opportunity to observe environmental considerations as well as other factors that bear on the health and well-being of the family. For example, the drive to visit the family creates a good opportunity to observe the extramural environment or community in which the family's home is located. The observable nature of that community provides clues to socioeconomic status, safety, and even overt health hazards, such as pollution and crowding. Specific assessment criteria relative to the concept of community will be discussed in detail in the next chapter. For now, it is sufficient to say that the family's potential for health is influenced continuously by its greater social, psychological, and physical environments.

Health Status of Each Family Member

The community health nurse should assess the physical and emotional health of each family member using an individual client assessment tool. As noted earlier, such an assessment provides opportunities for case finding and identification of anomalies that may affect the entire family unit. Types of information collected should include: name (including nickname); age; height and weight; habits and types of substance use or abuse including tobacco, alcohol, over-the-counter drugs, prescription drugs, and illegal substances; developmental stage; summary of health history; and current health status, including treatments and medications.

Additionally, if individual members have specific health problems, the nurse may want to complete a detailed, physical assessment, a mental-status examination, a Denver Development Test, or other specific or appropriate measurements. The health status of each member should be viewed in the context of the whole family unit. For instance, if a wage earner suffers a stroke, how can the other members be mobilized to care for the stricken member and begin assuming some of the ill member's roles and responsibilities within the family?

Family Health Practices

Family health practices include a multitude of health-seeking behaviors. Does the family make provisions for regular physical examinations, dental care and monitoring of individual health care problems? Additionally, the nutritional status should be determined to include variations such as obesity and the use of vitamin and mineral supplements. Recreation and exercise activities may include activities such as gardening and walking, as well as whatever the family defines as recreation. Finally, sleep patterns should be ascertained.

Family Lifestyle

The way a family organizes or experiences daily living can have a significant bearing on overall potential for health. When doing an in-depth family assessment, the nurse will want to ascertain how decisions are made, how the family defines and responds to crisis, and what overall attitudes the members have about health and well-being. Further, the nurse will want to determine how the family relates to the greater community. For example, is the family relatively isolated from the community, or do family members belong to community, professional, or religious organizations? Another question to ask is whether the community in question possesses resources needed by the family, and whether the family uses or values these resources.

Summary of Assessment Data and Formulation of the Nursing Diagnosis

After completing the family assessment, it is necessary to review and organize the data. (Refer to Curran's 15 traits of a healthy family earlier in this chapter.) How many of these traits can be identified? Identify specific strengths and weaknesses as they relate to the family's realization for maximum health potential. Specific risk factors that were identified as part of the assessment process can now be categorized under headings such as environmental risks, heredity, social/psychological, types and extent of substance abuse, acute/chronic disease or disability, developmental and interactional factors. One can now formulate a nursing diagnosis based on the assessment data. Essentially, the nursing diagnosis will reflect the following information.

- Family strengths
- Identification of specific health problems in family members
- Risk factors or potential for development of disease or dysfunction

Once problems are identified and categorized, they should be prioritized according to importance. The client's input (from the individual member and family as a whole) should be sought before priorities are finalized because it does little good for the community health nurse to centralize efforts and resources around a problem unless the family also assigns that problem high priority. When nurse and client jointly set priorities, the chance for successful intervention is heightened.[9,17]

Planning

Mutual goal-setting between the nurse and the client will help to identify possible resources and alternative approaches to be used in the intervention process. Goals should be acceptable to both the nurse and the client, and they should be clearly stated in behavioral terms so that ultimately they can be measured and evaluated. Goals then may be separated into (1) specific, immediate, and measurable short-term goals; (2) middle- or intermediate-level goals; and (3) long-term, more general goals that indicate the broad purposes that the nurse and family hope to achieve.[9(p 34)] During the planning phase, it may be important to consider what role(s) could be played by other members of the health care team, and then to consult these professionals as to the sequencing of their participation.

Implementation

In the home setting, the implementation phase involves any number of health professionals, including the community health nurse, and the client. Sometimes extended family members or significant others are also included. As the community health nurse works with the family, interventions are aimed at helping the family members change or modify their health behaviors. In reality, the nurse strives to enhance family skills and functioning so that higher family wellness or health is achieved. Thus interventions involving the family are aimed at helping the family to develop and expand its own problem-solving skills relating to health.[9]

Implementation requires the use of all one's nursing, public health and epidemiologic knowledge. Additionally, two methodologies have been identified that will increase the nurse's effectiveness when dealing with the family as a client. The first method is teaching, and the second is the use of contracts. Actually these skills should not be new, since they are used frequently in many types of nursing situations.

Teaching skills lie at the heart of public health nursing. In fact, as mentioned in Chapter 1, public health nurses were once called teaching nurses. Teaching skills are also a valuable method of prevention and control as indicated in the public health model for nursing practice. Teaching skills are used in the intervention phase to provide the family members with skills needed to meet their own health maintenance and promotion needs. Contracts are working agreements that specify client responsibilities as opposed to the responsibilities or functions of the health care team. The philosophy underlying these family-centered activities has been mentioned several times. In essence, use of contracts promotes client involvement which, in turn, increases the chances of the plan being carried out. Contracts include goals, length of time needed to accomplish the goals, and assignment of responsibilities to achieve mutually decided goals.[9]

Evaluation

The effectiveness of the plan of care is ascertained by examining family responses and outcomes and, like all other phases of family-centered nursing, the examination is a joint endeavor between the nurse and the family. If clear and behaviorally explicit goals have been written in the planning phase, evaluation of the plan is expedited. The evaluation phase is a time when the community health nurse assesses the realism and accuracy of the goals. Because all phases of the nursing process involve both the family and the nurse, it is important to determine the client's perceptions as to whether problems have been satisfactorily resolved.[9]

■ *Demographic Overview of the American Family*

Thus far, this chapter has focused on the qualitative traits, definitions, and characteristics of the family, and the nursing process applied to the family. Even though it is important to understand the qualities of a healthy family, it is often illuminating to explore quantitative descriptions as well. The demographic or statistical study of the size and distribution of American families or households is conducted every 10 years by the United States Bureau of the Census. The data that follows was gathered in the mid-1980s, and it provides a type of composite picture of the American family. It should be noted that the term "households" is further differentiated into family households and nonfamily households. A nonfamily household is one in which a person is living alone or with one or more persons who are not relatives.[8]

Although the number of households in the nation increased to 85.4 million by 1984, real increases in the number of separate households has been gradually declining since 1980. The decline in the rate of increase seen in past years is due partly to changes in the age structure of Americans. For instance, the population in the 20–34-year-old age group, the period when most persons form households for the first time, grew very rapidly during the 1970s as the baby-boom generation reached young adulthood. But the birthrate has been declining since 1960, and thus, fewer people belong to the 20–34 year group in the 1980s.

The second reason that there is a slower increase in the number of separate households is that the divorce rate in America has stabilized in recent years. When people remain married, the two spouses retain one household. The third factor behind the decline in new households is that more young adult offspring appear to be living with their parents, many marrying later in life (Table 5-1).

The data in Table 5-1 show an increase of nontraditional family units in that almost half (47%) of all households added since 1980 have been nonfamily households (according to the Census Bureau; one's definition of family may include most or all of these people). It is noteworthy that there were 20 million one-person households and about 2 million heterosexual, unmarried couples living together. A look back at data from the 1970s shows that there were only about 523,000 unmarried couples of opposite sexes identified by census data; however, there may have been more reluctance to report such relationships in the 1970s.

Although mentioned earlier, for clarification, the Census Bureau publishes figures on three types of family households. These are (1)

T A B L E   5 - 1
Specific Data on Households Reported by the 1984 Census

1. Total number of households in 1984: 85.4 million
2. Percent increase, 1980–1984: 5%
3. Average annual increase, 1980–1984: 1.2 million
4. Number of families in 1984: 62.0 million
   Percent with female householder (no husband present): 15.9%
5. Average family size in 1984: 3.24 persons
6. Number of nonfamily households in 1984: 23.4 million
7. Percent increase, 1980–1984: 10.3%
8. Percent of nonfamily households living alone in 1984: 85.2%

(U.S. Bureau of the Census, Current Population Reports, Series P-23, No. 145, *Population Profile of the United States*: 1983–84, Washington, D.C., U.S. Government Printing Office, 1985).

married-couple households (50.1 million in 1984); (2) families with a female householder where no husband is present (9.9 million in 1984); and (3) families with a male householder where no wife is present (2.0 million households in 1984). The number of families maintained by women with no husband present began to increase markedly in the 1970s and has continued through the 1980s. Thus, the number of nontraditional family units clearly is increasing.

Another notable trend that deserves attention is that the average family size in the United States reached a record low mark in 1984. The average number of family members under 18 years of age was also at a record low. The following are the underlying factors associated with this trend: (1) the age structure of the population is changing in that there are now more people in the older age groups; (2) crude mortality rates are continuing to decline since people are literally living longer; and (3) the fertility rate has decreased markedly due to a number of pharmacologic and sociologic changes.

The age distribution in America has considerable ramifications for health care delivery and for nursing. From this information it can be extrapolated that the proportion of aged clients will be increasing while overall family size will decrease. Further, since it is known that there is a strong relationship between chronic illnesses, such as heart disease and diabetes, and increased age, one can expect to see an increase in these health problems as the number of older people increase in the population.

■ *Living Arrangements and Marital Status*

As noted earlier, the number of single-parent families has increased dramatically in recent years. In fact, one out of four (22.6%) of the nation's 62.1 million children under the age of 18 years lived with only one of their parents in 1984. Over half of all black children (53%) lived with one parent in 1984, compared with 17% of white children. Despite the relatively new trend for some divorced fathers to accept custody of their children, only 2% of American children lived with their father in 1984.

Larger Proportion of Young Adults Live With Parents

Throughout the 1980s, there has been a quantifiable increase in the number of young adults who live in their parent's household. For example, in 1984, one half (52%) of men 20 to 24 years old lived with their parents compared with only 43% in 1970. For women aged 20–24 years, 32% lived with their parents in 1984 compared with 27% in 1970. Further, about 16% of men and 8% of women 25–29 years old were living with at least one of their parents in 1984. These increases are partly due to the tendency of young adults to delay marriage and to the occurrence of divorce when young adults may return to their parent's residence. The tendency to delay marriage is reflected in the fact that 75% of men aged 20–24 years in 1984 never married compared to 55% in 1970. Further, the median age for the first marriage has risen during the 1970 to 1984 period from 23.2 years to 25.4 years for men, and from 20.8 years to 23.0 years for women.

Nearly One Third of the Elderly Live Alone

In 1984, 53% of the nation's 26.3 million people 65 years of age and over (excluding those in institutions) were living with a spouse, and another 14% were living with other relatives. The remaining one third of the elderly population (8.6 million people) did not live with persons related to them, and the majority of these people (7.9 million) lived alone.

Following declines from 1980 to 1982, median family income increased 1.6% to $24,580 in 1983. Even so, the 1983 median was more than $2000 below the median income for 1978. For all age and household groups, increased education was associated with increased earnings.

The median income of white families increased by 1.4% between 1982 and 1983, whereas the increases for black and Hispanic families were not statistically significant. Part of the continuing difference between black and white families is due to differences in family composition, with blacks having a much higher proportion of families maintained by women.

To further illustrate the income differences between men and women in the United States, families maintained by women who worked full time throughout the year with no husband in the household had a median income in 1983 of $18,620. In contrast, family households maintained by men who worked full time throughout the year with no wife in the household had a median income of $28,330 during that same year. In March, 1984, about 15% of the nation's 85.4 million households consisted of women living alone. The median income of these women was $9,140 in 1983. In contrast, men living alone at that time accounted for about 9% of all households, but their median income was substantially higher at $14,120 (Table 5-2).

Although it would be risky to predict which federal government programs will be in effect in 1990, it is useful to look back at a period of time in a year past to examine what percentage of Americans qualified for and availed themselves of federal assistance. For example, as illustrated in Table 5-3, Social Security, Medicare, and Medicaid were the most frequently used benefit programs. Because persons 65 years of age and older are the single fastest growing component of the United States population, that trend is likely to continue unless the system undergoes drastic changes which could conceivably occur out of economic necessity.

Forty-eight percent of all Americans, or 31.7 million people receiving benefits from governmental programs (14% of the total population) used Medicare or Medicaid resources in 1983. The Medicare system was used heavily because of the number of elderly Americans, and also because an American citizen can qualify for Medicare regardless of economic need.

Programs such as food stamps, Medicaid, and Aid to Families with Dependent Children require that the individual or family meet a

T A B L E   5 - 2
Family Income: **The 1983 Median Income:**

All families	$24,580.
Married-couple families	$27,290.
Married-couple family, wife in paid labor force	$32,110
Families with a female householder, no husband present	$11,790.
Families with a male householder, no wife present	$21,850.
Women living alone	$ 9,140.
Men living alone	$14,120.

(U.S. Bureau of the Census. 1983–1984.)

T A B L E   5 - 3
Percent of Nonfarm Persons Receiving Benefits from One or More Government Programs, Third Quarter, 1983: 29.6%

Type of benefit	% of Persons receiving	Total number
Social Security	14.1%	31.7 million
Medicare	11.9%	26.7 million
Food Stamps	8.3%	18.7 million
Medicaid	7.8%	17.5 million
Aid to Families w/ Dependent Children	4.2%	*

*Not Calculated. U.S. Bureau of the Census. 1983–1984.

specified level of need. These are called means-tested programs. As shown in Table 5-3, the two largest programs were food stamps and Medicaid. This sort of data has meaning for the community health nurse in that they are partial barometers of poverty among the population.

As might be expected from reviewing the information on median family income, there was a large difference in race, marital status, and sex in those receiving federal benefits. For example, 13% of white households received such benefits, compared with 42% of black households and 35% of Hispanic households. Similarly, 55% of female householders with children and no husband present received one or more kinds of federal assistance. For added impact, that 55% benefits utilization rate can be compared to a 19% benefits utilization rate among married-couple families. One in three families receiving benefits was maintained by a woman who had children under 18 years of age and no husband present in the household.

Summary

*B*ecause community health nursing is family-centered, it is important to understand the myriad ways in which a family affects and is affected by an individual member's health status. However one defines family, there are certain characteristics that are universal, such as the notion that every family has its own cultural values and rules. The goal of community health nursing is to equip family units with knowledge and skills that will ultimately allow them to promote and maintain health. The nursing process applied to families is interdisciplinary and involves the family unit in all phases. Although entry into any given family may be initiated by a referral to a sick member of the group, the ultimate goal is *family* health.

1. Burgess W, Ragland EC: Community Health Nursing: Philosophy, Process, Practice, p 247. Norwalk, CT, Appleton-Century-Crofts, 1983
2. Jarvis L: Community Health Nursing: Keeping the Public Healthy, 2nd ed, p 152. Philadelphia, FA Davis, 1985
3. Helvie C: Community Health Nursing: Theory and Process, p 64. New York, Harper & Row, 1981
4. Farber B: Family and Kinship in Modern Society, p 2. Glenview, Il, Scott, Foresman & Co, 1973
5. Murdock GP: Social Structure, p 1. New York, Free Press, 1965
6. Mauksch H: A social science basis for conceptualizing family health. Soc Sci Med 8:522, 1974
7. Clements IW, Roberts FB (eds): Family Health: A Theoretical Approach to Nursing Care, p 8. New York, John Wiley & Sons, 1983
8. U.S. Bureau of the Census: Statistical Abstract of the United States, 106th ed. Washington, D.C., U.S. Government Printing Office, 1986
9. Friedman MM: Family Nursing: Theory and Assessment, 2nd ed, p 8 Norwalk, CT, Appleton-Century-Crofts, 1986
10. Leavitt MB: Families at Risk: Primary Prevention in Nursing Practice, p 6. Boston, Little, Brown & Co, 1982
11. Jordheim AE: Alternate lifestyles and the family. In Reinhardt AM, Quinn MD (eds): Family-Centered Community Health Nursing in a Sociocultural Framework, vol 2, p 61. St Louis, CV Mosby Co, 1980
12. Spradley BW: Community Health Nursing: Concepts and Practice, 2nd ed. Boston, Little, Brown & Co, 1985
13. Syme SL, Berkman, LF: Social class, susceptibility, and sickness. In Conrad P, Kern R (eds): The Sociology of Health and Illness. Clinical Perspectives
14. Kitagana EM, Hauser PM: Differential Mortality in the United States. Cambridge, Harvard University Press, 1973
15. Curran D: Traits of a Healthy Family. Minneapolis, Winston Press, 1983
16. Yura H, Walsh MB: The Nursing Process, 3rd ed. New York, Appleton-Century-Crofts, 1978
17. Burgess W: Family health and risk assessment. In Burgess W, Ragland EC (eds): Community Health Nursing: Philosophy, Process, Practice. Norwalk, CT, Appleton-Century-Crofts, 1983

References

Community as Client

LEARNING OBJECTIVES

After reading and understanding the contents of this chapter, the student will be able to:

1. Explain the difference between territorial and relational communities.

2. Adapt or create a definition of community that is consistent with practice philosophy.

3. List five characteristics of a healthy community.

4. Differentiate between geopolitical communities, territorial communities, and communities of interest.

5. Analyze the relationship between individual and family health and the overall health status of the community.

6. Name the indications for and purposes of community assessment, and contrast the qualitative and quantitative aspects of community assessment.

7. Identify at least two methods for determining the population at risk (p.a.r.) for purposes of community assessment.

8. Cite at least one use for the proportional mortality rate and the case fatality rate.

9. Calculate simple summary and specific rates, and identify numerator and denominator information.

10. List five types of information required for any complete community assessment.

Introduction

*T*he preceding discussion and analysis of the family according to the nursing process provides a logical foundation for discussion and analysis of a larger societal unit called the community. Just as the family influences individual potential for well-being, there is constant reciprocity between a community and the individuals of which it is composed. Not only is individual and family well-being affected in numerous ways by the community, but the community is shaped and influenced by its inhabitants, their behaviors and attitudes. Analysis of the community as client is a functional example of the union between nursing and public health practice since clinical practice in nursing usually focuses on the health of individuals, but public health practice focuses on the health of population in which the family is the unit of concern. Family and community are basic constructs in the public health model discussed in Chapter 2.

■ *Nursing Approach to Community*

Obviously there are different sizes and types of communities, and most people belong to or function within several different communities in the process of daily living activities. Although there are numerous ways in which communities can be categorized, one way to describe or differentiate communities is according to the nature of the bond between people comprising the population. One type of bond between members in a community is called territorial, while another type of bond is called relational.[1]

Territorial bonds are defined by boundaries of the community. There are three subdivisions of communities in which the inhabitants experience territorial bonds, geographical, problem ecology and solution.

1. A geopolitical community that has defined special boundaries such as schools of nursing, towns, cities, and countries. For example, the geopolitical community to which we belong is the earth. A geopolitical community may be either intramural (within walls) or extramural (outside walls, the greater community beyond institutional or agency walls).
2. Communities of problem ecology—These communities consist of a locale in which a particular problem exists although the actual territorial boundaries may overlap into more than one geopolitical community. For example, water or air pollution may actually be produced in one city limit (geopolitical community), but may

have the most adverse effect on a separate city downstream or downwind.

3. Community of solution—This type of community may be created in response to a problem ecology. This area, however, defined in geopolitical boundaries, is one in which the resources necessary to solve the problem are found.

Community may be defined by relational bonds. These groups or communities are those in which the bond between individuals exists in the form of a commonality of relationship rather than specific geographic or political boundaries and consist of community of interest and feeling community.

1. Community of interest: In this instance, the community is formed by a relational bond of shared interests or goals between and among the individuals. Here the members share a common interest or concern which is fostered through participation in the group. An example of a community of interest is a professional organization such as the American Nurses' Association.
2. A feeling community: In this instance, the bond between individuals who comprise the community is an emotional feeling of belonging, and examples include one's own neighborhood, or the Class of 1990.

    It is important to realize that none of these types of communities is mutually exclusive. That is, an individual or family may belong to any combination of these communities, even at the same time. Further, some groups and communities are formed by a mixture of intrapersonal bonds. For example, Alcoholics Anonymous may be considered a community of solution with vaguely-formed geographic boundaries, or it may be considered a community of interest that has no identifiable geographic boundaries.

▌ *Definitions of Community*

By the preceding discussion, one can see that community can be visualized according to physical, social or emotional parameters. Just as was true of family, it is possible to define community in various ways, depending on individual understanding and experience. Several definitions are exemplified. A community is

1. "... a complex combination of social units and systems that perform the major social functions having locality relevance."[2]
2. "... a complex, interrelated structure of interaction patterns on the basis of which certain locality relevant functions are performed."[2]

3. " . . . a defined geographic area characterized by social, cultural, and environmental factors."[3]
4. " . . . a group wherever the needs of the individual are being met."[4]
5. " . . . a group of individuals who have a centered focus or binding force."[5]
6. " . . . a collection of people who share some important feature of their lives."[6]
7. " . . . an aggregate of individuals who have in common one or more personable or environmental characteristics."[7]
8. " . . . a relatively autonomous political system and a relatively autonomous social system."[1]
9. " . . . a place, a collection of people, a social system, or a community of solution."[8]
10. " . . . a social group determined by geographic boundaries and/ or common values and interests. Its members know and interact with each other. It functions within a particular social structure and exhibits and creates norms, values and social institutions. The individual belongs to the broader society through membership in family and community."[9]

■ *Sources and Types of Data on the Community*

There are numerous sources of data that reflect the relative health state of any community's population and enable the community health nurse to arrive at a nursing diagnosis. In general, we can characterize community data as either quantitative or qualitative. The various morbidity and mortality rates as well as calculations relative or comparative health status of any given community. But a community's potential or realization of health can also be qualified. For example, Spradley has identified ten subjective criteria of a healthy community.[6] A healthy community is one that

1. " . . . prompts its members have a high degree of awareness that 'we are a community.' "
2. " . . . uses its natural resources while taking steps to conserve them for future generations."
3. " . . . openly recognizes the existence of subgroups and welcomes their participation in community affairs."
4. " . . . is prepared to meet crises."
5. " . . . is a problem-solving community; it identifies, analyzes, and organizes to meet its own needs."
6. " . . . has open channels of communication that allows information to flow among all subgroups of citizens in all directions."
7. " . . . seeks to make each of its systems' resources available to all members of the community."

8. " . . . has legitimate and effective ways to settle disputes and meet needs that arise within the community."
9. " . . . encourages maximum citizen participation in decision making."
10. " . . . promotes a high level of wellness among all its members."

When communities lack a sense of identity as an entity of a whole, (whether the bonds are territorial or relational), it is difficult for the community to react in a cohesive or collective fashion to common problems. When there is no sense that "we are a community," it may be very difficult to solicit sufficient individual participation for the common good of all because people who do not feel a sense of belonging are also apt to feel little sense of responsibility for maintenance or improvement of the community.

The second quality of a healthy community is that the inhabitants use natural resources endemic to the region in a conservative fashion. Additionally, the viable community makes concerted efforts to allocate resources among its members in an equitable fashion. Public recreational and educational facilities are evenly distributed and comparably equipped and staffed. The natural resources, whether agricultural or geophysical, are developed sufficiently to provide for esthetic as well as economic necessities among the population. Health care facilities and clinicians offer a variety of services, ensure quality of care and maximum accessibility for all socioeconomic levels. The political structure, whether formal or informal, is responsive and representative of all subgroups within the community and assures adequately-trained police and firefighters who function to meet basic safety needs of the population.

A healthy community is one that is capable of problem-solving and crisis resolution. Although it is desirable to involve as many citizens in the problem-solving process as possible, various formal and informal leaders can make emergency decisions in the interest of continued community viability. The community should be sufficiently organized to afford mechanisms whereby disputes can be resolved with minimum disruption of daily living. Efficient problem-solving and resolution of disputes requires that there be a level of trust between and among various community factions, and that the channels of communication function in both directions. In other words, communications should arrive intact whether originating from an individual or special-interest group upwards to political or official levels, as well as downward from government or other central authority to individual citizens.

It is important that community health nurses realize that the great majority of communities will have identifiable or partial weaknesses in one or all of these criteria that describe a healthy community. But since the notion of health is relative, weaknesses in any of these areas does not necessarily connote an unhealthy community.

The community health nurse can facilitate a community's understanding of their strengths and weaknesses, as well as assist the community in mobilizing its human and physical resources to achieve its maximum health potential.

■ *The Nursing Process Applied to the Community as Client*

The concept of community is the most difficult to put into practice probably because of the multifaceted nature of community and the overlapping nature of community affiliation. The concept of community is basic to public health practice and is a distinguishing feature of community health nursing. A sense of the meaning of community, geopolitical, territorial, or interest, is essential to carrying out the mandate to promote and maintain the health and safety of the public. The ability to identify and circumscribe the community of concern is the first step in meeting the needs of groups.

The health status of an individual is assessed through the application of the nursing process. When a group requires nursing services or when a population needs a review of its weaknesses and strengths, the community becomes the client. An individual patient is made up of characteristics or attributes. The physiological component is derived from assessment of the organs or members of the body. The psychological components are spiritual and emotional attributes of the patient. The sociological characteristics are basic values from which the sense of identity arises. Nursing assessments include all characteristics and, therefore, nursing care is described as holistic. When the community is client its components have the same attributes; thus the community has physiological, psychological (often referred to as group psychology) and sociocultural aspects. The community of concern assumes group characteristics and the population often acts together much like an individual composed of myriad "organs" or "members." Consensus produces joint action to solve problems. A diseased aggregate or an unhealthy community is without identity and in conflict with itself. It will fail to employ strategies to promote its own healing; it will be unable to marshal its strengths to become productive and maintain its health, just like a diseased patient.

Nursing Assessment

Community assessment is the first step in the nursing process for aggregates. The purpose of the nurse's role in assessment is to help the community identify and solve its own health problems. Assessment of community can be a qualitative procedure. Applying the criteria of a healthy community to the group of concern is a qualitative method of identifying needs and goals of the community. The knowledge of attributes of a healthy community assists assessment by focusing on desirable group characteristics; however, first it is necessary to identify the community requiring assistance in order to set priorities, to target populations for services, and to identify communities at high risk. This identification procedure locates the community of need.

These two major concepts, the community of need and the community of solution (mentioned previously), summarize two important approaches to community assessment. The first, the community of need, is identified and circumscribed to define the target population or group with a problem. The weaknesses of the aggregate, both physiological and psychosocial, are determined, and the most emergent problems of the community are prioritized. The second, the community of solution, is identified by recognizing the strengths of the community relevant for helping the group solve its own problems. The major role of the public health nurse is to identify and assess the community of need and community of solution and intervene to promote the health of the community as client.

Qualitative assessments require clinical expertise: quantitative data requires epidemiologic perspectives to substantiate subjective judgments and observations. Quantification is equally important for the nursing assessment of individual patients or clients because the nurse uses clinical inference and objective measurements, often highly technical in nature, as part of the nursing process. When the community is the client, clinical inference must be made from a community perspective. This requires the identification of the limits—geopolitical or relational—of the community of concern. Without the recognition of the boundaries of the group, clinical inference and epidemiologic quantifications may be in jeopardy. Quantitative as well as qualitative information are as necessary to the nursing assessment of community as they are to the nursing assessment of an individual or a family. Assessment of a community can be made using several processes such as a managerial mode, assessment by objectives or systems analysis, and a systematic review of interactions in groups recommended by sociologists. The process may also include an epidemiologic approach which requires epidemiologic quantifications, such as rates and statistics, to supplement more subjective measures.

The basic idea behind community assessment is to determine the occurrence and distribution of selected environmental, socioeconomic, and behavioral conditions that affect disease control as well as promotion of health. For example, many factors such as immunization levels, the incidence and prevalence of disease, health care utilization patterns, population demographics, and housing characteristics can be measured through epidemiologic parameters.[10] Attitudes, health care practices and beliefs, and a multitude of other factors affect the health potential of any given community.[11]

Even when a given community has been assessed sometime in the past, it may be necessary to update the assessment for several reasons. First, health problems change as the population changes.[12] For example, in an old, deteriorating urban neighborhood, the major health problems may be associated mostly with poverty, such as high infant/maternal death rates and/or a high prevalence of chronic disease associated with an aging population. However, when old homes are torn down to build new middle-class townhouses, the shift in demographics to young, child-bearing families can change the health needs of the same location markedly.

■ *Nursing Diagnosis*

Once the assessment data are obtained and organized, a clear statement of the problem should be formulated. This diagnostic statement consists of two segments. The first segment identifies the problem such as "potential lack of understanding." The second part of the statement clarifies the problem statement by describing the circumstances or reasons for the problem occurrence. For example, the second segment is connected to the first with transitional words such as "due to" or "secondary to."[13] It may be possible to form several nursing diagnostic statements, and each is updated as new information is obtained. In community health nursing, the diagnosis will refer to "lack of awareness as community", or "inability to meet crises" due to lack of leadership. High levels of illness or unemployment related to community needs require objective measures, such as rates, and must relate what is usual or endemic to what is hazardous or epidemic.

Planning

As with all phases of the nursing process, community health nurses collaborate and consult with the people in the community. Community leaders, formal and informal, should be sought out and included in the first assessment attempts. Since it is in the planning phase that problems identified from the assessment are categorized, the nurse may want to categorize various risk factors that have been identified according to (1) demographic characteristics such as age, sex, and socioeconomic status: (2) inherited or biological characteristics such as genetic traits and physical conditions such as obesity or hypertension; (3) environmental exposure factors that include physical or psychological aspects of the environment such as toxic substances or social isolation; and (4) behavioral characteristics such as the use of cigarettes or alcohol.[12] Problems should then be prioritized into short-range, mid-range and long-range goals and objectives according to a timetable approved by community representatives.

In the planning phase, program objectives are formulated that clearly specify the extent to which the plan is expected to change the health problems, among what group of people, where, and over what period of time.[12] Objectives specify not only the period of time required for the change, but also specify how much change is desired.

Although the importance of involving representatives of laity and professionals from the community has been mentioned several times, it is worth stressing once more. When all is said and done, each community must arrive at a plan to meet its own health needs. This plan must also fit the community's own politics and power structure through extant or realistic resources. Also, that plan must be congruent with the community's unique personality for it to be successful.[14]

Implementation

In the implementation phase, the community health nurse has an opportunity to be creative, within limits, and to share professional knowledge and judgment while working with others to bring about change that will contribute to the health status of the community. The implementation phase can be satisfying, but it can also be frustrating.[14] Even when the most detailed assessment has been conducted and the plan seems realistic, the change process involved in implementation can be anxiety-producing to the residents. Thus the nurse will need to remember some basic contents of the change process since some resistance to change is inevitable and must be anticipated. But again, one way to minimize resistance is to involve the residents throughout the process and keep them informed of the facts. Careful preparation for change, conscientious maintenance of effective channels of communication, and provision for continuing respect for differing points of view, as well as reward in the form of recognition will help to minimize resistance to change while it contributes to the overall success of the plan.

Evaluation

Because of cost-containment concerns in the health care industry, all programs to improve health care must be evaluated in terms of financial efficiency. One epidemiologist has gone so far as to say that evaluation should always include dollar costs as one criterion, and that the new program should reduce costs while it increases benefits or improves effectiveness.[11] Often some form of evaluation, using both qualitative and quantitative measures of the change process, can be provided to verify the accomplishments of group actions.

By now, it should not be surprising that there are numerous ways to approach evaluation. For example, there are structure, process and outcome evaluation, formative and summative evaluation, and a goals and systems model, among others.[14] Evaluation efforts at the bachelor's level of preparation will most likely revolve around referring back to the goals and objectives formulated in the planning stage, and then determining if the goals were accomplished and to what degree they were accomplished. Epidemiologic facts often can be helpful, and successful intervention can be classified through epidemiologic quantifications. Understanding epidemiologic parameters assists the nurse in describing the needs of the community. Rates and other facts provide objective measures of the attainment of group goals. Interpretation of community quantifications not only provide reasons for change but can show the effects of the change process.

As in every application of the nursing process, the diagnosis, planning, and implementation depend on the careful assessment of the patient. When the community is client, the assessment must be carefully quantified and must be representative of the total group identified as the target population. It must be inclusive, that is, some information on all aspects of the health of the community must be collected. Data to answer the specific questions related to clinical judgments, which made the assessment necessary, must be collected to answer the initial questions that promoted the need for assessment of the community of concern.

The database compiled by the community health nurse must include some information on each of the following five community assessment criteria shown in Table 6–1. This list of information, recommended by Woolsey and Lawrence, is applicable to any method chosen for the community assessment process, whether it is qualitative or quantitative.[15] It is all-inclusive and assures the public health nurse that all relevant information has been gathered as part of the assessment of the community. The use of this comprehensive summary is invaluable for the epidemiologic approach, for it guarantees

T A B L E 6 - 1
Information Required for Community Assessment

- Counts of people, including compilation of vital statistics such as marriage, divorce and family size, and an accurate estimate of the total number of persons in the population.
- Measures of health status, or rates, including estimates of major health problems and causes of morbidity and mortality.
- Identification of problems and causes of morbidity and mortality.
- Identification of health services received by the population.
- Identification of health services and resources in the community, including the numbers of health care professionals and facilities.
- Assessment of the environment, including social, emotional, physical and political aspects.

(Leavell and Clark, 1965).

that all the information needed to generate rates has been collected and all public health issues are being addressed.

For the community, rates can be viewed as a measure of acuity—of the severity of illness or problems of a group. Rates of illness, morbidity, and death, mortality are physiologic parameters. Rates of mental illness, alcoholism, delinquency, and drug abuse are examples of measures of sociopsychological problems; and rates of unemployment, overcrowding, and economic issues are examples of political and sociological parameters of the community as client. Thus, the community health nurse approaches the aggregate from a holistic orientation.

■ *Assessment of the Community Through Epidemiology*

Epidemiologic methods of the process of community assessment will not be detailed in this book. It includes methods of sampling the community to provide a representative test population of the total community. The information collected during an assessment and how that information can be interpreted and applied towards understanding and evaluating the community of concern for public health nursing will be explained.

A community assessment is descriptive epidemiology.[16] It is also called a cross-sectional survey or prevalence study. Information is collected on the target population or population at risk (p.a.r.) to describe its characteristics as well as problems that are postulated or expected to respond to nursing services. This information will be used for the numerators of proportions and rates. The target population or community of concern involved in the community assessment will form the denominator. If the area is a census tract, a county, or a state, figures for the denominator can be found in census data. If the area or the community is small, such as a school, an industry, or a hospital, estimates of the p.a.r. will be available from their internal records. Often nursing needs are directed to a community of special interest such as veterans with disabilities, Cambodian refugees, or low-income mothers. In these situations, considerable ingenuity is required by the nurse epidemiologist to estimate the numbers of people to include in the assessment. The identification of the population at risk or target population is indispensable for making meaningful nursing diagnoses of community needs.

In a cross-sectional or prevalence study, the information is collected as swiftly as possible from the target population. If the community is extensive, a random sample may be taken to identify a smaller group to represent the larger population. A team of nurses may decide to gather information in which the baccalaureate nurse will be involved. The team, probably led by a nurse-epidemiologist, will use a "collection tool," consisting of a questionnaire where the answers to the questions can be quantified for computer analysis. The structure of the questionnaire is important. The questions must be clearly stated in terms easily understood by the target audience and the choice of answers must be mutually exclusive or unequivocal. The intention of a prevalence survey is to make a cross-sectional analysis of what prevails in the community at the time of the inquiry, and thus collect information for planning and implementation of nursing care.

■ *Information Required for Community Assessment*

Woolsey and Lawrence identified five basic types of information. They are as follows: (1) counts of people; (2) measures or indices of health; (3) health services received; (4) health resources of manpower and facilities; and (5) the state of the environment.[15] When doing a community assessment, all five of these information groups in varying degrees must be included to ensure a comprehensive assessment of community needs. Descriptive epidemiology using a cross-sectional design is a commonly applied public health method used for community assessment; however, regardless of the process chosen, the information requirements remain the same in order to diagnose the health of the community. The first two requirements of counts and indices ensure that data is available from which the rates can be calculated to estimate the severity of problems in the community.

The Target Population (the p.a.r.)

When a group within the community is suspected of having special needs, problems or demands, the identification of this, the initial problem, is made through many channels. It may be a result of several observations made during delivery of services to families in the home; in other words, it may be a result of constant surveillance of families in the community. The problem in the population may be targeted through the public health department, and the need to assess the community may be a multidisciplinary decision. Local and national media may have covered the problem as a news item or it may be a managerial request from a hospital with a home health care agency. Whatever the suspected hazard, the target population must be circumscribed and must be quantified, for it will form the p.a.r. for the denominator of the rate that will be used as an acuity measure of the health status of the community.

The size of the p.a.r. must be assessed. Many state and county agencies keep population counts of the catchment area they serve. Hospitals record admissions and discharges at their facilities. Voluntary as well as public agencies may be able to give estimates of the size of a selected group. A resource, which is acknowledged as an accurate count of population size, is the *Statistical Abstracts of the United States*. The abstracts contain information from the census, and the federal government is responsible for counting of the population—a huge community assessment done every 10 years. The abstracts contain data that are not always directly associated with health; the census provides information for administration and government, industry, actuarial work, and public health services; however, it is the census that provides the basic counting mechanism for populations. In the *Statistical Abstracts of the United States,* information is available for geopolitically defined communities called standard metropolitan statistical areas (SMSA), but these data are used mainly for commerce as each area includes at least one city with more than 50,000 and the SMSAs are not necessarily contiguous with each other. They appear on the map as isolated areas defined to include large urban sections of the states. A more useful partition for public health is the division of the United States and protectorates into 11 geographic regions. For instance, Region 10 includes Washington, Idaho, Oregon, and Alaska. These areas have community needs in common and thus the administration of these needs for nursing and other services is facilitated.

The smallest area included in the census is the census tract (CT). The CT is a geographic area not exceeding 6000 people but not less than 4000 people and has homogeneous characteristics with respect to housing and education—components of socioeconomic status. The boundaries of the CT are not fixed: every 10 years during the census they are checked for homogeneity and size. When these factors change, the CT is split as long as the number of inhabitants is large enough to maintain at least 4000 in the new tracts. The number of splits is reflected by the addition of a decimal point to the identification number of the CT. For example, CT number 33.3 is a result of dividing CT #33 three times. Many public health nursing agencies organize the delivery of their services by CT, and the numbers in the CT populations for community assessments are readily accessible from census information.

The modern census includes varied and extensive information. Demographics are collected, such as age, sex, and marital status, and information is collected and stored about the head of the household, place of birth, citizenship, mother tongue, housing, and other information. When a community assessment for nursing care needs is made, the statistical abstracts can supply information on birth and death rates and population sizes by demographics. At the very least, the abstracts provide a framework for the area served by nursing services and may actually give a number for the population targeted for nursing service. Often, the community of concern for nursing is so specific that data is unavailable, and the needs of the defined community, or p.a.r., must be assessed without benefit of census or registration records. The basic population information must be collected to estimate the p.a.r. for the denominator so that the measures of health, another name for rates, can be computed carefully. In order to do this with validity and reliability, the target population must be clearly defined so that counts can be made. This is a basic requirement in order to make nursing decisions to serve the community as client.

Numerator Information

Woolsey and Lawrence recommend that counts of people and measures or indices of health are included as part of a community assessment. The counts of people are made to enable the rates, the basic measures of health acuity in the community, to be completed accurately for both numerator and denominator. Descriptive epidemiology for community assessment also requires data about the demographic variables of the chosen group or target population. Demographic variables are those characteristics held in common by all persons and thus can be used to describe group characteristics; basic demographic variables must always be included in the community assessment so that the community health nurse can describe the group receiving services. The famous trio of demographic characteristics are age, race, and sex, closely followed by the fourth variable of socioeconomic status (SES). The association of these four variables for nursing requires but little elaboration: the two ends of the continuum of age will demand increasing nursing care as high technology allows premature infants to survive. The elderly population is increasing as the expectation of life increases. Babies and the elderly require skilled nursing in institutions, in homes, and in the community. The next demographic variable, race, is closely associated with culture. Not only does an ethnic background indicate the mores that affect health care behaviors (as one will see in Chapter 7), it also predicts genetic illnesses. The sex of clients influences psychosocial and physical needs of clients, and some nursing services in the community, such as women's clinics, are directed specifically towards the needs associated with gender. SES, a composite measure of education, income, and occupation, influences access to care as well as attitudes towards healthy lifestyles. A community assessment is incomplete without the inclusion of these basic parameters. Demographic counts may be used as numerators or denominators.

Numerator data is included on the abstracts. Information is summarized from registration from which are generated vital statistics. This is the recording under law of births, marriages, divorces, and deaths. Morbidity and mortality information is provided by the federal government, which supplements the census by conducting national health surveys on a regular, periodic basis.[17] The health examination survey is the most rigorous and is taken in cycles by age group from 6000 people chosen as a random sample. Each volunteer receives a thorough clinical examination, sometimes through a mobile laboratory staffed by physicians, nurses, and technicians. A second type of survey done by the federal government to obtain numerator data for health indices of morbidity is a hospital records review called the Federal Hospital Discharge Survey. There is also a volunteer program, the Physicians Activities Survey (PAS), started in 1954 through a W. K. Kellogg Foundation grant to the University of Michigan.[18] The PAS survey runs concurrently with the Federal Hospital Discharge Survey.[19] The third method of gathering information on the health of the community is to conduct health interviews on random samples of the population, the Health Interview Survey. During the interviews, utilization of health services, self-perception of illness experienced in the last two weeks, and a history of sickness not requiring hospitalization is taken. It is obvious that the interview survey is conducted to assess illnesses that have occurred but have not required the use of hospitals, clinics, or medical and nursing services.

Prevalence surveys are community assessments from which rates are compiled. Rates are the barometers of health in the population and measure the degree of severity of physiologic and psychosocial problems of the group. Community assessment can also be used to evaluate public health services *after* the implementation of community intervention. Surveys can be used to augment the nursing process not only for assessment, but also for evaluation of change. Before discussing some special rates used to evaluate the effectiveness of public health services, the attributes and definitions of the most commonly used public health statistics will be reviewed. Definition of the numerator and denominator are crucial to accurate interpretation of rates. To illustrate the importance of definitions to describe the group situation, the following example is given. In Figure 6–1, the infant, neonatal,

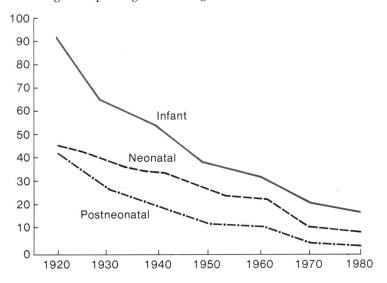

FIGURE 6 - 1

Infant, neonatal, and postneonatal mortality, in the United States, 1915–1980.

and postneonatal mortality rates for the United States are compared for the era from 1920 to 1980.[6] It can be seen that mortality associated with the perinatal period has been graphed over time. It is known that since the turn of the century, public health services have become increasingly targeted to prenatal and infant care. Figure 6–1 shows that infant, neonatal, and postneonatal rates have steadily declined from 1920 to 1980. In trying to assess these figures to determine where nursing services are needed, it becomes immediately apparent that the definitions of infant, neonatal and postneonatal are essential to accurately interpret the information. These crucial definitions are given in Table 6–2.

Table 6–2 shows the data from which the graph in Figure 6–1 was drawn. It is now obvious that an age less than 1 year is defined as infant, under 28 days is defined as neonatal and from 28 days to 11 months refer to postneonatal death. The infant mortality rates are a total of neonatal and postneonatal events. Without accurate definition of the terms in the graphs, explanations are obscured and planning and implementation of nursing interventions is obviated. In brief, the graph shows that the greatest risk of dying as an infant is in the crucial first month of life. The rates are quantified, objective evidence showing the success of all public health services for maternal and child care. The gradual decline of all rates for all infants is objective information for evaluating the success of public health services during this time period. Maternal and child care are mandated services in public health. The community health nurse offers and continues to play a significant part in promoting health and preventing disease in the very young.

T A B L E   6 - 2
Infant Mortality Rates by Age   United States 1950, 1960, 1965, and 1970–1980*

Year	Under 1 year (infant)	Under 28 days (neonatal)	28 Days to 11 months (postneonatal)
1980 (est.)	12.5	8.4	4.1
1975	16.1	11.6	4.5
1970	20.0	15.1	4.9
1965	24.7	17.7	7.0
1960	26.0	18.7	7.3
1950	29.2	20.5	8.7

*For 1979 and 1980, based on a 10% sample of deaths; for all other years, based on final data, rates for 1000 live births. Based on a 50% sample of deaths.

(Adapted for National Center for Health Statistics. Vital Statistics of the U.S. Vol. II A. Government Printing Office, Washington, D.C. Selected Years and Vital Statistics Rates in U.S. 1940–1960. No. 1677, Government Printing Office, Washington, D.C., 1978[20])

Another thing that is interesting about the example in Table 6–2 is that the deaths are reported by units of 1000 live births. The denominator denoting the true population of infants at risk of death would be the number of infant deaths plus the number of infants who did not die; but for many reasons, only live births have been included in the denominator. The use of only live births depends on several factors: the tables show that the risk of death is greatest in the first month of life and since 1970, the postnatal rate has been between 4% and 5% of live births. Actuarial or life table analysis supports the fact that the force of mortality or the odds of not surviving is greatest during the first month of life; therefore, risk of death is unevenly spread throughout the infant's first year. Another reason for using live births in the denominator is the under-registration of very small infant deaths in some parts of the country with tiny fetuses, where the problem in identifying stillbirths from live births is exacerbated. The World Health Organization defines a live birth as any indication of life after complete expulsion or extraction from the mother, such as beating of the heart, pulsating of the umbilical cord, or definite movement of voluntary muscles. Once this classification is made, a live birth requires registration: if death follows, a death certificate and burial are required. But the identification of a birth as "live" is not always easy. Often it is the nurse who has to make this judgment. The combination of a difficulty in defining a live birth and the uneven spread of mortality results in fluctuating information about neonatal deaths. To compensate, the number of infant deaths is not included in the denominator. The number of live births is used as a more stable and dependable denominator.

Another rate using live births in the denominator is the maternal mortality rate. The true denominator should include all pregnancies, that is, all mothers who conceive as well as mothers who die for reasons associated with pregnancy. Not only is it impossible to annotate the number of conceptions, but again, the definition of fetal death, usually defined as death occurring after a 20-week gestation period, is not easy to apply. It is customary to use live births as a more stable index of the p.a.r. Fortunately, the effects of public health services on the maternal death rate have been so successful that this rate is reported as per 10,000 live births rather than 1000 live births per year. Infant mortality and maternal mortality are important measures of the effectiveness of public health services to the community. They are a critical index of community health and influence the political and social environment. It is well known that legislation to legalize abortions affect maternal mortality rates favorably, and prenatal care reduces both infant and maternal mortality rates.[21] Community assessment using health indices are a method of objective evaluation of health policy.

Changes in the terminology used for rates occur over time and are reflected in the use of fetal death to replace the old terms of abortion and miscarriage. A comparatively new rate is the perinatal mortality rate which covers deaths occurring after 28 weeks of pregnancy and 7 days after birth. Losses in late fetal life and early infancy are quantified by the perinatal rate; thus the rate spans the total perinatal period. The perinatal mortality rate has the advantage of fostering collaboration between nurses from different specialty areas associated with the perinatal period. It also bypasses the need to identify any products of conception that may be defined as viable between 20 and 28 weeks during this very uncertain time period. Other rates measured by units of 1000 live births are the fetal death rate, a "true" rate with deaths and non-deaths in the denominator (Chapter 4), and the fetal death ratio, comparing live births to fetal deaths. The fetal death ratio is a "true" ratio that is also measured per 1000 units of live births. As one may guess, the ratio is preferred because it reduces the error from fetal death reports.[22] At the risk of endless repetition, it is emphasized that all rates and ratios must relate to a time period. Some of the most important measures of community health and effects of public health services are summarized in Table 6–3.

Rates are a measure of acuity or the degree of severity of problems in a community; however, there are also important ratios measuring community events, such as the fetal death ratio included in Table 6–3, and the proportional mortality ratio (PMR). The PMR relates the number of deaths from a specified cause to all causes in the same time period. The PMR may relate deaths from cancer to all cases of death, or deaths from cases of cancer at a specific site related to all cancer deaths. The ratio quantifies the proportion of deaths attributable to a specific cause or the proportion of all cancer deaths attribut-

T A B L E   6 - 3
Some Important Death Rates Used to Evaluate Efforts of Public Health Services

Fetal Death		
(Old terms: stillbirth, abortion, and/or miscarriage)	=	Registered as deaths after 20 weeks' gestation (per 1000 live births)
Perinatal mortality	=	Fetal deaths after 28 weeks of pregnancy and deaths up to 7 days (per 1000 live births)
Maternal mortality	=	Number of deaths associated with puerperium (per 10,000 live births)
Fetal death rate	=	$\dfrac{\text{Fetal deaths}}{\text{Fetal deaths + live births}}$
Fetal death ratio	=	$\dfrac{\text{Fetal deaths}}{\text{Live births}}$

(Definitions from Mausner and Bahn: An Introductory Text. Philadelphia, WB Saunders, 1974)

able to a specific cancer and is always expressed as a percentage. It is important to note that the PMR is not a statement of probability because there is no population at risk in the denominator. The PMR is useful because it can estimate the number of lives to be saved from a specific cause of death through the eradication of factors contributing to that death.

Another ratio of interest to nursing is the case fatality ratio (CFR), often mistakenly called a rate. The CFR is a measure of virulence. It is calculated by relating the number of deaths from a disease to the number of cases of the same disease. In toxic shock syndrome, the CFR was just over 8% of all cases, or 1 in every 12 cases died. In acquired immune deficiency syndrome (AIDS), the case fatality rate is causing extreme concern because it is over 60% for a 1 year period, or 1 in 3 cases will die within 1 year of diagnosis. The case fatality ratio illustrates the virulence of the infection by relating the cases to the number of deaths.

■ *Measures on Indices of Community Health*

Many rates are used to describe a community. The rates collected in a survey depend on the needs suspected or known when the community assessment is undertaken. There are many other measures of community health, such as life expectancy, years left to live, disability rates, and life table analyses. The public health nurse needs to know the most commonly used measures of community health so that some judgments can be made about the need for public health nursing services and to evaluate nursing interventions. To complete a community assessment of the health of the community, the public health nurse often requires special measures of general mental and socioeconomic well-being as well as physical health measures. Some of these indices are marriage, divorce, and illegitimacy rates, the proportion of babies with no prenatal care, rates of unemployment, crime and substance abuse, or other measures which may be relevant to the particular problem of the defined communities. Utilization rates in hospitals, clinics and agencies and the proportion of people in substandard housing or with incomes at or below poverty level may be relevant information. These and many more measures can be used to assess the health and needs of a community.

Rates are selected to answer the initial purpose of the assessment. Woolsey and Lawrence's information list ensures the inclusion of basic information required to make nursing judgments, including the utilization and availability of health services so that nursing services can be prioritized. To complete the information required during community assessment, resources for health care in the community should be counted and noted, not only for nursing care but for other services such as use of self-help groups and counseling centers. Client utilization of clinics, hospitals, and medical services are important to prevent overlap or duplication in delivery of services. Some notation of the environment will also be of assistance. Many homes and offices do not ensure safe ambulation of clients or provide for the mobility of the disabled. Sanitation and ventilation may be inadequate. These are part of the community problems that will affect nursing care assessments and interfere with healthy living; therefore, assessments must include all information that provides a total understanding of community needs and will answer the questions formed during the original inquiry. Community strengths or the ability to meet the demands of the groups must be categorized so that solutions for nursing care will utilize existing resources to solve the identified concerns.

■ *Validity of Measures of Health*

On the whole, registration data and census data is accurate. In 1980, several studies were done to verify the validity of census data. David established that very low birth weight babies, defined as less than 1500 grams at birth, were not being registered as live births in the state of North Carolina.[23] He also showed that gestational age, as estimated from the death certificates, and deaths in high-risk, rural, non-white populations, were under registered. McCarthy discovered 21% underregistration of very low birth weight babies in the same high-risk population in Georgia.[25] Frost also studied race-specific mortality rates in Washington State by linking death records to birth records.[24] He found that infant deaths increased for the non-white races and recalculated the infant mortality rates in Indians to show that little, if any, effect had been made by public health services on the infant mortality rate in Indians during a 20 year period. What this means for nursing is that rates from the statistical abstracts used to estimate the impact of nursing services on increasing the length of gestation or reducing race-specific mortality in high-risk groups will *not* be accurate. Studies must be done through specially designed nursing assessments rather than using census data. On the whole, though, in the United States, registration of births occur in 95% of the population and registration of deaths is even more complete, probably over 96%. They are reliable indices of community health as long as the rates are used to describe the total community rather than culturally defined subsections with special needs.

Summary

Communities are complex social systems that may be intramural or extramural. The role of the community health nurse is distinguished by the ability to define communities within communities and to use group characteristics to promote healthy, functioning populations. Communities can be defined by the geographic, political, or consensual boundaries. They can be defined by their ability to provide solutions or by their needs and demands. The community health nurse assesses, diagnoses, plans, implements, and evaluates communities as clients. Planning and implementation depend on effective qualitative and quantitative assessment of a community's needs. Community assessment can also be used not only to define problems of groups, but also to evaluate public health nursing interventions. Many methods of assessment are available, such as system analyses and management approaches. An epidemiologic approach uses cross-sectional or prevalence surveys to perform in-depth analyses of targeted populations. Using a list of information first identified by Woolsey and Lawrence assures public health nurses of a comprehensive assessment of community needs and resources.

The epidemiologic approach also guarantees the collection of information necessary to quantify community needs through rates, objective parameters utilized by all public health personnel to measure the severity of physiologic and psychosocial problems. The rates and ratios most often used to assess the community are reviewed to assist community health nurses in interpreting rates when applying the nursing process to the community. Some basic sources of statistical information on population size, demographic distribution, and counts of people are included to assist the public health nurse in obtaining accurate information to describe the community of concern for public health nursing.

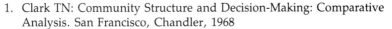

References

1. Clark TN: Community Structure and Decision-Making: Comparative Analysis. San Francisco, Chandler, 1968
2. Warrant R: The Community in America, p 9. Chicago, Rand McNally, 1963
3. Cohn H, Tingle J: Manual for Nurses in Family and Community Health, 2nd ed, p 2. Boston, Little, Brown & Co, 1974
4. Wigley R, Cook JR: Community Health, Concepts and Issues, p 4. New York, Van Nostrand, 1975
5. Jarvis L: Community Health Nursing, Keeping the Public Healthy, p 5. Philadelphia, FA Davis, 1981
6. Spradley BW: Community Health Nursing, Concepts and Practice, 3rd ed, p 5. Boston, Little, Brown & Co, 1985
7. Williams C: Community health nursing—what is it? Nurs Outlook 25 April, 1977. 250–254

8. Ruybal SE, Bauwens E, Falsa MJ: Community assessment: an epidemio-logic approach. Nurs Outlook 2154–2170, June 1955

9. World Health Organization Expert Committee on Community Health Nursing: Community Health Nursing; Report of WHO Expert Committee. Geneva, WHO, 1974

10. Mausner JS, Kramer S: Epidemiology—An Introductory Text, 2nd ed., p 7. Philadelphia, WB Saunders, 1985

11. Dever GE: Community Health Analysis: A Holistic Approach. Germantown, Maryland, Aspen Systems Corporation, 1980

12. Watson NM: Community as client. In Sullivan JA (ed): Directions in Community Health Nursing. Boston, Blackwell Scientific Publications, 1984

13. Chavigny KH. In Higgs ZR, Gustafson DD (eds): Community as a Client: Assessment and Diagnosis, pp 109–117. Philadelphia, FA Davis, 1985

14. Tinkham CW, Voorhies EF, McCarthy NC: Community Health Nursing: Evolution and Process, 3rd ed. New York, Appleton-Century-Crofts, 1984

15. Woolsey T, Lawrence P: Moving ahead in health statistics. Am Public Health 59 (10):1820, 1969

16. McMahon B, Pugh TF: Epidemiology: Principles and Methods. Boston, Little, Brown & Co, 1970

17. National Health Surveys, National Center for Health Statistics (NCHS) USPHS

18. Professional Activity Survey. Length of Stay by Diagnosis, United States, 1984, p 1. Ann Arbor, Commission on Professional and Hospital Activities, October, 1985

19. Hospital Discharge Survey: NCHS USPHS

20. Vital Statistics of the U.S. Vol 11A, NCHS No. 1677. Washington, DC, Government Printing Office, 1978

21. Mausner JS, Baum AK: Basic Medical Statistics. New York, Grune & Stratton, 1982

22. Elandt–Johnson RC: Definitions of rates. Am J Epidemiol 102:4:267–269, 1975

23. David RJ: The quality and completeness of birthweight and gestational age data in computerized birth files. Am J Public Health 70:9:964–969, 1980

24. McCarthy: The Underregistration of Neonatal Deaths: Georgia. Am J Public Health 70:9:970–973, 1980

25. Frost F, Shy KK: Racial differences between linked birth and infant death records in Washington State. Am J Public Health 70:9:974–976, 1980

Kenny Mallow
Williamson

Joan G. Turner

Katherine H.
Chavigny

Sociocultural Communities

LEARNING OBJECTIVES

After reading and understanding the contents of this chapter, the student will be able to:

1. *Define culture, cultural stereotyping, acculturation, and ethnocentrism, and explain how each is related to health provider and consumer behavior.*

2. *Explain why knowledge of culture is necessary in order to deliver individualized community health nursing care.*

3. *Discuss the various nursing implications of Warner's descriptions of discrete social class.*

4. *Analyze the following cultural aspects that are relevant to the community health nurses' plan of care for any given family:*
   - *Nutrition*
   - *Family relationships*
   - *Health beliefs*
   - *Education*
   - *Religion*

5. *Determine how practices such as pica and kuru affect health.*

Introduction

Socioculture combines factors of group relationships with patterns of belief and customs of racial and religious classes. Culture identifies and circumscribes communities of concern geopolitically as well as within larger populations. The bonds that are forged by ethnic and religious learning and are passed from generation to generation are strong and compelling. The values and customs of communities are critically important to public health nursing. Sociocultural factors must be integrated into the total nursing process to serve groups and families in the community.

The United States is truly a matrix of many sociocultural groups. Massive waves of immigrants have continued to shape the character of the country throughout the last two centuries. It was not, however, until the social protest movements of the 1960s that Americans began to reaffirm the acceptance of cultural diversity in society. Today, the melting-pot myth largely has been rejected. Immigrants and members of cultural groups do not have to discard their own traditions and values in order to gain acceptance in the workplace, school, or community. This reemergence of cultural unity permeates the actions of individuals, families and social groups. Its consequences are pervasive and implications for practice are broad.[1,2]

The purpose of this chapter is to explain the meaning of culture as it relates to the practice of community health nursing, and to provide a means for assessing cultural variables in order to provide culturally relevant care. Cultural differences are often at the root of poor communication, interpersonal tension, and poor assessment of health problems. Successful nursing care for clients of various backgrounds depends on accurate assessment of cultural beliefs and values.

■ Culture Defined

Culture may be viewed as a blueprint for living that guides the thoughts, actions, sentiments, and even health behaviors of individuals, families, and communities. Through socialization with others, people learn cultural patterns of behavior resulting in specific ways of solving vital problems. Goodenough maintains that "culture consists of standards for deciding what is, what can be, how one feels about it, and how to go about doing it."[3] Thus culture forms a basis for identifying what is and is not acceptable in a given situation. Additionally, these culturally based responses may be made subconsciously, and if unrecognized, may contribute to a breakdown in interpersonal relationships among those from culturally different orientations.

Just as there are significant differences between cultures, there are variations within cultures. Much of the cultural variation seen in public health nursing is related to the degree to which the client subscribes to the American culture, regional differences in the native culture, social class differences, and/or simply idiosyncratic variations.[4] Since effective nursing care is based on individualized client needs, it is important to take into account the diversity of individuals within various cultural groups. However, there is a tendency to oversimplify the assessment of cultural needs through stereotyping. Cultural stereotyping involves the nonacceptance of individual or group diversity. In a stereotypic situation, everyone from a particular culture is viewed as fixed in their personal, social, and intellectual characteristics.[5] Nurses must realize that cultures change, as do individual members and their families within given cultures.

One of the major causes of change within a given culture is a phenomenon known as acculturation. In acculturation, the influence of the original or native culture is diminished as people live and become interested in another cultural environment. As time passes, some of the native cultural values and behaviors are subsumed by mores intrinsic to the new cultural society.[6] For example, when Irish or Italian immigrants arrived in this country, they were more or less culturally distinct from other ethnic groups. However, as time passed and generations became more removed from the motherland, the influence of old cultural mores lessened and subsequent generations adopted more and more of American values and beliefs. Acculturation does not necessarily equate with a total loss of cultural identity because many culturally based customs continue, such as those related to food, religion, music, and dance. Many times, these culturally based activities become the major cultural difference between groups.[7]

As indicated in sociology, "culture shock" occurs when a person or groups experience confusion, immobilization, or a sense of loss in dealing with a new culture that is completely unfamiliar.[8] Varying degrees of culture shock may be experienced by community health nurses when dealing with clients from different cultural backgrounds. However, the phenomenon of culture shock can be minimized when caregivers allow themselves time to become acquainted with various beliefs and customs particular to a given cultural subgroup. The nurse's own cultural background colors individual perception of clients from different cultures. Therefore, personal feelings, beliefs, and attitudes relative to culture must be identified, discussed, and accepted in order to assist culturally diverse clients seeking health care.[9]

■ *Cultural Diversity in Nursing Practice*

Leininger refers to cultural diversity as "the overt and covert differences among people of different population groups with respect to their values, beliefs, language, physical characteristics, and general pattern of behavior."[10] Cultural differences between the client and nurse can affect the client's response to health service. Variation in cultural expectations are found in almost every nursing situation. The nurse must be aware of both personal and client culture systems in order to ensure the development of optimal nursing intervention.[11,12]

There are at least three reasons to study cultural influences on health care. First, when caring for culturally diverse groups, nurses tend to be ethnocentric in their approach to health care delivery, to believe that their own professional, scientifically based practices are superior to those of other cultural groups.[13] Usually, this ethnocentrism is not evident until the nurse encounters other cultural beliefs. Once nurses are exposed to other cultures, they can appreciate why certain norms and values have been effective in that culture and move beyond ethnocentric behaviors.[14,15] Second, studying different cultures helps nurses to better understand their own culture. In studying new types of behavior, the nurse is able to identify both differences and similarities between cultures. All too often, differences alone are identified, resulting in interpersonal tension.[16] Recognition of similarities provides a common ground for interaction and can serve as the first step toward greater sensitivity toward others.[17] Increased cultural sensitivity is achieved through examining the life patterns of people in other cultures. Cultural sensitivity refers to respect for different cultures, recognition of culturally different health beliefs and values, incorporation of those practices that are not life-threatening, and acting on behalf of people who are being denied safe, culturally appropriate health care. Cultural sensitivity requires concern, time, and a sense of advocacy.[18,19] Third, the relevance of cultural diversity to the practice of public health nursing becomes clear if the nurse accepts the idea that cultural patterns are an integral part of safe, effective nursing care. Leininger recognized that "if culturally specific care is not realized, clients may show displeasure with nursing care services, remain uncooperative, refuse to carry out nursing expectations and withdraw from the helping relationship."[10]

■ *Social Class Assessment*

The second prime molder of lifestyle, particularly in the United States, is social class. Individual and family lifestyles and associations with the external environment of neighborhood and community vary greatly from social class to social class. This variance may be explained partly by differences in preferences and perspectives; however, more importantly, these variations arise from the different demands on and conditions of living in the various social classes. Social class combined with cultural background exerts the greatest overall influence on lifestyle including socialization, role expectations, value development, and behavior.[2]

Social class may be defined as the relationship between educational level, occupation, and income. Each social class is composed of groups of individuals who occupy broadly similar positions on a prestige scale.[25] Occupational position, weighted with education and income, is generally used as the index of social class in the United States. The occupations deemed to be of the greatest value to society receive the greatest rewards, including money, power, prestige, and autonomy. All societies differentiate or rank people, lifestyles, possessions, and work based on what attributes are viewed as most valuable. Status consciousness is present in all cultures, even among children who begin at a young age to recognize their own place in society and the places of others.[2]

In the early 1950s, Warner developed six descriptions of discrete social classes in the United States.[26] These class definitions are still in use today and often form the basis for descriptions of client systems, communities, and individuals. However, there is a great deal of blurring between social classes. Within each of the groupings, there are variances in values and perceived status.[27] Additionally, other factors within the group, such as cultural and religious orientation, create diversity within each social class; therefore, the following discussion of Warner's schematization only provides a guideline for examining patterned relationships, lifestyle differences, and value differences between and within social classes (Table 7-1).

The upper class, according to Warner, is divided into two groups: the established upper class and the new rich (*nouveau riche*) or lower upper class. Families or individuals who have possessed wealth for three generations or more are classified as the established upper

T A B L E   7 - 1
Warner's Descriptions of Social Classes in the USA

Upper Class		
	Upper-upper	Established affluent
	Lower-upper	Newly affluent or *nouveau riche*
Middle Class		
	Upper-middle	Community leaders
	Lower-middle	Small business, para-professionals
Lower Class		
	Upper-lower	Blue-collar workers
	Lower-lower	Culture of poverty

class, while persons of recent affluence are classified as new rich.[26] Members of the upper-upper class are firmly entrenched in a close extended family relationship specifically designed to guard against exposure to other social classes. Financial and occupational security are provided by the extended family or through inheritance.

In contrast, members of the lower-upper class are much less likely to inherit their wealth or social position; they have a larger percentage of earned income and exhibit a pronounced difference in the values they place on family relationships. The *nouveau riche* tend to socialize with prominent individuals rather than forming close ties with extended family, resulting in a nuclear family structure where members act independently of kin.[26]

The middle class is considered to be the dominant group both numerically and socially. Warner identifies two distinct subgroups that make up the middle class, each with its own values and expectations. The upper middle class is generally composed of substantial business persons and professionals who are also the civic leaders in the community. The majority of these persons are college graduates with strong career orientations. The family unit tends to be nuclear in structure with weak ties to the extended family.[28]

The lower middle class family is composed primarily of the owners of small businesses, clerical workers, paraprofessional workers, and some highly skilled craftsmen or service workers. There is a wide variety of cultural and religious backgrounds among the members of this group. Socially, the kinship group is close and major social activities often take place within the extended family.[29]

The lower class is also divided into two groups: the blue-collar worker or upper lower class and the lower-lower class. The blue-collar group is made up primarily of skilled workers, semiskilled workers in factories, and service workers paid at minimum or below minimum wages. For many members of this group, economic instability related to swings in the business cycle is common. Employment choices are frequently based on economic necessity rather than a desire for a career. Multiple family stresses are associated with this economic uncertainty.[28] When the family needs assistance, relatives are more likely to be called than public agencies, and if agency assistance is required, it is often met with suspicion.[30] The extended family, the neighborhood peer group, and the informal work group provide the majority of socialization opportunities for members of the blue-collar group as well as actual assistance with problems.

Members of the lower-lower class live at the most impoverished level of existence. Wide variations in lifestyle exist due to variations in the environment (rural versus urban, or regional differences); however, there are four common social characteristics of this group. The amount of formal education attained by the members of this group is usually 8 years or less. The most likely occupation is that of unskilled worker with long periods of unemployment. Because of unemployment and low wages, these individuals are more likely to receive public financial assistance. The majority of the lower-lower class group live in substandard housing with few, if any, safety- or health-related features such as fire alarms, adequate sanitation, or rodent control.[31] Lewis has termed this class "the culture of poverty." Inherent in this notion is the recognition that the lower-lower class lifestyle is a direct result of poverty, not simply an American phenomenon, and represents values and behaviors found across many cultures.[32]

In contrast with other social classes, the lower-lower class is generally stigmatized, and its members are stereotyped as lazy, shiftless, or unnecessarily dependent on others. Rodman identified the sources of this stigmatization as an inability to meet the cardinal requirement for success in American culture productivity.[33] Indeed, even the term lower-lower class imposes a negative connotation based on the values of other groups, leading Russell to coin the phrase "underclass," implying a lack of sufficient resources to meet human needs.[34] Rodman proposed that this negativism is related to judgmental attitudes on the part of individuals who have studied the underprivileged.

> It is possible that the problems of the lower class identified by middle class sociologists . . . early marriages, failure to complete school, emphasis on fighting ability . . . are actually solutions or coping behaviors utilized to deal with other issues faced by the lower class.[33]

More jobs and better education are clearly needed if new coping behaviors are to be formed. In an achievement-oriented society, employment is not only a source of income, it is a source of stability and promotes acceptance from the community at large. With increased acceptance and economic stability, the underprivileged can "afford" such values as long-range planning and achievement orientation, and can pass these values along to their children.

Members of the underprivileged population are in need of multiple health care services. However, these individuals frequently fail to use the health resources available to them. Suchman proposed that poorly educated persons with limited professional contacts did not develop the sophistication necessary to negotiate the complex medical service system. The majority of health services used by the lower socioeconomic group were crisis-related and were in life-threatening situations.[30] This crisis intervention approach to health care was related to a failure to recognize or implement health promotion practices and an inability to respond to medical crisis. The nurse who understands and analyzes variations in culture can help the client avoid cultural conflicts, miscommunication, and unneeded stress.

▉ *Cultural Assessment*

Certain cultural components are present in every social group. Subtle as well as obvious differences exist since cultural patterns will be followed by individuals to varying degrees. A cultural assessment will provide valuable keys to a client's cultural identity and should be a part of a routine assessment procedure. Fong's CONFHER system, Table 7-2, identifies the key variables of a cultural profile that may influence a client's health care beliefs and practices.[20] This system provides a means of assessing cultural background and gathering data required to develop a culturally appropriate plan of care.

Communication Style

Communication style, both verbal and nonverbal, is fundamental to any valid cultural assessment. Effective communication between a public health nurse and a client is essential to safe nursing care. The language and dialect preference of the client must be noted. Does the client speak fluent English? If not, is the client able to understand common health terms such as fever, pain, or nausea? Is the client able

T A B L E 7 - 2
Confher System for a Cultural Profile

Cultural component	Variable
Communication style	Language and dialect preference Nonverbal behaviors Social customs
Orientation	Cultural identity Acculturation Value Orientation
Family relationships	Family structure and roles Family dynamics and decision making Lifestyle and living arrangements
Health beliefs	Alternative health care Health, crisis, and illness beliefs Response to pain
Education	Learning style Informal and formal education Occupation and socio-economic level
Religion	Preference Beliefs, rituals, and taboos

(Fong CM: Ethnicity and nursing practice. Top Clin Nurs 7(3):10, 1985)

to communicate a need for assistance. If necessary, the choice to engage an interpreter should be made by the client.

The meaning of nonverbal behaviors in various cultures must be recognized. Gestures, body language, facial expressions, and the use of personal space may have significant meaning to various cultural groups. The nurse can consciously increase an awareness of nonverbal expressions by considering the following questions. Are there cultural styles of communication that the client adheres to, such as the Japanese custom of bowing the head to show respect? Does the client mean what is said or does any question elect a noncommittal answer? How much physical touch is appropriate in that culture?

Orientation

Nurses must allow clients to identify their own cultural values, beliefs, and priorities. Choosing for a client is, for the most part, a form of stereotyping that prevents the client from developing a unique identity. The following questions may be used to help delineate a client's cultural orientation. Does the client identify with a particular group (Chinese, Jewish, Native American)? Where was the client born? Where has the client lived and for how long?

It is essential to understand intercultural variations based on generational differences within groups. For example, first-generation Vietnamese may have more traditional cultural values than third-generation Vietnamese Americans due to acculturation with the dominant American society. Similarly, frequent contact of younger generations with older relatives, who are the chief source of cultural transmission of traditional values, affects the rate of acculturation.[21] Appropriate questions related to intercultural variance may include: How long has the client or the client's family been in America? How closely does the client adhere to the values of the cultural system?

Kluckholm and Strodbeck identified five values that need to be assessed in the area of cultural orientation. The public health nurse should assess the client's beliefs regarding human nature, the relationship between humans and nature, the value of time in the culture, the main purpose of life, and the nature of peoples' relationships to one another.[22] For example, a male Chinese client may say that the most important events that guide his life happened in the past (ancestor worship), that he lives in harmony with nature, and that he values his extended family relationships, with the group's goals having precedence over the individual's goals.

Nutrition

Dietary habits that are symbolic, meaningful, and cherished by cultural groups for many generations should be assessed and left unchanged as much as possible. Inversely, a client should not be expected to prefer certain foods just because of cultural heritage. The following questions addressed to the client may help determine preference and taboos. Are there foods that you prefer? Are there foods you are encouraged to eat when you are sick? Are there foods you must avoid? For example, traditional Chinese postpartum clients generally avoid fruits and vegetables and usually eat only rice, eggs, and chicken.

Family Relationships

Three interrelated aspects of family relationships should be explored in cultural assessment. First, questions related to family structure and roles are essential. Who is a member of the family? How does the client define the family? Is the family nuclear, extended, or tribal in nature? Who is the head of the household? What are the roles of the various family members—mother, father, eldest son, daughter, and grandparent? Who is responsible for the rearing of children?

Second, family dynamics must be considered. How are decisions made in the family? For example, in the patriarchal orientation of the Middle Eastern family, all decisions are made by the male head of the household. Who is responsible for the management of finances? What is the role of the family in caring for the client's illness? What are the major social customs or taboos? For example, the Navajo culture places great emphasis on pausing before responding to a question or statement and considers a rapid response an indication that little thought was given to the answer. What are the goals of the family? Are there great values placed on having many children and on children who complete college, or are financial securities the major area of emphasis?

Finally, questions related to lifestyle will assist the nurse in developing a culturally appropriate plan of care. Where does the family live? For example, to say that members of a Mexican-American family are urban residents is not sufficient. Does the family live in an area where all the other residents are also Mexican Americans or have they been isolated from their culture through a move? What social and recreational facilities are available?

Health Benefits

Clients from all cultures have specific folk health beliefs. In fact, the nurse must be aware that these beliefs often take precedence over scientific knowledge, especially when there is a conflict between the two.[23] Questions related to client beliefs and practices on health, illness, and crisis situations are necessary to avoid conflict in nurse-client expectations. Does the client rely on any self-care or folk health practices? Is the client currently receiving treatment from a cultural healer such as a shaman (witch doctor) or faith healer? How does the client explain the nature of illness—as a curse, bad spirits, or an imbalance with nature? Whenever possible, beliefs regarding health and illness and folk medicine should be included in the client's plan of care. Indeed, the power of such beliefs cannot be underestimated. In East Africa, researchers have documented evidence indicating that tuberculosis (TB) patients who believed they were under a curse were extremely hard to treat and frequently experienced more untoward reactions from the prescribed treatment.[24]

Education

In planning for the care and education of clients in the public health setting, it is important to identify how the client learns. Orque, Bloch, and Monrroy state that identification of a client's learning style is the most important factor in the successful implementation of health education for culturally different patients.[21] To assess a preferred method of learning, the nurse may ask the following questions. Does the client prefer printed literature or audiovisual presentations? Does the client learn best from trial and error or didactic methods? What is the client's informal and formal education level? Using this information, the nurse can tailor a program to meet the learning needs of the client and family with a minimum of wasted effort.

Religion

Religious beliefs and practices may have a strong influence on a client's physical and emotional health. Does the client believe in a god or many gods? Does the client have a religious/denominational preference? What religious rites are necessary in the treatment of illness? What clergy or religious advisors will be involved in the client's health care?

In the practice of public health nursing, much of the nurse's effort is concentrated on helping those in lower socioeconomic groups attain and maintain optimal levels of health. It is only through understanding attitudes and beliefs regarding health and illness that nurses can even begin to assist these clients with the resolution of their health care needs.

Cultural and social class are assessed as part of the nursing process when delivering public health nursing services to families and communities. Measuring cultural values is a subtle, often qualitative process and requires special methods. Socioeconomic status is quantified by epidemiologist as SES, a combination of education, income, and other variables, usually occupation as denoted by Hollingshead.[39] The difference between some ethnic groups and SES is (regrettably) so consistent that Green's SES index includes race as a weight for quantifying socioeconomic status for public health purposes.[40] This index measures the mother's education as a more accurate measure of sociocultural impact. Qualitative assessments by nurses are often based on expert clinical judgments; however, quantifications are useful for setting priorities and are indispensable for measuring community parameters. Integration of observations for delivery of nursing care requires professional judgments that are keenly sensitive to the needs of different cultural groups.

The combined efforts of customs, beliefs, and social class can be beneficial or harmful to health. This is particularly true when rituals and mores influence nutritional behaviors (many cultures orient religious beliefs around eating habits). In some cultures, these customs have promoted community survival. For instance, Jewish law has banned food such as shellfish and pork that are now known to have a high potential for harboring infective organisms causing disease. The religious beliefs of the Moslems include the cleansing of the hands before meals, using sand, if necessary, when water is in short supply. But all rituals are not beneficial. Choice of food and the customs surrounding social actions where food intake is formalized can sometimes be detrimental to the health of the group. When social status, either from poverty or from ranking within groups, restricts food choices or is associated with food privileges, the results may be disastrous. Epidemiology can assist in identifying behaviors associated with societal values that cause disease. To emphasize the importance of the effect of food choices and social behaviors, two examples will be reviewed. The first is a discussion of pica, the consumption of nonfood items found all over the world but mainly associated with family and group habits. The second is kuru, a neurological, degenerative disease, first discovered in New Guinea. The latter is a dramatic example demonstrating anthropo-epidemiology as a method of identifying causal association between sociocultural factors and disease.

■ *Pica as a Cultural Phenomenon*

The food habits of individuals are deeply influenced by the society and culture in which they live.[41] In fact, common dietary items in one culture may not even be considered as food in another. A variety of dietary curiosities come to mind such as iguana in Central America, squid and octopus in the Far East, and blood pudding in Great Britain. Regional dietary differences occur also in the United States, as a visitor to the South may find when served grits, turnip greens, or hush puppies for the first time.

Perhaps one of the strangest eating habits worldwide, however, relates to consumption of nonfood items such as laundry or corn starch, clay and dirt, charcoal, soap, ashes, plaster, paper, and hair. This phenomenon, known as pica, has been documented in many areas, including the United States. Pica is described as "a physiological craving for abnormal food constituents, or for substances not commonly regarded as food."[42]

The historical records of pica date from 10 B.C. to the present and point out that pica is practiced in widely separated geographic regions, and by some animals as well as humans. The earliest forms of pica reportedly include clay lozenges that were ingested to treat illness and poisoning, as well as earth eaten in bread dough.

Throughout the ages, a variety of explanations for pica have been offered including heredity, food allergy, and stress. Likewise, the reported physiologic effects of pica on humans include dwarfism, hypogonadism, hepatosplenomegaly, iron deficiency syndrome, intestinal obstruction, parotid enlargement, and perinatal casualties. Pica is thought to be age-related, with the majority of cases occurring in children and pregnant women. However, recent data and actual case reports indicate that pica is not limited to any age, sex, or racial group: it can occur anywhere among any people.

Pica may also involve other substances in addition to those already listed, as the case studies below illustrate:

1. One young pregnant woman developed an appetite for blocks of toilet-bowl freshener (paradichlorobenzene). This client presented with anemia and was treated with iron and folic acid. Neither medication improved her hemoglobin level, however, and her pica practice continued.[43]
2. A nonpregnant woman ate handfuls of tomato seeds. She presented with anemia that resolved following parental administration of iron.[44]
3. One mentally retarded adolescent consumed up to two packages of cigarettes a day. He presented with low plasma zinc levels, elevated copper levels, and wounds that would not heal, but showed a reversal of all signs after oral administration of zinc sulfate.
4. A 74-year-old black woman presented with severe microcytic hypochromic anemia without blood loss. She was consuming 60–180 grams of magnesium carbonate daily.[45]
5. Other cases of pica in pregnant women have involved cigarette ash, burned matches, peanuts (gooberphagia), hair (trichophagia) and lettuce (lectophagia).

Physical findings in subjects who practice pica vary to some degree with the type of substance consumed. For instance, one type of pica (cravings for grass, leaves, and insects) is associated with normal plasma values of metals and minerals. Overall, nutritional status may be influenced by pica in several ways. First, the consumption of the craved substance can reduce the intake of normal dietary sources of nutrients. Second, pica can reduce the bioavailability of minerals. On the other hand, some clays can be sources of minerals such as magnesium, potassium, iron, zinc and calcium.

Pica practices have been associated with cultural and familial factors. Clay eating was encouraged among the male youths of Greece because it was believed to produce a desirable complexion and a slender, effeminate body. Further, symbolic geophagy (earth eating) occurs in many cultures, and earth eating, irrespective of cravings, has frequently been associated with religious belief.

In African cultures, the consumption of earth during the first trimester of pregnancy is reportedly believed to suppress nausea. Young girls are taught in childhood that during pregnancy, the consumption of earth is desirable. Some researchers consider the eating of clay to be deeply ingrained in black culture in the American South. There, clay is sometimes fed as a pacifier for the infant. That same practice has also been observed in Africa. However, individuals in the United States may have acquired pica practices either from Europe or from the indigenous Indian population in the New World since geophagy has been documented in both cultures.

In a research study conducted in Alabama in 1984, 63% of subjects, (N=148) reported practicing pica either as children or young adults. All subjects in the study were female, and a majority were black and earned less than $3000 per year. Half of the subjects never completed high school, and the great majority were between 15 and 26 years of age. When subjects were asked why they ate pica, 32% said they did so because of the taste and 22% cited familial reasons, such as "I saw my mama do it, so I did it too." Slightly more than 90% of the subjects reported having seen other people eating the particular nonfood item ingested. Frequencies of pica practice varied, but the greatest percentage reported weekly ingestion (34.1%). The amount of substance consumed at one time ranged from pinches to handfuls.[46]

Although both the underlying cause and the psychological/physical effects of pica are not totally understood, we can assume that the phenomenon is associated with cultural experiences. Pica consumption is a salient example of how cultural background influences health behaviors and beliefs.

■ *Kuru*

Any discussion of the effects of beliefs and mores on health behaviors from an epidemiologic perspective would be incomplete without a review of a famous anthropo-epidemiologic investigation in New Guinea in the 1950s. This study has fascinated subsequent generations of public health professionals. The epidemic of a disease known as kuru was insoluble until the cultural rituals of this community were taken into consideration. The study remains a dramatic example of the need to know the belief structure of families, community, and society in order to understand health behaviors and intervene effectively for health promotion. The community health nurse delivering care in homes and facilities must include the values underlying the standards of behavior held by ethnic and religious groups to engage families in meaningful change of health care practices when necessary. Solutions to group problems may be evasive and inadequate unless the appropriate hypothesis can be developed to consider cultural factors. These caveats are not limited to local customs and identifiable groups within the United States but apply equally to Third World countries. Understanding sociocultural factors influences the success of public health interventions, such as the activities of the Peace Corps. The famous example now presented underscores the relevance of mores to group health and the role of epidemiology in solving culturally associated problems.

The first evidence of a new disease emerged early in 1957, and it was labeled as endemic to New Guinea.[47] It was publicized in the press as an illness where patients "laughed themselves to death." These unscientific reports were received with deserved skepticism.[48] Later in the same year, a lucid, clinical article was published concerning a degenerative disease of the central nervous system where the illness and its history were described in more detail.[49] The first symptoms of the disease were commonly observed as an episode of severe tremors or an unsteadiness of gait. As the illness progressed, the shaking episodes intensified and became more frequent. The progressive motor ataxia slowly developed into paralysis, although it was assumed that in most instances cerebration remained intact. The disease was fatal mostly within 1 year. Only occasionally did kuru first present with fits of uncontrollable laughter. When it did, it alternated with episodes of severe depression.

Kuru, a native term meaning trembling due to fear or cold, was observed in a limited region in the eastern highlands of New Guinea. This inland, mountainous area, romanticized as Shangri-la, had been impervious to exploration until 1930. The initial penetration of the area was followed by the establishment of missions and government posts, and the inevitable prospectors looking for the chance to get rich. The invasion of the Japanese in 1934 put an end to European infiltration, and after World War II, New Guinea became an Australian Trust Territory. After 1945, organized attempts were made to open up the area to deliver medical and nursing services into the region and provide organized government control. Consequently, anthropologists from all over the world became interested in New Guinea as the primitive cultures living in the area became increasingly accessible. The first observance of "shivering and shaking sickness" among the highland tribes was observed by anthropologists, who found the condition was "fairly common"—a qualitative estimate.

Anthropologists who investigated the native cultures found that the villagers differentiated kuru from sorcery and from the disease causing death. It became evident that these interpretations were recognized to be deeply embedded in the tradition and magic of the Fore people, a tribe where 80% of the cases of kuru occurred. Anthropologists investigated the shaking ascribed to sorcery. They found that it takes only a short time to develop magical explanations for strange illnesses in primitive societies. For example, bacillary dysentery, a disease introduced into the area at the time of World War II, had evoked a similar reaction invoking evil.

In 1958, a team of health scientists went to New Guinea in response to world concern about kuru.[50] The geographic region where kuru occurred was in the highlands. The community consisted of about 35,000 people living in 160 villages called census units. The people spoke a dozen different languages and had as many different cultures. Deaths from the disease were found to be preceded by an illness which never lasted more than 2 years, and once the symptoms appeared, kuru was invariably fatal. Cases occurred mainly in the women. The female–male ratio in adults was 14:1, and although 60% of cases were adults, when it occurred in children the sex ratio was 1:1. The Fore suffered most from the disease, but there were some scattered cases among other tribes with whom they occasionally intermarried. Laboratory studies did not reveal any striking abnormality, and no gross pathology was found on autopsy. There were no seasonal variations in disease occurrence and no memory among the people of any epidemic of encephalitis.[49]

Careful inquiry revealed that at least 300 deaths from kuru had occurred in the 5 years previous to the investigation, although the disease was known among the natives before government control of the region 25 years before. As in any native society, a complex kinship existed and information on childbearing was readily obtainable. As the investigation continued, it was found that in over half the cases, close relatives had died of the disease, and 43% of cases had occurred in parents and siblings. The disease had an unusual sex and age distribution with high familial prevalence in a closely intermarried community. In fact, it seemed impossible to find any extended family without a case of kuru.

The first hypothesis was to associate the illness with genetic factors and label it as hereditary. Environmental influences were not ruled out, especially when therapy for treating the illness was found to be ineffective. The investigation intensified. The neurological degeneration suggested a toxic factor, perhaps in the diet; therefore, pica, smoke, material used for skin painting, and other organic and inorganic agents were investigated. Finally, questions of cultural mores and social customs were raised to find answers to the epidemic.

It was known that before 1930, the society of the Fore was described as close to the Stone Age. Married men did not live with their wives, and sexual activity was restricted to daylight hours in secluded places. At puberty, males were initiated into manhood through elaborate ceremonies. For the rest of their lives they lived with the men in housing separate from the women and children. Women were responsible for cooking and preparing meals cooked in pits, with steam made from pouring water on hot stones. Food was often packed into bamboo cylinders and placed in hot ashes. The meals were low in protein, and it was a tradition for families and communities to feast on the occasional surfeit of pork, the only available livestock. But there was another source of meat. It was a tradition of the Fore to eat members of the same family or tribe who had died. The ritual is called endocannibalism. The rituals occurred for two reasons. The first was that it was used as a method of detecting sorcerers who had inflicted kuru on a victim, most often a wife, valued among the Fore as the most prized possession. When the victim died, the men would eat her body and watch the unknown sorcerer ingest the victim.[49] Subsequently, if disease occurred in one of the men attending the ritual, it was believed to reveal the identity of the man who had cast the spell and, at the same time, inflict punishment. The other reason for endocannibalism occurred as part of the rites of mourning, the rituals surrounding a death in the family. The deceased was eaten apparently to preserve the spirit and wisdom of the one who had died. In preparing the body for the meal of mourning, the women were assisted by their children, and the body was prepared according to the customs of their ancestors. The top of the skull was removed, and the brains were smeared on parts of the bodies of the women and children and eaten without cooking during preparation of the ceremonial meal. The rest of the flesh was packed into bamboo cylinders for cooking over the fire for the family meal.

With this information, the hypothesis that endocannibalism was spreading the disease was an obvious postulation, and the disease was thought to be associated with an infectious agent in the tissues of the brain. These associations were supported by epidemiologic evidence that the frequency of cases increased in women and children and clustered around tribal families. Moreover, the hypothesis was confirmed by subsequent facts, such as the decline in the incidence of kuru with decreased cannibalism. Today there are only a few scattered cases in the area, and they occur where endocannibalism has been practiced surreptitiously.[51]

This unusual epidemic was identified at its peak. The causative organism of kuru is now known to be a retrovirus confined almost entirely to the brain tissue. There is a long period of time between the invasion of the body and the onset of symptoms. Kuru is a well-known anthropo-epidemiologic study not just because it is dramatic, but because it emphasizes the influence of belief and ritual on disease and its counterpart, health. It raised the important question of the role of viruses in chronic degenerative diseases of the central nervous system. The investigation of kuru demonstrated that extended incubation periods can occur between the exposure to a viral agent and the onset of disease. Kuru was also the first epidemic thought to be caused from a viral mutation. Research stimulated by this epidemic has been of assistance in the investigation of AIDS and may contribute to knowledge about Alzheimer's disease.[52]

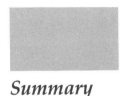

Summary

*C*ultural and socioeconomic variables impact greatly on the practice of public health nursing. Indeed, nurses who are knowledgeable about and sensitive to the cultural needs of clients, families, and groups have found a new satisfaction, which has replaced burnout, negative viewpoints, and stereotypic beliefs. More importantly, nurses are aware that socioculturally appropriate care can make a difference in the quality of nursing services, the restoration of health, and in ongoing, interpersonal relationships.

While many advances have been made in developing an awareness of the need for culturally sensitive health care, much remains to be done. Nurses as leaders in the field of public health practice must serve as advocates for those individuals who do not have access to culturally oriented care and must educate other health care providers in the sociocultural needs of the individual families.[38]

The qualitative and quantitative assessment of families and communities must include sociocultural factors. Epidemiology provides a framework for pursuing the effects of values and beliefs on the occurrence of illness and assists in the evaluation of changes in norms that influence health. It is through the practice of public health nursing that the solutions to the challenge of socioculturally sensitive health care can be identified and implemented.

References

1. Lipson JG, Meleis AI: Culturally appropriate care: The case of immigrants. Top Clin Nurs 7(3):48–56, 1985
2. Friedman MM: Family Nursing: Theory and Assessment, 2nd ed. Norwalk, CT, Appleton-Century-Crofts, 1986
3. Goodenough WH: Cooperation in Change. New York, Russell Sage Foundation, 1966
4. Koshi, PT: Cultural diversity in the nursing curricula. Nurse Educ 15:14–20, 1976
5. Kay MA: The Mexican American. In Clark AL (ed): Culture, Childbearing, and Health Professionals, pp. 227–254. Philadelphia, FA Davis, 1978
6. Kroeber AL: Anthropology. New York, Harcourt and Brace, 1948
7. Kobrin FE, Goldscheider C: The Ethnic Factor in Family Structure and Mobility. Cambridge, MA, Ballinger Press, 1978
8. Aamodt AM: Culture. In Clark AL (ed): Culture, Childbearing, and Health Professionals, pp 48–53. Philadelphia, FA Davis, 1978

9. Leininger M: Transcultural nursing: An essential knowledge and practice field for today. Can Nurse 80(10):42–45, 1984

10. Leininger M: Transcultural Nursing: Concepts, Theories, and Practices. New York, John Wiley & Sons, 1978

11. Brink PJ: Value orientations as an assessment tool in cultural diversity. Nurs Res 33:198–203, 1984

12. Louis KB: Transcending cultural bias: The literature speaks. Top Clin Nurs 7(3):78–84, 1985

13. Reinhardt AM, Quinn MD: Family Centered Community Nursing. St Louis, CV Mosby, 1973

14. Tripp–Reimer T: Research in cultural diversity. West J Nurs Res 6:353–354, 1984

15. Tripp–Reimer T, Brink P, Saunders JM: Cultural assessment: Content and process. Nurs Outlook 32:78–82, 1984

16. Cannon RB, Gilead MP, Haun E, Johnson MJ et al: A value clarification approach to cultural diversity. Nurs Health Care 5:161–164, 1984

17. Weeks WH, Pedersen PB, Brislin RW: A Manual of Structured Experiences for Cross-Cultural Learning. Chicago, Intercultural Press, 1982

18. Belloc R: The relationship of health practices and mortality. Prev Med 2:67–81, 1976

19. La Fargue JP: Mediating between two views of illnesses. Top Clin Nurs 7(3), 70–77, 1985

20. Fong CM: Ethnicity and nursing practice. Top Clin Nurs 7(3):10, 1985

21. Orque MS, Bloch B, Monrroy LSA: Ethnic Nursing Care. St Louis, CV Mosby, 1983

22. Kluckholm FR, Strodbeck FL: Variations in Value Orientations. Evanston, Row and Peterson, 1978

23. Johnson M: Folk beliefs and ethnocultural behavior in pediatrics. Nurs Clin North Am 12:78–86, 1977

24. Kegley CF, Saviers AN: Working with others who are not like me. J Sch Health 53:81–85, 1983

25. Williams RM: American Society: A Sociological Interpretation, 3rd ed. New York, Knopf, 1960

26. Warner WL: American Life. Chicago, University of Chicago Press, 1953

27. Kohn ML: Class and Conformity: A Study of Values. Homewood, IL, Dorsey Press, 1969

28. Eshleman JR: The Family: An Introduction. Boston, Allyn and Bacon, 1974

29. Schultz DA: The Changing Family. Englewood Cliffs, NJ, Prentice-Hall, 1972

30. Suchman WA: Social factors in medical deprivation. Am J Public Health 65:1725–1733, 1977

31. Bell R: Marriage and Family Interaction. Homewood, IL, Dorsey Press, 1971

32. Lewis O: Children of Sanchez. New York, Random House, 1961

33. Rodman H: Marriage, Family, and Society. New York, Random House, 1965

34. Russell G: The American underclass. Time, pp 16–19. August 29, 1977

35. Mare RD: Socioeconomic effects on child mortality in the United States. Am J Public Health 72:168–176, 1982

36. Markland RE, Durand RE: An investigation of socio-psychological factors affecting infant immunization. Am J Public Health 66:168–169, 1976
37. Leininger M: Transcultural nursing: An overview. Nurs Outlook 32:72–73, 1984
38. Leininger M: Transcultural care diversity and universality: A theory of nursing. Nurs Health Care 6:209–212, 1984
39. Hollingshead AB, Redlich FC: Social Class and Mental Illness. New York, 1958
40. Green WL: Manual for scoring socioeconomic status for research on health behavior. Public Health Rep 85(9):815–827, 1970
41. Krause MV, Mahan LK: Food, Nutrition and Diet Therapy. Philadelphia, WB Saudners, 1979
42. Danford DE: Pica and Nutrition, p 303, Annu Rev Nutr 2:302–322, 1982
43. Campbell DM, Davidson RJ: Toxic haemolytic anemia in pregnancy due to a pica for paradichlorobenzene. J Obstet Gynaec Brit Comm 77:657–659, 1970
44. Coleman DL, Greenberg CS, Ries CA: Iron-deficiency anemia and pica for tomato seeds. N Engl J Med 304:848, 1981
45. Leming PD, Reed DC, Martelo OJ: Magnesium carbonate pica: An unusual case of iron deficiency. Ann Intern Med 94:660, 1981
46. Willard AA: Concept Clarification of Pica in Women. Unpublished Thesis, University of Alabama at Birmingham, 1984
47. Gajdusek DC, Zigas V: Regenerative disease of the central nervous system in New Guinea. N Engl J Med 257:30:974–979, 1957
48. Editorial. Kuru Med J Austr 2:21:765–766 Nov 23, 1987
49. Editorial. Kuru Brit Med 2:5059:1480–1481 Dec 21, 1957
50. Gajdusek DC: Unconventional viruses and the origin and disappearance of kuru. Science 197:9:943–960, 1977
51. Medicine around the world (editor). In Papua, New Guinea, health aides carry medical burden. Hosp Pract 90–101, 109, 1976
52. Fenner FJ: The Australia aborigines, the Fore of Papua, New Guinea and the 1976 Nobel Prizes for medicine. Med J Aust 2:64:73–74 July 16, 1977

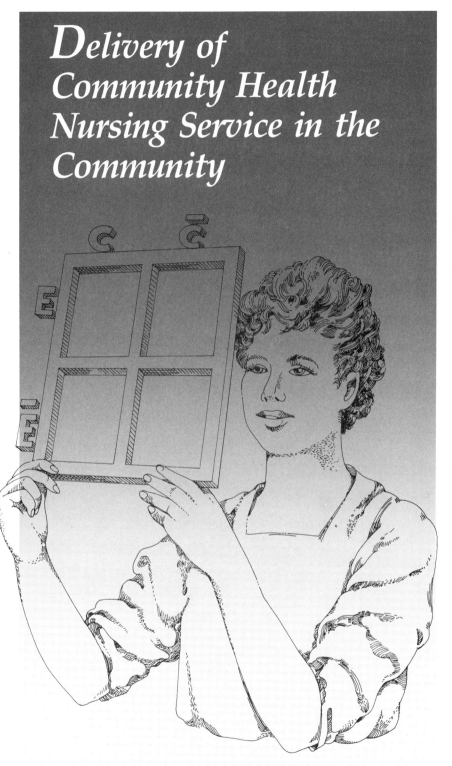

Delivery of Community Health Nursing Service in the Community

Epidemiology provides tangible evidence of the impact of nursing services and promotes the use of end points of quality that are recognizable and acknowledged by the public health system.

Epidemiology for Nursing Services in the Community

LEARNING OBJECTIVES

After reading and understanding the contents of this chapter, the student will be able to:

1. Adapt or create a definition of epidemiology that will help guide the use of epidemiologic principles in nursing practice.

2. Explain how the epidemiologic process relates to the nursing process in various clinical situations.

3. Analyze why it is necessary that community health nurses be able to read and understand graphic displays of numerical distributions.

4. Cite at least one instance in which it would be appropriate to display data in a bar graph, a polygon configuration, a histogram format, or a pie chart.

5. Identify 5 to 8 basic rules for assessing the quality of tables and graphs.

Introduction

We have been discussing epidemiology and how it augments community health nursing; but we still have not yet defined epidemiology. We have examined the characteristics of epidemiology and its relationship to public health. We have outlined its methods and its model, but we have yet to say what epidemiology is. Before we can gain an epidemiologic perspective on delivery of services, we need to define epidemiology and discuss the structure of the health delivery system.

▌ *Defining Process*

On reflection, definitions should logically precede explanations of how to use a science for nursing care. Definitions operationalize applied professions, that is, they show in the most general terms how the discipline is used for practice. The reasons for not defining epidemiology until halfway through the text are several. No definition of epidemiology is totally acceptable to all public health workers; epidemiology is a process and a method, therefore it is difficult to define. The content of epidemiology depends on the problem of the moment; it will vary according to whether the illness is chronic or acute, or whether the need is to evaluate or to assess nursing services. This requires a definition applicable to all situations that could occur. These are some of the reasons why, up to this time, we have described the characteristics of epidemiology and definitions so that the essential features of epidemiology could be identified regardless of the problem. In other words, we have concentrated on how to recognize epidemiology and how to use it rather than on its nature.

The difficulty of defining a discipline based on methods is a familiar one in nursing. Epidemiology and nursing have basic processes. Nursing has problems in agreeing to a definition that is universally acceptable within the profession. Nurse theorists have produced several definitions, all of which have merit but none that have general acceptance. Henderson has defined nursing as doing for patients what they would, under ordinary circumstances of health, for for themselves.[1] Orem defines nursing as a continuum of progressive care along which nursing moves the patient/client towards independence. In the social statement of the American Nurses Association, nursing is defined as the diagnosis of human responses to actual and potential health problems.[3] There are many other definitions of nursing, all with their own singular strengths and contributions to the profession.

An assessment of the merit of defining nursing has been outlined by Fitzpatrick and coworkers, and their approach is most useful for graduate nurses. From a simplistic but practical point of view, any definition of nursing must include and, above all, must indicate what nursing does. A working definition guides administrators, assists in interfacing nursing into new situations and importantly, provides a baseline for political and legislative action. It is of assistance in the nursing of aggregates to be able to define the scope of nursing practice, especially when services demand a community team composed of many disciplines.

All the observations just made about nursing can and do apply to epidemiology. It is just as desirable to have definitions that are understandable and practical for epidemiology as it is for nursing. Operational definitions of epidemiology facilitate its use in a multidisciplinary context. Epidemiology is motivated by principles of the public health mode. Community health nursing is based on the same concepts; therefore, any definition must be consistent with the concepts of community, delivery of services, and prevention and control. Before nurses can effectively utilize the principles and methods of epidemiology for health care, it is preferable and easier to know how to define epidemiology. An operational definition can summarize what epidemiology can do to contribute to the scope of practice of nursing and assist the community health nurse in integrating an epidemiologic perspective into the daily activities of delivery of care to communities. An adequate definition must reflect the concepts of public health and the characteristic features of epidemiology.

We have given only a few examples of the many definitions of nursing to illustrate the complexity of defining a process applied to many situations for meeting the needs of patients and clients. Now we will review nine definitions of epidemiology and assess them by comparing them to the public health model and the characteristics of epidemiology that we know are typical of its process and method. Some of these definitions have arisen from the traditional use of epidemiology over several years. Others have been derived from the roots of the word "epidemiology." Some are the attempts of famous epidemiologists to express what epidemiology is in a succinct and all-inclusive way.[4-6] These definitions are listed in Table 8-1.

▪ *Definitions of Epidemiology*

We will now consider the first three definitions of epidemiology appearing in Table 8-1 and assess their adequacy by comparing them to the concepts used in the public health model and the characteristics described in Chapter 4. The first definition is that epidemiology is an inductive method applied to large groups; the second is that epidemiology is a research method for public health; and the third is that

T A B L E   8 - 1
Definitions of Epidemiology

Epidemiology is
1. An inductive method applied to large groups.
2. A research method for public health.
3. The science of public health.
4. The study of statistics of diseases in populations.
5. A quantitative science. The measured quantities and descriptive terms are used to describe groups.[4]
6. The measurement of risk of disease in communities.
7. The study of epidemics—of hazards to large groups.
8. A method of diagnosing the condition of the people.[6]
9. The study of health of populations in relation to their environment and ways of living.[5]

epidemiology is the science of public health. Essentially, these three definitions say the same thing. The inductive method is intrinsic to research and is the method used by science. In the inductive method, observations are collected, and from them conclusions are drawn. Induction is the process of going from specific observations to a generalization. Research operationalizes the inductive method to test hypothetical associations, but the process used to test hypotheses is inductive and collects specific observation from which conclusions can be drawn. This research method is a process of inductive thinking rather than deductive thinking and is a scientific method. These three definitions refer to the epidemiologic method or process.

Another concept shared by the first three definitions is community. All three refer to aggregates implied in the word "public." In short, all three definitions incorporate the concepts of the group. It is clear that inductive, research, or scientific methods are all part of a scientific approach to safeguard the health of the public, and all three definitions refer to a method of drawing conclusions from observations. When scientific method is confined to the laboratory, the independent variable may be totally controlled by the researcher. In epidemiology, total control over people is never achieved. Populations are aggregates of people with rights, privileges, and concerns. Epidemiology is a research method developed as an alternative to laboratory research and uses methods of analysis, such as statistics and research, designed to compensate for lack of control. Nevertheless, the careful observation and collection of facts and the formulation and testing of hypotheses are scientific methods synonymous with epidemiology and have produced the epidemiologic process, which is similar to the nursing process for clinical situations.

Let us now look at the next triad of definitions of epidemiology. A fourth definition of epidemiology is the study of statistics of diseases in populations. In the fifth definition, epidemiology is described as a quantitative science where measured quantities and descriptive terms are used to describe groups. The sixth definition defines epidemiology as the measurement of risk of disease in community. These three definitions emphasize another attribute of epidemiology—to quantify observations in groups. The focus of epidemiology on services to populations is also included, but all three definitions draw attention to the function of epidemiology to describe and quantify risk of disease. We have already discussed, perhaps endlessly, the rate as the basic statistic of public health and how it quantifies disease. The rate is an acuity measure of risk in communities. This quantification is used to describe groups by studying health and disease in populations. Inherent in definitions four through six is the attribute of making comparisons between and among communities and using quantifications to estimate risk. These three definitions incompletely describe epidemiology, but they emphasize two characteristics of epidemiology, the measurement of observations to quantify risk to aggregates and the outcome event of health and disease.

The first three definitions emphasized scientific methods and the second three emphasized the quantification of risk. Now let us look at the final three definitions of epidemiology in Table 8-1, which emphasize the condition of the people in relationship to their environment. The seventh definition of epidemiology is that epidemiology is the study of epidemics—of hazards to large groups. The eighth definition is that epidemiology diagnoses the condition of the people, and the final definition is that epidemiology is the study of the health of populations in relationship to their environment and ways of living. Once more, none of these definitions adequately described epidemiology because each omits some basic characteristics necessary to fully operationalize what the discipline can accomplish. Instead, the definitions emphasize an important component or feature of this public health science.

In these last three definitions, people, the environment, and epidemics are related so that the results of people living together in groups can be analyzed. These three definitions relate diagnosing hazards to studying the relationship of the environment to healthful living. The interaction of people with problems encountered in adjusting to their world are so important to epidemiology that the epidemiologic or natural history of disease model has been formulated. The model consists of the interactions among three concepts: the host, the agent, and the environment, as discussed in Chapter 3. The epidemiologic model is based on diagnosing the condition of the people in relationship to their environment and ways of living. The interactions are intrinsic to studying and understanding the source of epidemics and to estimating the condition of the people regarding their health.

Understanding the components of the model and the relationship among the host (population), the environment, and the agent (or exposure) is critical to directing nursing assessment and intervention. These last three definitions invoke the basic epidemiologic model and are more inclusive definitions of epidemiology. They omit, however, reference to the characteristic of epidemiology to quantify observations. They also inadequately referenced the outcome of concern of epidemiology with disease and health.

A review of these nine definitions of epidemiology show that none are considered totally adequate. By comparing these definitions to the characteristics described in Chapter 4, it is possible to see whether all the attributes of epidemiology are included and to recognize the strength of each definition. Using the same approach, let us analyze the advantages of the most commonly accepted definition of epidemiology in use today. Although even this definition is not totally inclusive, it is clearly an operational definition, that is, it defines epidemiology by showing what can be expected as an outcome of practice. The most often used and widely accepted definition of epidemiology is shown in Table 8-2.

Epidemiology is the Study of the Frequency and the Distribution of the Determinants of an Infective Process, a Disease, or a Physiological State and Their Precursors in a Community

This definition is the one most frequently used in epidemiology and is the most comprehensive and applicable to nursing practice. Let us examine this definition with some care. In saying epidemiology is the study of the frequency of various phenomena, frequency is simply a count of people and/or events occurring to people. This is the same counting information requested by Woolsey and Lawrence for assessing the community. The rates are more complex statistics, but rates are also a measure of frequency to measure health and disease. As a

T A B L E   8 - 2
A Definition of Epidemiology

Epidemiology is the study of the frequency and the distribution of the determinants of:

• An infective process

• A disease

• Or a physiological state and their precursors in a community

measure of health, rates are also part of the basic information needed for community assessment of the need for nursing services.

Epidemiology is not only a study of the frequency of events but is also the study of distribution or patterns of occurrences associated with the health care system impacting on community health care. The concept of distribution is important. A distribution may be defined statistically as a table, a graph, or a mathematical expression giving the probabilities with which a random variable takes different values or sets of values.[7] An example of a mathematical expression is as follows:

$$\frac{1}{\sqrt{2\pi\sigma^2}} \cdot e^{-\frac{1}{2}\left(\frac{x-\mu}{\sigma}\right)^2}$$

This formula is, of course, the computation for the area under the normal curve.[8] Different values of the x variable can be entered into the formula to give an instantaneous rate of change occurring for a phenomenon. These successive values can be graphed on a bell-shaped curve (Fig. 8-1).

Tables are also distributions. In epidemiology, the classic table is the two by two showing the relationship of disease to the exposure event (Chapt. 4). In Figure 8-2, the column marked C represents cases, the column marked $\overline{C}$ represents the non-cases. In the two by two table, the rows are labeled as E for exposed populations and $\overline{E}$ for populations not exposed to a hazard or a therapeutic agent. In biostatistics, the columns are usually labeled j and rows are labeled i. A table consists of the sum of the rows and columns. Σ_{ij} the only difference between Figure 2-3 and Figure 8-2 is that biostatistical annotations have been included.

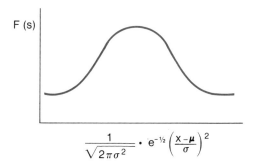

$$\frac{1}{\sqrt{2\pi\sigma^2}} \cdot e^{-\frac{1}{2}\left(\frac{x-\mu}{\sigma}\right)^2}$$

F I G U R E   8 - 1
A mathematical formula as distribution. (Remington RD, Schork MA: Statistics with Applications to the Biological and Health Sciences, p 125. Englewood Cliffs, NJ, Prentice-Hall, 1970)

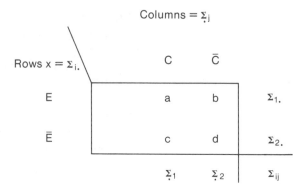

**F I G U R E
8 - 2**
*A 2 × 2 epidemiologic
table with statistical
annotations.*

The total in Figure 8-2 is represented by the Greek letter
(summa) Σ_{ij}, meaning the rows *(i)* and the columns *(j)* have been added together. This is the usual biostatistical notation. The cell showing
the frequency of cases due to exposure is the *a* cell and is of the utmost importance to the nurse epidemiologist. The *a* cell of the two by
two table is called the *cell of concern* because it relates the outcome of
disease to the exposure event. This cell shows how the exposure,
which might be an infectious agent, a toxicological agent, or some intervention method, relates to disease occurrence. It shows the results
of the interaction between host, agent, and environment. This *a* cell
shows the counts of a disease, complications, or episodes of recidivism occurring in response to the exposure to a hazardous experience. The number of cases of infection or frequency of remissions or
readmissions to the hospital may be the events of concern reflected in
the *a* cell. Thus, the distribution of values in the table relates to delivery of services and clinical practice as well as the effects of hazards
occurring among people in the community. A two by two table is the
model display of a distribution for nurse-epidemiologists.

Graphs are also distributions. They take the form of polygons,
bar graphs, histograms, and line diagrams as well as many other variations. They are quick, unequivocal ways to communicate problems
occurring in groups and the effects of services in prevention and control. It is useful for the community health nurse to be able to interpret
graphs. Public health graphs are fast and effective methods of communicating group events.

Distributions are used by all public health workers and constitute part of the common language of public health. They can be of
great assistance in health policy decision-making and in establishing
the credibility of nursing observations in communities. Therefore, it is
important for public health nurses to be able to read and understand
graphs for interdisciplinary communication and for documenting
group problems and solutions to clients in the community.

Graphs as Distributions: Their Use and Interpretation

Graphs are a function of the nature of the data they represent. To put it another way, information is graphed according to whether the data can be classified as nominal, ordinal, and interval (continuous). The choice of graphs should relate to these classifications. Bar graphs are used for nominal data. What this really means is that if there are several different groups with different names or classifications, the best way to depict them is to use bars because this method clearly indicates the separateness of the categories. For instance, bar graphs are used for graphing mortality by different diseases. Each disease is treated as a discrete entity, one from another. Bars may also be used for ranked or ordinal data. Nominal and ordinal data are both called discrete information (Fig. 8-3).[9]

A polygon is used for continuous or interval data. Interval data has the attribute that in the space between any two observable values there is the possibility of inserting another observable value. Mathematically, interval data or continuous data is information that can be quantified so that it can be divided into any number of values measured on a continuum. The independent variable, x, is usually placed on the horizontal axis of the graph (the abscissa). The perpendicular axis, or ordinate, is for the dependent variable 'y', which is a function of or depends on the independent variable x, expressed as $f(x) = y$. The polygon is very useful in contrasting rates over time from two or more populations. Overlay is possible and allows easy and accurate comparisons to be made. Figure 8-4 shows the effects of the introduction of the vaccine on the rates of rubella. Figure 8-5 shows a comparison of rates of hepatitis A and B and unspecified hepatitis as parts of the total rates and is an example of overlaying several polygon graphs to make easy comparisons for the same time period.[10]

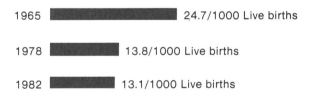

1965   24.7/1000 Live births

1978   13.8/1000 Live births

1982   13.1/1000 Live births

FIGURE 8-3
Infant mortality in the U.S. (National Center for Health Statistics: Advance report of final natality statistics, 1983. MVSR 34[6] Supp DHHS Pub. No. [PHS] 85-1120. Public Health Service, Hyattsville, MD, 1985)

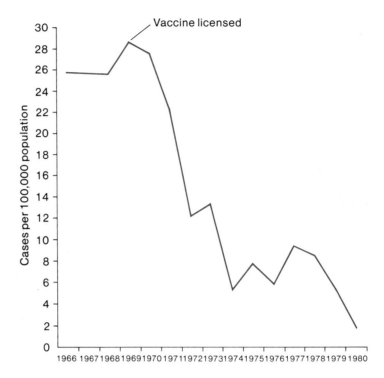

F I G U R E
8 - 4
Rubella—reported as rates by year, United States, 1966–1980.

The histogram is a graph used most often for showing the distribution of cases during an epidemic. It has certain advantages over the polygon, even though instead of rates the histogram uses cases over time. The advantages of a histogram are many. It shows relationships between the number of cases occurring within an epidemic time period. The cases are denoted by blocks so that the number of cases is

F I G U R E
8 - 5
Hepatitis reported case rate by year, United States, 1955–1980.

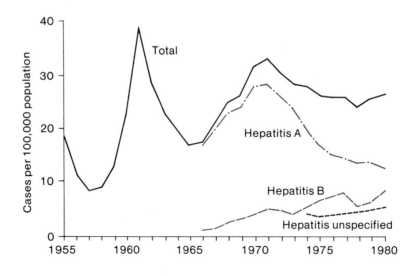

indicated clearly by the number of blocks. The histogram allows gaps in case occurrence to be displayed to show time periods when no cases occurred. The use of frequency of cases in a graph does *not* adjust for the size of the population as shown by a rate, but histograms are usually chosen to graph an epidemic circumstance where time is understood to be confined to the epidemic period for a fixed or known population base where comparisons to other populations are unnecessary. In Figure 8-6, the number of cases of malaria occurring in San Diego, California is indicated clearly by the number of blocks in the histogram.[11] This histogram allows gaps in case occurrence to be displayed to clearly show that no cases occurred in the first weeks of June, the first 2 weeks of July, nor in the first and third weeks of September, 1986.

Another graph that is confined to cases, not rates, is the timeline graph or, more simply, the case-line graph. This is used when only a few cases are involved in the problem, as indicated in the self-learning module in the appendix.

One other simple graph will be discussed. The pie graph is used to depict the proportion of a whole. It may be used to show relationships between classes or ranks for discrete data, as long as there are a limited number of categories. An example is shown in Figure 8-7 using information on nurse manpower for 1985.[12]

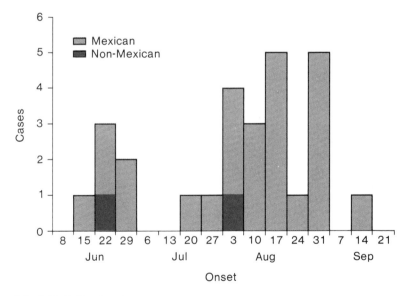

F I G U R E   8 - 6

Example of a histogram. Cases of Plasmodium vivax *malaria, by week of symptom onset—San Diego County, California, June 8–September 21, 1986. (Centers for Disease Control:* Plasmodium vivax *malaria—San Diego County, California. MMWR 35[43] 679–681, 1986)*

	%	Numbers of RNs
Associate degree or diploma graduates	63	1,134,000
Baccalaureate degree graduates	30	540,000
Master's degree graduates	6	108,000
Nurses with Ph.D. preparation	1	18,000

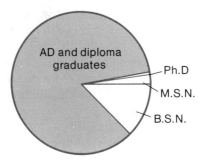

F I G U R E   8 - 7
Example of a pie graph. Approximate number of RNs by type of education, 1985.
(Mauchk I: Presentation to Association of Rehabilitation Nurses. Philadelphia, PA,
October 1986)

Tables are probably the best way of relating the information that
is extensive and detailed. What is important to remember is that tables, as well as graphs, are distributions of quantified observations of
communities. Some basic rules for assessing the quality of tables and
graphs which are simple and informational are the following.

Basic Rules for Assessing the Quality of Tables and Graphs

> a. Graphs or tables must be complete and able to stand alone—
>   the graph must be self-explanatory.
> b. The graph and tables must be clearly titled and summarize the
>   contents precisely.
> c. Axes of graphs must be labeled so that the information is clear.
> d. Observations must be assigned units of measurement as
>   appropriate.
> e. Groups or classes of information should be equal within the
>   graph or table, i.e., blood pressure classifications should all be
>   5mm Hg (or be 10mm Hg, and so forth) apart.
> f. Scales should relate to zero and scale breaks should be clearly
>   indicated on truncated (scales not starting at zero or breaks in
>   unit measurement) data.
> g. Entries of zero should be shown in the table because zero is a
>   quantity. A dash indicates unavailable information.
> h. Numerical entries should not begin with a decimal point;
>   instead, a zero should be used.

All graphs and tables in any text, journal article, or display should comply with this simple codification.

We have been discussing the definition of epidemiology as the study of the frequency and distribution of many events concerning the well-being of the community. The definition includes other phenomenon, such as blood pressures and blood antibody levels as physiological phenomenon, which form patterns in populations. This is a more comprehensive definition that specifies observations that emphasize the outcome events of concern of disease and health. Distributions reflect the attribute of epidemiology to quantify observations and display them. The definition includes the concept of community and emphasizes comparisons between groups and the major characteristic of epidemiology as a public health science. It is clearly operational and shows the analytical approach that can be utilized effectively by public health nurses in the delivery of services. Distributions may be graphical, tabular, and mathematical. Examples of distributions are summarized in Figure 8-8.

▉ *Analysis of a Table*

In community health nursing as in all public health professions, the use of epidemiology must include quantifications. The epidemiologic perspective includes an appreciation of the excitement of measuring significant causal associations as well as concern and compassion for

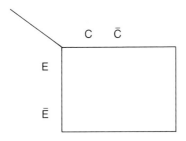

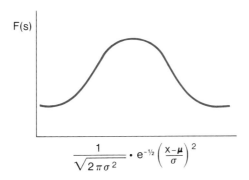

FIGURE 8 - 8
Definition of a distribution. A distribution is a table, graph, or mathematical expression giving the probabilities with which a random variable takes different values or sets of values.

the extent of human suffering. Epidemiologic tables contain frequencies that describe groups and associate events with the rise and fall of disease, tragedy and, (happily) accomplishment through community services. Tables show patterns. They evaluate the progress of community activities. They are warning signals of hazards. Tables tell the story of people, of human beings who form a community, albeit the groups may sometimes be temporary. The following example illustrates how a table can be used to extrapolate the story behind the numbers in a table.

First examine Table 8-3 and read it critically using the following steps.

1. Look at the title and decide the type of quantifications used for the observations (counts, rates, or proportions).
2. Examine the title to denote the reason for the table and the information collected.
3. Look at the total number of observations, the N.
4. Examine the marginals—the row and column totals—to identify subgroups.
5. Compare and contrast subgroups within the table.
6. Analyze the relationships shown in the table.

The data given in Table 8-3 are taken from an actual human experience. The deaths occurred during a short period of time in a completely isolated population. What can be inferred from the information provided about the nature of the experience, the cause of death, and the attendant circumstances?

First it is necessary to review and summarize the information given in the table. The title shows that these are mortality data and the purpose of the table is to provide an educational experience. The

T A B L E   8 - 3
Analysis of a Table: Mortality by Sex, Socio-economic Status and Age

Socio-economic status	Adult males			Adult females		
	No. in pop.	Deaths No.	Percent	No. in pop.	Deaths No.	Percent
High	183	125	68.3	144	5	3.5
Medium	160	147	91.9	93	15	16.1
Low	454	399	87.9	179	81	45.3
Unknown	865	676	78.2	23	2	8.7
Total	1662	1347	81.0	439	103	23.5

frequencies show the totals of subsets within the groups as well as the total population. On inspection, we can see that the population at risk of death (the p.a.r.) is equal to 2206, the total number of observations. We also note that 1503 or 68% of all the people in this community died! What kind of calamity can cause such a serious disaster?

Inspection of the subpopulations are shown in the margins, the totals of columns and rows. The smaller groups are formed from dividing the p.a.r. into specific groups, are labeled by three demographic variables of sex, socioeconomic status (SES), and age. Demographic characteristics are held in common by all human beings and are used to describe a group of people. Age is dichotomized into adults and children, but these categories are not further defined. "Children" could be under 21 years, under 18 years, or under 12 years of age—we do not know. Sex is divided into two categories, male and female; in contrast, SES is divided into three groups: high, medium, and low. But we notice to our dismay that there is a lot of "missing values" regarding SES—888 to be precise, almost a third of the population. The total group is mostly male (1662 out of 2206 or 75%) with about one child to every four females. In order to compare subgroups, the percentages or rates of death are used to show where the highest and lowest rates of death are occurring. Using only the information that is known to us in the table, we find that deaths are highest in males (81%) compared to females (23.5%), but half of all the children died (50.5%). The high rate in children is associated with the lowest stratum of SES even though there were some upper and middle class children in this community. As we look more closely at the mortality rates by social class, we find that due to extensive loss of information in this category, the most one can say is that deaths probably occurred with least frequency in the highest SES band (39%).

Children both sexes			All		
No. in pop.	Deaths		No. in pop.	Deaths	
	No.	Percent		No.	Percent
5	0	—	322	130	39
24	0	—	277	162	58
76	53	69.7	709	533	75
0	—	—	888	678	76
105	53	50.5	2206	1503	68

We can now describe this completed, isolated population. A tragedy has occurred as shown by the extremely high death rate. Although the information on age and sex is almost complete, SES specific rates are computed from data on 60% of the community. Given this caveat, we can safely say that the population is mainly composed of adult males who also suffered the highest death rates. All of the children who died and most of the women were probably in the lowest economic group and even the deaths in males were higher in the lowest economic stratum or band.

We now must consider the kinds of circumstances that fit all these observations. Three conceptual hypotheses will be advanced and tested by applying the observations to a postulated association.

Hypothesis #1.   A sudden eruption of a volcano on an isolated island has caused death and destruction to the population.

An island population would be a small community, as in the table, especially if the island was remote and tiny. A volcanic eruption is a sudden occurrence creating an epidemic of deaths. The pattern of distributions of the deaths by demographic variables is less easy to explain through this hypothesis. Why would an island population be predominantly male? Perhaps the island was a site for a prison, but then children would not be present and the prison population would be unlikely to differentiate groups by SES. If it were an isolated colony of infected people, such as those suffering from Hansen's disease, the sudden surge of deaths from other causes would have to be explained because the disease does not attack men more than women. This hypothesis does not quite fit the data.

Hypothesis #2.   A sudden calamity in a mining community has caused death and devastation in the population.

We know that the event has taken place in a totally isolated population. It is possible that a mining community might grow around gold mines in Alaska or copper mines in Africa. We also know that although this assumption is possible, it is more likely that mines are found in more populated areas. This hypothesis explains the preponderance of deaths in males who are a majority in the mining industries and fits the composition of this popoulation as unusually male-dominated.

It is reasonable to associate male deaths with low economic status in a mining community; however, the high rate of deaths of low socioeconomic women and children are less easily explained. It is possible that a major explosion from a mine would also demolish homes and offices near the mine shaft causing the deaths of some women and children, but it seems unlikely. Also it is feasible to suggest, despite the unknown values, that there are too many high and middle class people for a mining community. The hypothesis does not quite fit the data, although it would be a better explanation than the first postulation.

> *Hypothesis #3.* A ship has fondered at sea snd sunk before adequate rescue could be accomplished.

As we recall from Chapter 6, a community may be defined in many ways. A group on board a ship forms a felling community—a community with a common goal. To regard a ship as a community that is completely isolated is also logical because, despite naval communication systems, the ship is spacially separated from land. The increased number of men may be explained by the fact that crews on ships are predominantly male. Presence of women and children may imply that the ship was not used for military purposes, and the vessel could have been a pleasure cruiser. The SES distribution suggests differences in classes of tickets and accommodations, which would explain the proportions of middle and upper class passengers. Drowning would also explain lack of information on SES for so many passengers. The higher death rates in men not only reflects the number of males in the group, but suggests that women and children were saved first. The highest rates of death in the lowest SES category implies deaths in the lower part of the ship, in the steerage class, where it would have been more difficult to make an escape in a sudden calamity. These facts are supportive of the hypothesis of a disaster at sea. These data are, in fact, derived from the sinking of the Titanic early in this century.

This example illustrates that epidemiologic tables tell stories. Tables speak of human disasters and human accomplishments. For community health nurses, tables, graphs, and mathematical expressions are commentaries on the public domain. Understanding them is necessary to interpret graphs and tables for groups and families in the community and is an important perspective for the public health nurse.

Summary

*T*he nursing process and the epidemiologic process do not lend themselves easily to comprehensive definitions. A few definitions of nursing have been examined to illustrate the problem of arriving at a statement about nursing that is all-inclusive and operational. Similar experiences are applicable to epidemiology, which is also a process or method. Process requires content. Process is a structure that can be applied to promote health, to prevent diseases, and to control health problems that cannot be prevented. For public health nurses, these areas of concern can be divided into four substantive areas similar to epidemiologic concerns: acute communicable diseases, chronic diseases, psychosocial problems, and delivery of health services. All areas interact because even acute communicable diseases may have chronic illnesses as sequelae. All areas involve all levels of prevention, including the promotion of health.

Definitions of epidemiology have been examined in order to assist the community health nurse in understanding how to translate epidemiologic perspectives into nursing practice or in other words, to operationalize epidemiology for nursing care. The definitions have been briefly assessed according to the characteristic features of applied epidemiology. The most often quoted definition of epidemiology, that is, the study of the frequency and distribution of illnesses and their precursors in the community, have been examined in detail. Some fundamental concepts concerning the presentation of distributions or patterns of community problems through tables and graphs have been discussed. Staff nurses in public health need familiarity with reading and interpretating graphs in order to counsel families and groups in communities. Finally, a table and its concepts have been analyzed to illustrate their relevance to people and human disaster.

References

1. Henderson V: The Nature of Nursing. New York, Macmillan, 1966
2. Orem DE: Nursing: Concepts of Practice, 2nd ed., New York, McGraw-Hill, 1980
3. American Nurses' Association: Nursing: A Social Policy Statement, p 9. Kansas City MO, American Nurses' Association, 1980
4. Friedman GD: Primer of Epidemiology, 2nd ed., New York, McGraw-Hill, 1980
5. Lilienfeld AM: Foundations of Epidemiology. New York, Oxford University Press, 1976
6. Hill AB: The environment and disease: Association or causation? Proc R Soc Med 58:295, 1965
7. Remington RD, Schork MA: Statistics with Applications to the Biological and Health Sciences, p 99. Englewood Cliffs, NJ, Prentice-Hall, 1970
8. Remington RD, Schork MA: Statistics with Applications to the Biological and Health Sciences, p 125. Englewood Cliffs, Prentice-Hall, 1970
9. National Center for Health Statistics: Advance Report of Final Natality Statistics, 1983. MVSR 34(6) Supp DHHS Pub No (PHS) 85-1120. Hyattsville, MD, Public Health Service, 1985
10. Center for Disease Control: MMWR. 31(6):69, 1982
11. Centers for Disease Control: *Plasmodium vivax* Malaria—San Diego County, California, MMWR. 35(43):679–681, 1986
12. Mauchk, I: Presentation to Association of Rehabilitation Nurses. Philadelphia, PA, October, 1986

Structure and Organization of Public Health Agencies

LEARNING OBJECTIVES

After reading and understanding the contents of this chapter, the student will be able to:

1. Identify the branch of government that has the responsibility for carrying out the provisions of the United States Constitution.

2. Name the functions of the executive, judicial, and legislative branches in relation to government-related health matters.

3. Report on different types of environmental health activities performed by federal, state, and local governments.

4. Describe the major functions of the United States Public Health Service and the Centers for Disease Control.

5. State the major responsibilities of the Department of Labor, Occupational Safety and Health Administration (OSHA).

6. List and describe some of the major types of private agencies that provide health care services.

Introduction

*P*erhaps because American societal needs are multifaceted, public health services are multidimensional. In this instance, our discussion of public health services includes all those organized attempts to meet the plethora of human needs related to promotion, maintenance, or restoration of health. These services can be categorized in many ways, but essentially fall into those under governmental auspices, or those organized and offered by the private sector. Community health nurses must have a basic understanding of the evolution and status of various public health services so that informed and appropriate client referrals may be made.

The availability, quality, and type of community or public health services vary according to locale. Many different national directories exist that can be consulted to ascertain which services can be obtained in any given area. Additionally, individual states, counties, and cities have compiled their own resource directories. When these directories exist, they should be utilized and systematically updated. Because some services are location-specific, such as local churches or shelters for the homeless, effort should be expended toward compilation of a resource directory when none exists.

▋ *Government Provision of Public Health*

Role of the Branches of Government in Public Health

Although health per se is not mentioned in the United States Constitution, the basis of public health on a federal level is embedded in the Constitution.[1] The powers vested in the federal government by the Constitution are numerous and essentially allow both the opportunity and the responsibility to exercise leadership in developing and implementing health matters based on changing concepts, philosophy, and community needs. Over the years, the interpretation and application of both the Constitution and the Bill of Rights have changed, and these changes have come about through Constitutional amendments and Supreme Court decisions in response to societal change.

It is the executive branch of government, headed by the President and special agencies, such as the Department of Health and Human Services, that has the responsibility to carry out the provisions of the Constitution, its amendments, and all other national legislation, including the affecting health and welfare.[2] The executive branch of government (federal, state, and local) has multiple health services functions such as those listed below.[3]

- Acts as a provider of personal and public health services
- Helps finance provision of personal and public health services as well as education for health care professionals.
- Licenses individuals and agencies/institutions that provide health services
- Regulates the provision of health services
- Helps finance biomedical and health policy
- Operates (or delegates) public health services like quarantine, national health promotion programs, and efforts directed against problems such as alcohol and drug abuse
- Collects, compiles, and publishes vital and health statistics

In some countries, there is a central authority called the Ministry of Health. However, in the United States, no single agency at any level of government has the primary responsibility for conducting the previously listed health service functions of the executive branch. Instead selected tasks are accomplished by federal, state, or local agencies and public health personnel.

The judicial branch of government at all three levels (federal, state, and local) have important powers relative to public health. Together, the judicial and executive branches constitute civil and criminal justice systems which are vital supports to both private and public sector public health programs. The legislative branch of government, represented by the Congress, enacts national laws and appropriates tax money for support of government activities, including those germane to health and welfare.

Federal Versus State and Local Levels of Government

Although states have broad powers to organize their own government in response to societal needs, all state and local laws must be compatible with American constitutional provisions. In turn, the federal government intervenes in state activities when foods, drugs, and biologic agents are sold through interstate commerce or when certain problems arise that are beyond the control of an individual state. In short, the federal government has the power to intervene for mutual protection of all its population groups.[2]

In most instances, general health policy and procedures on the state level are aligned or modeled in a manner that is congruent with the philosophy and intent of the national level. However, no two states have the same mechanism for resolution of problems related to health and social needs, and few states are consistent in the application of their sovereign powers to specific issues, or even in how they name their agencies. For example, not all states call their principal governmental health agency a health department.

> In fact, the exercise of these powers has resulted in 50 different state sanitary codes, 50 different requirements for marriage and divorce, legal adoption, education, and employment of children, licensure of practitioners of the healing arts, safety of buildings, eligibility for public assistance and medical care, procedures for handling the mentally ill and retarded, and so on.[2]

The state then allocates authority to local government. Additionally, the local government usually adopts ordinances but may also mandate supplemental rules and regulations so long as these supplements are congruent with state statutes. Minimum public health laws on the local level include some legal provision for the reporting of vital statistics such as births and deaths, for reporting certain communicable diseases, for food and milk control, and for environmental sanitation. However, many large, local health departments include the following divisions or departments: (1) health statistics and records, (2) sanitation, (3) sanitary engineering or environmental health, (4) maternal and child health, (5) public health nursing, (6) epidemiologic service, (7) communicable disease control, (8) mental health, and (9) health education.[1]

New state and local health laws and/or amendments are enacted annually. These laws then become a part of the health and safety codes of the state or locality. Most of the time, these laws are generated in an effort to develop health legislation that is in the best interests of state and local residents. But occasionally, health enactments result from an attempt on the part of the state or locality to permit participation in federal funding. For example, if a given community wishes to obtain federal funding support to assess or clean up a given environmental pollution problem, they might have to enact stricter laws relating to monitoring and documenting the extent of the problem. By the same token, states that wished to continue to partake of federal highway development/improvement funds found it necessary to make highway speed limits 55 miles per hour.

Looking at the numbers and types of employees at the state level gives some insight into functions and/or services offered by these agencies. According to a 1981 survey,[4] over 120,000 people worked in various state health departments, and the vocational categories cited most often were:

- Registered nurses (16,000)
- Engineers, sanitarians, and related employees (7200)
- Professional and technical laboratory employees (5600)
- Administrative and managerial employees (5300)
- Licensed practical nurses (4500)
- Physicians (3500)

Forty-seven percent of state health departments' staff were in institutional and noninstitutional personal health programs, 7% in health resources programs, 4% in laboratory programs, and the balance in general administration or programs not specifically identified. According to that same survey,[4] most state agencies reported providing programs in maternal child health, communicable disease control, public health nursing, chronic disease control, mental health, public health laboratory services, and dental health. Another 80% operated programs for handicapped children, 75% operated home care programs, and about 89% had one or more programs in speech, occupational, or physical therapy. Interestingly, although public health services are in theory designed to meet the needs of the general population, most programs were targeted toward persons with low incomes.

In the representative year of 1981, state health agencies spent a reported $323 million on environmental health activities.[3] Those activities related to environmental control are listed below.

1. Consumer protection and sanitation including substance control and product safety, facility sanitation, and vector and zoonotic disease control
2. Water quality services, including portable water and sewage disposal
3. Radiation control
4. Occupational health and safety, accident prevention, and noise pollution control
5. Solid and hazardous waste management
6. Environmental health personnel training
7. Environmental health planning, design, and impact studies

Local Level Government Activities in Public Health

It is difficult to report accurately on the particular structure and function of local health departments because there is little standardization among these agencies. According to one rather dated survey, about half of all local agencies provide one or more of the following services.[5]

- Immunization
- Environmental surveillance
- Tuberculosis control
- Maternal and child care
- School health care
- Sexually transmitted disease control
- Chronic disease control
- Home health care
- Family planning
- Ambulatory care
- Health code enforcement

Governmental Organization of Public Health Services in the United States

The numerous federal agencies that have responsibility for public health in the United States generally fall under the executive branch of government. According to Hanlon and Pickett, federal agencies that have responsibility for some aspect of public health fall into four categories. The first category could be called broad health interests such as the United States Public Health Service (USPHS). The second is concerned with special groups in the nation's population, such as the Administration on Aging and the Bureau of Indian Affairs, to name two. The third category of federal agencies consists of those that address special problems or programs such as the Bureau of Labor Statistics, the Office of Education, the Federal Trade Commission, and many bureaus within the Department of Agriculture such as those involved in entomology, human nutrition, and animal industry. The fourth category is concerned with international health interests of the country and includes the Office of International Health of the Public Health Service, among others.

The Department of Health and Human Services

The largest federal government department in terms of budget and number of employees is the Department of Health and Human Services (HHS). HHS is the successor of the Department of Health, Education, and Welfare (HEW). In 1979, HEW was split into the Department of Education and HHS, which retained the bulk of the health service responsibilities.

Both HEW and HHS have a history of reorganization. As of 1985, the two principal HHS health agencies were the Health Care Financing Administration (HCFA) and the USPHS. The USPHS contains public health agencies, and the primary responsibility of HCFA is to oversee the operation of Medicare and Medicaid (Fig. 9-1).[3]

■ The United States Public Health Service

1. History

The history of the USPHS dates back to 1798 when its historical forebearer, the Marine Hospital Service, was established by Congress. Various responsibilities for control of communicable diseases were assigned by Congress over the years, but the first public health function involving foreign quarantine activities occurred in 1878.

The Commissioned Corps was created in 1889 and in 1912, the agency's name was changed to USPHS. The USPHS was actually a part of the Treasury Department until 1939, when it was transferred to an antecedent of HEW. In 1981, the USPHS hospital system that

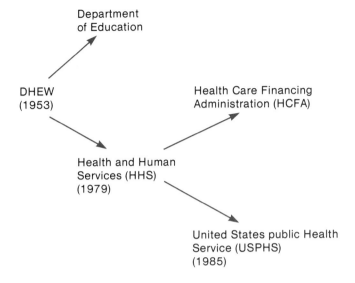

Department
of Education

DHEW
(1953)

Health Care Financing
Administration (HCFA)

Health and Human
Services (HHS)
(1979)

United States public Health
Service (USPHS)
(1985)

*FIGURE
9 - 1
Reorganizational
history of the U.S.
Department of Health
and Human Services.*

began with the Marine Hospital Service was discontinued although the PHS agency remains to this day.[3]

As can be seen in Table 9-1, the overall USPHS houses seven health-related agencies or offices, and in Table 9-2, it can be seen that the Office of the Assistant Secretary of Health, for instance, heads a number of subordinate offices that address specific public health concerns. Some of these office titles bespeak specific concerns, and there are others, such as the National Centers for Health Statistics (NCHS), which has been referred to in previous chapters as the agency responsible for outing and analysis of statistics on morbidity, mortality, and their relationship to population segments.

2. Health Resources and Services Administration

Another principal component of the USHPS (as shown in Table 9-1) is the Office of Health Resources and Services Administration (HRSA). The HRSA operates a variety of direct health program support services, and its beneficiaries include American Indians, Eskimos, and federal prisoners. Additionally, the HRSA is the agency responsible for supporting health sciences education, health planning, health facilities construction, the National Health Services Corps, and Health Maintenance Organization development. Finally, it is the HRSA that administers health services block grants to individual states.[3]

3. Centers for Disease Control

The Centers for Disease Control (CDC) serves as the principal public health agency for both the USPHS and the HHS (Fig. 9-1). Although CDC has ten regional offices, it is headquartered in Atlanta, Georgia. Formerly titled the Communicable Disease Center, CDC was

T A B L E   9 - 1
The Principal Components of the USPHS as of 1985

- Office of the Assistant Secretary for Health (OASH)
- Centers for Disease Control (includes 10 Regional Offices: Boston, New York, Philadelphia, Atlanta, Chicago, Kansas City, Dallas, Denver, San Francisco, and Seattle)
- Food and Drug Administration
- Agency for Toxic Substances and Disease Registry
- Health Resources and Services Administration (HRSA)
- Alcohol, Drug Abuse, and Mental Health Administration
- National Institutes of Health

T A B L E   9 - 2
Federal Public Health Functions in the Office of Assistant Secretary for Health as of 1985

- Offices of Disease Prevention and Health Promotion
- Population Affairs
- Smoking and Health
- International Health
- President's Council on Physical Fitness and Sports
- National Centers for Health Statistics (NCHS)
- National Centers for Health Services Research (NCHSR)

established primarily to prevent and control communicable disease, to direct foreign and interstate quarantine operations, and to improve the performance of clinical laboratories all over the country.[3] However, CDC's functions and responsibilities have expanded greatly with the passage of time and now include:

Serving as the national focus for developing and applying disease prevention and control, environmental health, and health promotion and health education activities designed to improve the health of people in the United States.

To accomplish its mission, CDC identifies and defines preventable health problems and maintains active surveillance of diseases through epidemiologic and laboratory investigations and data collection, analysis and distribution; serves as the PHS lead agency in developing and implementing operational programs relating to environmental health problems, and conducts operational programs relating to environmental health problems, and conducts operational research aimed at developing and testing effective disease prevention, control, and health promotion programs; administers a national program of research, training, and technical assistance to assure safe and healthful working conditions for every working person; develops and implements a program to sustain a strong national workforce in disease prevention and control; and conducts a national program for improving the performance of clinical laboratories.[6]

Additionally, CDC remains responsible for controlling the introduction of infectious diseases as well as providing consultation to other nations to assist in improving their disease prevention and control, environmental health, and health promotion activities.

4. *Agency for Toxic Substances and Disease Registry*
The Agency for Toxic Substances and Disease Registry was created in 1983 by assigning some services previously assigned to CDC and the Office of the Assistant Secretary for Health (OASH). Essentially, this agency is responsible for interventions designed to protect the nation's population against hazardous substances and toxic wastes.[3]

5. *Alcohol, Drug Abuse, and Mental Health Administration (ADAMHA)*
Treatment, research, and education related to mental illness, alcoholism, and drug abuse were grouped in 1983 under ADAMHA. Since that time, ADAMHA has exhibited a preventive emphasis in a range of programs that concentrate on both service and research of related problems.[3]

6. *The Food and Drug Administration*
The Food and Drug Administration (FDA) is responsible for protecting the public against electronic or radiologic hazards posed by various products of different manufacturers. The FDA ensures the safety and efficacy of drugs and the purity of food, regulates the production of animal feeds and drugs, and determines the safety of cosmetics.[3] The FDA is one of the better known USPHS agencies, and it is also one of the most controversial. As a unit of the FDA, the Bureau of Drugs, which has responsibility for assuring the efficacy and safety of all drugs, has sustained considerable criticism from private citizens and special interest groups who contend that the lengthy and expensive approval process denies the marketing of some products while the time required to review others is too extensive.

7. *National Institutes of Health*
The last unit of the USPHS, and a major national force in biomedical research is the National Institutes of Health (NIH). NIH conducts its own research, and it funds research in other public and private institutions through awarding of grants and contracts. The center for nursing research is part of NIH.

▌ *Public Health Responsibilities of Other Federal Agencies*

1. *Department of Defense*

The Department of Defense (DOD) runs its own health care facilities for members of the United States armed services. In fact, every military station in virtually all parts of the world where military personnel are assigned operates some kind of health care facility. These facilities range from shipboard hospitals to airborne "Flying Nightingales" to stateside care facilities ranging from outpatient dispensaries to sophisticated and specialized care settings like Brook Army Medical Center and Walter Reed Medical Center. Although the DOD has historically emphasized "sick care", in 1983, a comprehensive health promotion program for the armed services was begun that emphasized alcohol and drug abuse prevention, family advocacy (focusing on prevention of child abuse), smoking cessation, stress management, and control/prevention of sexually transmitted disease.

The United States Army established a community health nursing speciality in 1949. In 1968, the infection control nurse speciality was begun and various types of nurse practitioners were recognized by the United States Army Nurse Corps shortly thereafter. The objectives of the community health nursing program are found in the following quote.

> To provide a comprehensive Army community family-centered nursing service which will provide health care nursing continuity and contribute to the promotion and maintenance of military family physical and emotional well being . . . to reduce the military man-hours loss and improve military effectiveness by assisting in the prevention, control and rehabilitative aspects of disease and injury.[8]

2. *Department of Agriculture*

Besides being responsible for the health of animal, human, and plant life, the Department of Agriculture (USDA) is also active in various aspects of nutrition. It is the agency that administrates the National School Lunch Program and the Food Stamp Program. The USDA also supervises food safety regulations, along with the FDA, and has responsibility for grading meat and other food for consumers.

3. *Department of Labor-Occupational Safety and Health Administration*

The Occupational Safety and Health Act of 1970 affirmed that industrial management is responsible for providing a safe and healthful environment for its workers. The Department of Labor-Occupational Safety and Health Administration (OSHA) is the agency responsible for enforcing laws and policies as well as educational programs aimed at protecting the workers' health and well-being. For example, workers have a right to know about the safety and health hazards of their work environment as well as any precautions to be taken and the procedures to be followed in case of accidental high exposure to a toxic substance.

The responsibility for implementing OSHA's standards belongs to industrial management who, in turn, depend on health professionals like the occupational health nurse (OHN) to teach health and safety practices. Unfortunately, more than half of the labor force in America is employed by settings that employ less than 100 workers and do not employ a full-time OHN.[8]

When OSHA was created in 1970 and assigned to the Department of Labor, the National Institute for Occupational Safety and Health (NIOSH) was assigned to HHS. The responsibility for enforcing occupational safety and health standards rests with the Department of Labor. OSHA and NIOSH responsibilities are outlined below.

OSHA Responsibilities
- Conducts the inspections of workplaces and the investigations of working conditions
- Promulgates and modifies mandatory occupational safety and health standards
- Prescribes the regulations that determine what records and reports concerning work-related injury, illness, and death the employer must maintain
- Certifies and monitors state occupational safety and health programs
- Conducts, or has others conduct, educational and training programs to help employers and employees understand the Act and how to fulfill their responsibilities under the Act
- Maintains a system for collecting and analyzing OSHA statistics.[8]

4. *Environmental Protection Agency*

Unlike the other agencies discussed, the Environmental Protection Agency (EPA) is an independent (nondepartmental) federal agency that has responsibilities related to air and water quality, pollution control, solid waste disposal control, pesticide regulation, radiation hazard control, noise abatement, and toxic substance control.[3] The overall responsibility of EPA is to administer the Toxic Substance Control Act passed in 1976, which required toxicity testing on all new chemical substances before they are used in the production process.

▮ *Private Provision of Public Health Services*

Both governmental (official) and voluntary (unofficial) agencies have experienced sporadic growth since their inception in the late 1700s in this country. Actually, some official agencies, such as the local health departments in New York City, Boston, and New Orleans predate their private or voluntary cohort since the notion of organized charities was unpopular until the late 1800s.[1] As cited in Chapter 1, the 1886 founding of Visiting Nurses' Associations in Boston and Philadelphia probably constituted the first organized home health care services of any type in America.

Private (nonofficial, nongovernmental) agencies that deliver a variety of public health services are generally of two types. First, there is the commercial agency, and second, there is the charitable or voluntary agency. Examples of services offered in private agencies or companies include home nursing services, solid waste disposal, and pure water suppliers. Although many cities offer all three or these services as a municipal or tax-supported service, some cities require part or all of their citizens to contract with private firms for these services. However, the majority of private agencies providing public health related services are voluntary or nonprofit in nature.

Another aspect of the commercialism of public health services that will be discussed in more detail in a later chapter is the phenomenal growth of commercially based home health care agencies. In 1966, official health agencies (such as those operating out of public health departments) and visiting nurse associations (VNAs) were the major providers of home care services. By 1971, the VNAs had dropped to 24% of the market while newer, hospital-based programs gathered impetus. By 1975, it was evident that the private, nonprofit home care agencies were moving into the market. Between 1975 and 1977, the private, nonprofit home care agencies more than doubled their share of the total market as did proprietary or for-profit home health care agencies. By 1980, VNAs were down to 17% of the total market while commercial agencies continued to rise. For example, Upjohn Health Care Services started with 37 offices in 1969 and by 1977 had more than 200 throughout the United States and Canada. By 1981, the company was treating 10,000 patients a day and maintaining 270 offices.[9]

Voluntary Agencies

Voluntary home nursing began in 1886 and in 1904, the National Association for the Study and Prevention of Tuberculosis, now the American Lung Association, was the first nationwide voluntary health agency. Other agencies followed quickly. The National Society to Prevent Blindness was established in 1908, the Mental Health Association in 1909, the American Cancer Society in 1913, and the National Easter Seal Society for Crippled Children and Adults in 1921. Currently, directories of national voluntary health organizations of all types include listings ranging from 1200 to 1500 agencies.[1] These hundreds of national agencies fall into the following four main categories.

1. Agencies that are concerned with specific disease such as the American Cancer Society and the American Diabetes Association, among others.
2. Agencies that are concerned with certain organs or structures of the body, such as the Eye-Bank Association of America, the National Kidney Foundation, the American Lung Association, and the American Heart Association.
3. Agencies that are concerned with the health and welfare of special groups in society, such as the National Council on Aging and the National Society for Crippled Children.
4. Agencies that are concerned with particular phases of health and welfare, such as the National Safety Council and the Planned Parenthood Federation of America.[1]

Community health nurses need to be aware of the existence of various agencies either on the state or local level since the services offered are frequently valuable to individual clients. These agencies also typically produce either free or low-cost educational material that can be obtained by request for health profession or client use.

Ideally, the structure and function of voluntary agencies contribute to well-balanced community health programs that actually complement the work and resources of official agencies. By providing funds and/or facilities where gaps exist, voluntary health agencies can make the difference between a mediocre community health program and one which is superior in its range of resources and services. Survival of voluntary agencies depends on solicitation of corporate and individual donations. Additionally, voluntary agencies are operationally dependent upon the estimated 500,000 nonpaid persons who volunteer their time and expertise.[1]

Although we have said that voluntary agencies are nonofficial in nature, the one notable exception is the American Red Cross. With over 4000 chapters and 6000 branches in the United States alone, the American Red Cross can be called quasi-official since the President of the United States serves as its president, and the organization is regarded as the official disaster relief agency of the nation.[1]

Foundations

Ranking next to governmental and voluntary health agencies in their influence on America's health affairs are the philanthropic foundations. These foundations also constitute a second large group of voluntary organizations with one important difference. Foundations do not depend on individual donations, but are established and financed by private philanthropy. Prominent examples include the Rockefeller Foundation, the W.K. Kellogg Foundation, the Carnegie Foundation, and others.

Foundations tend to be somewhat less formal in their review procedures and granting operations. They function in a variety of ways and contribute to overall public health by promoting and subsidizing local health departments, supporting basic research and professional education, and in general, providing valuable stimulation to the health field in a fashion not always possible in government-operated agencies.

Professional Associations

Professional associations play an important role in the organization of the health affairs of the nation and constitute a third type of voluntary association. These organizations are generally national in character, with state and local affiliates. At every level, they function as sources of information for their memberships and provide a fulcrum to establish and improve standards and qualifications, further consumer education, and generate and disseminate research.

Summary

*T*he provision of public health services on the local or national level is undertaken by a plethora of official, nonofficial, charitable, and commercial service agencies. The bureaucratic maze that characterizes governmental public health services on the national level has taken more than 200 years to evolve to its present state. It fluctuates with party representation and philosophy of our nation's leaders, and to a lesser extent, in response to societal need and sentiment. It is altogether possible that major overhauls may be made in any official department described herein at any time, but especially after installation of a new presidential administration. For that reason, the purpose of this overview of governmental agencies was to provide some rudimentary understanding of their structure and function in relation to public health endeavors on the national, state, and local levels. To remain updated on agency titles and overall organization requires concentrated effort and an awareness that change can be expected.

Voluntary philanthropic organizations also play a significant role in the overall arena of public health services. With proper health planning, voluntary agencies, foundations, and professional organizations can help fill some of the gaps in the provision of services as well as serve as influential voices and consumer advocates on the national level.

1. Hanlon JJ, Picket GE: Public Health Administration and Practice, 8th ed, p 159. St Louis, Times Mirror/Mosby, 1984
2. Wilner DM, Walkley RP, Goerke LS: Introduction to Public Health, 6th ed, p 31. New York, Macmillan, 1973
3. Last JM (ed): Maxcy–Rosenau Public Health and Preventive Medicine, 12th ed, p 11624. Norwalk, CT, Appleton-Century-Crofts, 1986
4. The Association of State and Territorial Health Officials: Public Health Agencies, 1981. Kensington, MD, April, 1983, (cited in Last)
5. Miller CA, Brooks EF, DeFriese GH et al: A survey of local public health departments and their directors. Am J Public Health 67:931, 1977
6. Centers for Disease Control: Organization, Mission and Functions. Atlanta, Public Health Service, March 1983
7. Headquarters, Department of the Army: Medical Services Health and Environment, Army Regulation 3-14, September 25, 1974
8. Brown ML: Occupational Health Nursing: Principles and Practice. New York, Springer, 1981
9. Spiegal AD: Home Health Care, p 558. Owings Mills, MD, National Health Publishing, 1983

References

Delivery and Evaluation of Community Nursing Services

LEARNING OBJECTIVES

After reading and understanding the contents of this chapter, the student will be able to:

1. *Identify the interrelationships between the areas of content for nursing and for an epidemiologic approach to community health.*

2. *Describe how the care of persons with acute communicable diseases overlaps with the care for noninfectious conditions in community health nursing.*

3. *Explain the major concern(s) of quality assurance programs.*

4. *Differentiate the concepts of licensure, certification, quality assurance, and professional liability.*

5. *Name the two basic features of quality assessment.*

Introduction

Community nursing care is delivered for a variety of needs. Staff nursing in the community is generalist in nature in order to meet the diverse requirements of families and groups. Community health nursing requires the integration of skills learned at the bedside with concepts singular to public health, as outlined in the public health model. Epidemiology is a process whereby many of the concepts of public health, particularly the concepts of community, prevention and control, delivery of services, and multidisciplinary cooperation, are applied to practice situations. This is particularly true in the evaluation of services delivered to groups. Epidemiology has provided a method of quantifying outcomes of delivery of care. As such, it also provides some guidelines (by no means complete or exclusive) for evaluating the quality of services delivered to groups. An epidemiologic approach combined with parameters described by nurse researchers and nurse managers provides enriched methods of assessment of programs of nursing care for groups in hospitals, agencies, and the community.[1]

In the modern health care system, delivery of care is moving into homes, clinics, and ambulatory care centers. In the present environment, the need to ensure that safe and effective care is delivered both in and out of institutions is escalating as both the public and the government demand evidence of the quality of services. Methods have developed over time attempting to guarantee the levels of quality services. Quality assurance programs started in hospitals; however, evaluation of community services has become a necessary and important activity for all public health programs, especially nursing services in homes and agencies where care is intermittent and often requires isolated and independent judgments from providers.

An epidemiologic perspective hones the focus of community nursing and not only enhances the quality of nursing services but also facilitates methods of program evaluation for delivery to extramural and intramural communities.

■ *Program Evaluation or Estimating the Quality of Nursing Care*

The delivery of nursing services to groups is varied. The variety of needs in the community can be grouped into three main content or substantive areas. The first large classification of problems is the communicable diseases. The staff nurse in the community requires knowledge in the prevention and control of infections of all kinds and must be familiar with the services that are organized to accomplish the mandate to control communicable disease. The services usually involve the screening of populations to identify high-risk groups. The screening is accomplished through sero-surveys (e.g., for AIDS testing and skin testing for tuberculosis in high-risk groups). They also include immunization clinics for childhood diseases. Communicable diseases remain a major problem demanding increasing vigilance and constant surveillance. Delivery of services to ensure prevention and control of infectious diseases is the responsibility of nursing and other health care providers. But as life expectancy increases and the rates of the most common childhood diseases fall, nursing services to the chronically ill have become increasingly important. Community health nurses organize services for supervising and rehabilitating the chronically ill, a tertiary prevention approach. At the same time psychosocial issues and the impact of choice of lifestyle on health has evolved as an important responsibility of community health nurses. As education for health promotion has become even more compelling, the need for community health nurses to counsel and educate families and groups about the consequences of choice of behaviors has grown proportionally.

With the passing of time, populations became more dense, and urban sprawl covered the landscape making the delivery of services more comples. Communities of solution sought government action on health matters at state and federal levels. Legislation to protect the poor, the elderly, and the handicapped, was enacted in response to need. Taxpayers' money was spent to give care to these groups. At the same time, evidence that care was being delivered by competent care providers was demanded. It was not enough that programs were available: it became necessary to monitor the quality of care that was received by the consumer. Consequently, quality assurance programs were instituted in hospitals. As care in the 1980s is transferred to the home, the evaluation of quality of care remains a growing area of concern, particularly in the community. Quality assurance programs or program evaluation is still expanding as an area of concern.

■ *Epidemiology and Delivery of Nursing Services*

Nursing is a process.[2] It requires substantive areas to activate nursing methods. The substantive areas or areas of content for public health nursing may be summarized as communicable diseases, chronic diseases, psychosocial issues, and health services delivery for prevention and control of disease and the promotion of health. But epidemiology is also a process and requires substantive or content areas to activate its methodology. To meet the diverse problems arising in communities, the content areas of epidemiology are

1. Acute communicable disease
2. Chronic diseases
3. Health Services Research and Program Evaluation

Since World War II, the interest in psychosocial problems and psychiatric epidemiology has grown so fast that it has become another area of concern for epidemiology under the rubric of psychosocial issues. It is not accidental that the content area for community health nursing and epidemiology are similar. The two specialty areas depend on the concepts of public health. Both disciplines are dedicated to the same goals and both disciplines tend to the same needs.

Areas of content for community health nursing are interrelated. It is impossible to deliver services for acute communicable disease without the recognition of the possibility of chronic sequelae. For example, the association of infection from Herpes hominis virus type II (herpes simplex II) or HHVII with cancer of the cervix was first identified in the early 1970s. Before this time, although it was suspected that there were two viruses, it was impossible to distinguish between infections from the Herpes hominis virus type I (HHVI), and HHVII. A blood test was developed to identify the antibodies to HHVII in 1970. It was soon established as reliable enough to conduct serosurveys, and in 1972, Rawls and Gardner examined two populations in Houston and in a city in South America for the levels of antibody to both viruses to confirm the presence of previous infections in the population.[3] The distribution or patterns of antibody levels are shown in Figure 10-1.

Analyses of the data in Figure 10-1 show that the antibody levels for HHVI begin in early childhood whereas the onset of exposure to HHVII coincide with the menarche. A hypothesis of infection with

	HHV		HHV	
Age	I	II	I	II
0–4 yr	17	0	71	0
5–8 yr	45	0	93	0
9–12 yr	59	0	92	3
13–16 yr	70	9	85	14
17–20 yr	77	16	95	18
	Houston		South America	

F I G U R E   1 0 - 1
Patterns or distributions of positive antibodies to HHVI and HHVII in two populations. (Rawls WE, Gardner HL et al: Genital herpes in two social groups. Am J Obstet Gynecol 110[5]: 682–689, 1971)

HHVII viruses and venereal diseases seemed supportable. Ultimately the venereal spread of herpes II became acknowledged, and clinical counseling for prevention of spread of the disease and the management of palliative measures for infected clients became incorporated into community nursing activities.

With the discovery of a laboratory test confirming the difference in antibodies for the two herpes viruses, many other researchers began to use the test to identify groups where exposure seemed higher than average. Slowly a profile of subgroups with high rates of herpes infection was compiled. A high-risk profile is a summary of subgroups with higher than usual rates of disease. The high-risk profile for herpes virus II consists of populations where antibody levels are higher than usual (epidemic) according to defined criteria or attributes. These attributes include characteristics that are demographic variables, such as age, sex, and socioeconomic status (SES), and may include other behaviors or features. By pooling all the information from all sources, a profile can be developed which identifies populations at high risk for a disease or precursors to a disease. For HHVII this profile shows that infection with the virus occurs with increased frequency in female prisoners, in prostitutes, in those with a history of venereal disease, in those experiencing early coitus, and those of lower SES (Figure 10-2).

Examination of the patterns in high-risk populations for HHVII called to mind an identical high-risk population profile of another illness. The similar disease pattern of high occurrence is found in cancer of the cervix (Fig. 10-3). Through a comparison of the profiles and other data, the hypothesis of viral carcinogenesis was postulated.

For nursing, the hazard of venereal spread of herpetic infection is a matter of concern. There is a risk of death in primary herpetic infections to neonates; but the real hazard is the predisposition to early cancer of the cervix later in life. It is the community health nurse who can, through counseling, monitoring, and support over time, encourage clients to have regular Papanicolaou's smears for early detection of this life-threatening desease, especially if there is a history of herpes II infection.[4] In addition, observation of the occurrences of clusters of similar complaints or problems by the community health staff nurse may assist the nurse epidemiologist in the identification of high-risk populations with the community served by the nursing agency. This information is of great importance in the identification of populations for specific nursing services.

↑ Prisoners—female

↑ Prostitutes

↑ Early coitus

↑ Low socioeconomic group (occurs earlier)

↑ History of VD

FIGURE 10-2
High-risk profile of HHVII.

FIGURE
10-3
High-risk profile—
cancer of the cervix.

↑ Prisoners—female
↑ Prostitutes
↑ Early coitus
↑ Low socioeconomic group (occurs earlier)
↑ History of VD

This example illustrates that it is impossible in practice to deliver nursing care for communicable diseases without acknowledging their relationship to more chronic illnesses. Other viral infections produce life-threatening or disabling diseases. It has been substantiated epidemiologically that herpes viruses are associated with Burkitt's lymphoma and nasopharyngeal cancer. Recently Salahuddin identified a human B-lymphotropic virus in lymphoproliferative disorders.[5] Care for patients with acute communicable disease overlaps with care for noninfectious conditions.

Nursing services are organized and delivered to patients and clients with psychosocial problems and acute and chronic mental illness as well as to healthy groups of people. Chronic and acute illness results from social choices such as smoking, high cholesterol diets, and sexual habits. Health services are designed to meet all community needs for all areas of concern. In brief, communicable diseases, chronic illnesses, and psychosocial problems are linked to the need for services and to each other. These interactions are diagrammed in Figure 10-4.

▪ Quality Assurance, Quality Assessment, and Health Service Research

Quality assurance programs are processes established to maintain codified standards of care. These programs are systematic efforts to maintain and improve services through regulation. Quality assessment on the other hand is a method to evaluate the quality assurance program. Quality assessment is an organized way to evaluate the implementation of programs that are designed to assure quality of services. Health services research and program evaluation is a highly specialized area of epidemiology that is used to scientifically evaluate the impact of services, to compare and contrast systems or models of delivery of care, and to assess quality with sophisticated methods of measurement and inductive rigor. Basic to all methods of program evaluation is the selection of an important element of performance, setting standards for the performance of the element of service, and then comparing the expected standards to observed performance.

Methods for the assessment of quality control for health services do not always use epidemiologic approaches but involve systems analysis, assessment by objectives, and other management tech-

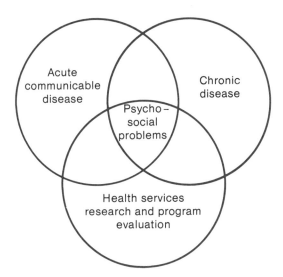

F I G U R E
1 0 - 4
Areas of concern for nursing services—an epidemiologic perspective.

niques. Surveillance of effectiveness of care has been increasing rapidly in the past 50 years.[6] Programs for the assurance of quality care was developed in the 1920s and their principal method was a review of hospital records. Ponton, a physician, was the orginator of the chart audit by peer review in 1929. Gradually during the 1930s and 1940s, evaluation of care became dominated by the philosophy of self-regulation and included other methods besides chart audit, such as accreditation of programs of education and certification of specialists. Nursing adopted its own methods of review. Self-accreditation of nursing schools was instituted in the 1950s as part of the National League for Nursing's ongoing activities. Credentialing through certification has been the hallmark of the 1970s spearheaded by the American Nursing Association and Specialty Nursing Associations. Peer review has been part of general procedures for over 20 years in hospitals and is now being rapidly incorporated into the activities of community health nursing services. In 1986, peer review organizations, or PROs, assumed increasing importance in an era of cost containment, utilization review, and litigation.

Several critical events have influenced the growth and intensity of program evaluation. Since 1953, the Commission on Professional and Hospital Services—the precursor to the Joint Commission on Hospital Accreditation (JCAH) initiated the Physician Activity Survey (PAS) funded through the W. K. Kellogg Foundation. This survey reviews the discharge records of patients who have been hospitalized. A little later the JCAH began a voluntary program of regulating the quality of hospital care. In 1965, Medicare and Medicaid legislation was passed. A utilization review of reasons for staying in a hospital longer than the average time established from the PAS records and other sources was mandated for reimbursement of patients receiving care through these programs. In the 1970s, the self-regulation of quality of care was challenged by some legal actions defining responsibilities for patient care. Some court cases, which affected accountability of nurses and the rights of the public to be protected from communicable diseases, are reviewed here very briefly.

1. *Tattersof v. Regents of the University of California.*[8] In this case, a psychiatric patient was discharged home. The medical diagnosis on admittance to the institution was paranoid schizophrenia, and the presenting symptom was a desire to kill his spouse. A short time after the patient's discharge, his wife reported that she feared for her life and requested review of her husband's case. Subsequently, the patient was readmitted into the hospital. Unfortunately, the patient escaped from the institution and after 3 days returned to his home and did, in fact, kill his wife. The family sued claiming that the wife should have been informed of her husband's escape so she could take precautions. The hospital claimed that the patient's right to privacy required their protection. The court argued that, as in the cases of communicable diseases, people who are regarded as a public hazard forego their privacy, and the law demands protection for the public good.

2. *Darling v. Charleston Community Hospital.*[9] In this case, a 21-year-old football player entered the emergency room for a fracture of the lower leg. The fracture was reduced and the leg placed in a plaster cast. The patient remained in the emergency room waiting for hospital admission for about 12 hours. During this time, he complained of discomfort and tightness of the plaster cast to both nurses and doctors. After 4 days, the cast was finally removed to relieve the constant, acute pain. The leg was gangrenous and required amputation. The hospital was sued. The hospital's administration pleaded that the nurses' and physicians' licenses attested to their professional expertise; thus the professions bore the responsibility for quality of care delivered in the hospital. The court ruled that the competency of employees of the hospital was the responsibility of the employer, regardless of licensure procedures.

3. *Gonzalez v. Nork and Mercy Hospital.*[8] In this case, the patient, Mr. Gonzalez, had such intense back pain that he was admitted into the hospital emergency room. Dr. Nork was taking emergency calls, and although he was not an orthopedic surgeon, nor had he performed a laminectomy before, he operated on Mr. Gonzalez the following day. The patient's condition, instead of being relieved, was exacerbated. The patient remained in constant pain and became depressed for which he was later hospitalized. When discharged from the psychiatric institution and 2 years after his operation, he committed suicide, still complaining of

acute pain. The family sued. The physician was ruled incompetent to perform the surgery after testimony to his lack of surgical knowledge in the operating room. The hospital and the physician lost the case. The court ruled that the hospital board must monitor the quality of service delivered within the hospital community.

These cases relate to quality care and its counterpart, liability for lack of care. In hospitals, the patients share the institutional environment with many health care providers who control living space. Nurses have many peers and other professionals easily accessible for consultation. In the community, the clients are in their own homes and their own environment. Providers enter the patients' environment to deliver care: they have been described as "guests".[10] Peer group support for health care providers is scattered and intermittent, and consultation has to be planned with clients and their families. As care moves into the community, quality assurance and program evaluation becomes imperative, and methods of surveillance have to be adjusted to accomplish the goal of safe, high-quality care.

An outcome of these court cases was not only definitions of the responsibility and accountability for patient care, but also governmental action to legalize the requirement for peer review (P.L. 92-603). As a result the PSRO, or Professional Standards Review Organization, was formed. It took only a short time before doubts about the effectiveness of these methods became evident. Standards were called into question and their validity and reliability became suspect.

The basic features of quality assessment are first to select an important element of performance and set standards, and second, to compare expected levels of observed performance. Standards are elusive and change with the times. For instance, it used to be a criterion of excellence to keep the newly delivered mother in bed for 10 days postpartum. This is no longer thought desirable or necessary, and early ambulation is now the norm. Many subtle circumstances affect standards of care and add to the difficulties of measuring for quality assurance. The philosophy and competency of leadership in administration, the availability of highly technical equipment, and the competency of personnel all affect the way standards are perceived. Normative standards have been based on two approaches in the past: empirical norms and consensual norms. Empirical norms are standards that are local; consensual norms are derived for consensus of experts. The PAS uses empirical norms, where the average hospital standards in a major geographical area are used as a comparison of the function of an individual hospital (Fig. 10-5).

Consensual norms, called optimal care criteria or OCC, have been used in the past. They are generated from panels of experts. In a study of medical care in Hawaii in 1972, the adherence rate to optimal care criteria was 71% in hospitals and 41% in offices in the com-

P.A.S. Study

1) Empirical norms

Each hospital is compared with grouped
standards found in geographic areas of
the individual hospital.

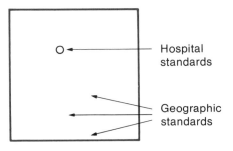

Hospital
standards

Geographic
standards

*FIGURE
1 0 - 5*
*Standards of quality
care.*

P.A.S. data is based on abstracts of patient
charts prepared by medical librarians.

munity. These observations stimulated research on the validity of empirical norms. In 1977, a study of PAS data was conducted to review
the reliability of the abstracts of information from the charts. There
was a discrepancy found in 35% of the diagnoses and 27% of the procedures defined as "commonly occurring" when compared to repeat
abstract data. It was concluded that surveys such as the PAS are suitable for utilization studies but not program evaluation through health
services research.

Consensual standards faired even worse than empirical standards when researched for reliability. In 1976 Wagner stated that standards differ according to the group selected as experts.[11] Brook, in
1973, said that optimal care criteria based on expert opinion were fu-
tile because management of the cases was found to be inadequate according to consensus even when patient outcomes were confirmed as
being of high quality.[12] In 1975, the JCAH recommended a Performance Evaluation Procedure based on the principles of outcome assessment. This meant that outcomes of patient care are assessed first.
For example, when the accuracy of diagnoses is confirmed by surgery
and the patient recovers, estimating the process can be made in view
of successful outcome. For nursing, the outcomes of nursing care,
such as satisfaction and ability for self-care, can be assessed; only
then should the nursing process be evaluated. Outcomes of patient
care are judged first in order to guide the assessment of patient management.

Assessment of outcomes was recommended by Sheps in 1955.[13]
He maintained that quality assessment must comply with the basic

principles of measurement and evaluation in epidemiologic health services research, especially reliability and validity. Subsequently, Donabedian took Sheps' three criteria and redefined them into structure, process, and outcome.[14] The standards for appointing staff as well as the physical nature of the facility are denoted as structure. Process is confined to the management of the case, the completion of charts. Nursing and medical diagnoses and procedures ordered for patient care are process variables. The third rubric of quality assessment is outcomes of patient health status. This is diagrammed in Figure 10-6.

Donabedian recommended that all morbidity and mortality rates, risk estimates, patient satisfaction, rate of return to work, and costs of care be outcome events. Other outcomes attributable to activities such as education, counseling, and client/patient self-management, and complications with medical and nursing regimens are measurable outcome events. This list of outcomes is not exhaustive, but these measurable outcomes are the *sine qua non* of the quality care in the community. All outcomes are influenced by the quality of nursing care delivered in families and groups (Table 10-1).

Studies have been done to assess the validity of structure and process by relating their criteria to outcomes. There has been very little to document that the structure has an influence on the outcome of care; however, standards for staff appointments sometimes have reduced the 7-day mortality after surgery. The effects on care through clinical nurse specialists has not yet been researched. As far as pro-

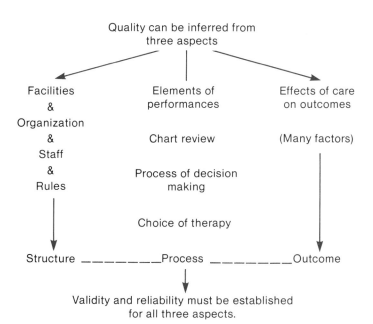

Quality assessment must comply with principles of measurement and evaluation—especially reliability

Quality can be inferred from three aspects

Facilities & Organization & Staff & Rules	Elements of performances	Effects of care on outcomes
	Chart review	(Many factors)
	Process of decision making	
	Choice of therapy	

Structure _____Process _____Outcome

Validity and reliability must be established for all three aspects.

FIGURE 10 - 6
Basic principles of assessment of quality of care. (Sheps CG, Taylor EE: Needed Research in Health and Medical Care: A Bio-social Approach. Chapel Hill, University of North Carolina Press, 1954)

T A B L E 1 0 - 1
Outcome: Sine Qua Non of Good Quality Care

Outcomes	Outcomes Attributable to
Mortality	Education
Longevity	Counseling
Change in disease rates	Self-Management
Risk of adverse effects	Compliance
	Patient Satisfaction
	Patient Adjustment to work and home
	Costs

(DONABEDIAN)

cess is concerned, the results are confusing. Too many times process has been found to have little relationship to patient outcome. Barkauskas recommends that community nurses concentrate on intervention designed to affect outcomes rather than confining their practice to assessment.[15]

Sheps' and Donabedian's criteria are directed at assessments of public health services. These clinical approaches to assessment of quality of care can be applied appropriately to institutional care when the hospital or nursing home is perceived as a community. There is a need in nursing to identify quality nursing outcomes. Many nurse researchers have contributed their efforts and progress has been made; however, outcomes for estimating the quality of nursing care in home health in agencies in the community and at the bedside remain challenging new areas for research in nursing and community health nurses in general.

Summary

*S*ervices in community health nursing are delivered for three main reasons: communicable disease control, chronic illness, and psychosocial problems. Epidemiologic profiles for identifying high-risk communities and families provide a method of targeting nursing services. The fourth area of concern for community health nursing is evaluation of the community nursing programs regarding their impact and quality. These areas of concern are also the focus of substantive areas of epidemiology which, through health services research, offers a rigorous scientific method of evaluating quality of care.

The delivery of nursing services in the community is now, more than ever, associated with establishing the safety and effectiveness of care. Historically, quality of care was monitored in institutions where quality assurance programs and their assessment were formalized through voluntary participation in accrediting systems using chart audit and peer review. Several events affected self-regulation and accreditability for quality of care: Medicare legislation required utilization review; legal cases promoted public interest; laws required peer review organizations; and standards of care were challenged.

All methods of assessing quality are based on identifying standards and comparing observed performance to expected performance according to the accepted rubrics. Epidemiology provides scientific assessment of standards associated with structure, process, and outcomes as defined by Donabedian. Outcomes are the *sine qua non* of measuring quality of care and include rates, risk estimates, and results attributable to education and counseling as well as many other community nursing activities. Epidemiologic approaches to health services evaluation is not the only method of assessment for the rapidly expanding programs in home and community; but epidemiology provides tangible evidence of the impact of nursing services and promotes the use of end points of quality that are recognizable and acknowledged by the public health system.

References

1. Lang NM: Quality Assurance in Nursing: A Selected Bibliography. Springfield, VA. US Dept of Health and Human Services, 1981
2. Hetrie C: Community Health Nursing: Theory and Process. New York, Harper & Row, 1981
3. Rawls WE, Gardner HL et al: Patterns of distributions of positive antibodies to HHVI and HHVII in two populations. Am J Obstet Gynecol 110:5:682–689, 1971
4. Nahmias AJ, Dowdle WR, Schinazi RF (eds): The Human Herpesvirus: An Interdisciplinary Perspective. New York, Elsevier, 1981
5. Josephs SF, Salahuddin SZ, Ablashi DV, Schacter F, Wong–Stall F, Gallo RC: Genomic analysis of the human B-lymphotrophic virus (HBLV). Science, 234:601–603, 1986
6. Sanazarro PJ: Quality assessment and quality assurance in medical care. Annu Rev Public Health 1:37–68, 1980
7. *Tattersof v Regents of the University of California.* 17 Cal. 3rd 425, 551 P. 2d 334 (Cal. 1976)
8. *Darling v Charleston Community Hospital.* 33 I11. 2d 326, 211 IV.E. 2d 253 (1966), cert denied 383 U.S. 496 (1966)
9. *Gonzalez v Nork and Mercy Hospital.* No 228566, Sacramento Co. Super. Ct., Calif., 1973, reversed on other grounds 60 Cal. App. 3d 835 (1976)
10. Freeman RB, Heinrich J: Community Health Nursing Practice, 2nd ed. Philadelphia, WB Saunders, 1981

11. Fletcher EH, Fletcher SW, Wagner EH: Clinical Epidemiology—The Essentials. Baltimore, Williams & Wilkins, 1982
12. Brook RH: Quality Care Assessment: A Comparison of Five Methods of Peer Review. Natl Cent Health Serv Res Dev US Dept of Health, Education, and Welfare, 1973
13. Sheps CG, Taylor EE: Needed Research in Health and Medical Care: A Bio-social Approach. Chapel Hill, University of North Carolina Press, 1954
14. Donabedian A: A Guide to Medical Care Administration. New York, American Public Health Association, 1965–1969
15. Barkauskas VH: Effectiveness of public health nurse home visits to primiparous mothers and their infants. Am J Public Health 73:5:573–580, 1983

Prevention and Control
A Community Health Nursing Responsibility

The careful observation and collection of facts, and the formulation and testing of hypotheses are scientific methods synonymous with epidemiology and have produced the epidemiologic process, which is similar to nursing process for clinical situations.

Applied Epidemiology

LEARNING OBJECTIVES

After reading and understanding the contents of this chapter, the student will be able to:

1. *Cite the overall goal of epidemiology as an applied science.*

2. *Discuss the ways in which an entry level community health nurse participates in the process of epidemiologic research.*

3. *Name and briefly describe the three main epidemiologic research study designs used to examine community problems.*

4. *State some factors that enter into the decision to select one epidemiologic study design in a given situation.*

5. *Debate the advantages and disadvantages of cohort or incidence studies, prevalence or cross-sectional studies, and retrospective or case-control studies.*

6. *Describe the steps in the epidemiologic problem-solving process.*

7. *Describe the activities associated with nursing responsibilities for each step of the epidemiologic method.*

8. *Explain how in-depth knowledge of any given community can alert the community health nurse to a threatened or actual epidemic.*

9. *Demonstrate how systematic examination of time, place, and person variables can help form hypotheses about health phenomena.*

Introduction

*E*pidemiology is an applied science used to identify acute hazards to communities and slowly evolving dangers to the quality of life in populations. Epidemiology describes communities, analyzes associations between exposure factors and hazards to health, and estimates the impact of public health interventions and services. Epidemiology can be descriptive to provide information on what exists. It can be analytic or etiologic to identify associations and cause; or it can be experimental to measure the effects of intervention for the health of the public or community. Regardless of applications, the goal of applied epidemiology is the prevention and control of hazards to health and the precursors to diseases such as accidents and physiological phenomena.

Epidemiology uses the scientific process to accomplish objectives. These inductive methods assume two forms. The first is population-based research, and the second is a more traditional and immediate problem-solving approach described in Chapter 2 as a ten-step process. The role of the community health nurse as a member of the staff in a public or private agency is to participate in the process of epidemiologic research by collecting information and participating in discussions using the epidemiologic language of public health problems and services, so that she will be able to cooperate meaningfully in the epidemiologic process, often as a member of a multidisciplinary health care team.

■ *Epidemiology as a Research Method*

Population-based research is applied epidemiology. For the study of community problems, three main research study designs are used. These designs or models are as follows.

- The prevalence study, a cross-sectional design or study
- The cohort study, a longitudinal or prospective study
- The case-control study, a retrospective model

The design or model of the study is chosen to accomplish the objective or purpose of the research.[1] Other factors enter into the decision about selection of study design such as economic considerations, the urgency of requiring information, and the need for accuracy and reliability. The prevalence or cross-sectional study is most likely used to describe the burden of disease in the community and for more detailed community assessments. It is possible to use a prevalence mode of design to observe and describe some associations; however, the prevalence study generates prevalence rates, and so the study results have all the limitations that apply to prevalence measures. A prevalence survey will capture old and new cases. If the objective of the study is to provide nursing services for all cases of illness or preventive services for a defined group, this model will be effective and is the method of choice for administrative purposes. It is possible to calculate estimates of risk from prevalence studies; but the risk will, again, refer to old and new cases, and this information is not a useful measure of probability of disease when exposure to risk has occurred. Sero-surveys, the collection of antibody levels in the community, are prevalence surveys, and the data they yield is useful to denote high-risk groups for infections such as acquired immune deficiency syndrome (AIDS). Sero-surveys assist in the organization of vaccination programs, services that are often managed and delivered by public health nurses. The advantages of prevalence studies are that they are economical and, comparatively speaking, quick to perform.

Cohort studies are longitudinal designs, and observations are collected for a specific time period, T_0T_1, in two populations—a control group and an experimental group called the "propositii" by Miettinen.[2] Cohort studies are used for both analytic and intervention studies in epidemiology. Cumulative incidence rates are collected from cohort studies, and observations are made on new occurrences of a phenomenon and the factors that precede the onset of problems. This is the design of choice for establishing risk, for identifying the probable cause of hazards, and for measuring the effects of interventions for prevention and control.

Now let us consider using two designs at once. This sounds very complex but only refers to using a prevalence survey to precede a cohort study. The prevalence survey is used to identify a cohort experiencing an exposure such as smoking or special diets for preventing hypertension or heart disease. The prevalence survey will also locate people in a cohort who have no risk factors or protective behaviors. Then, with the permission of each participant, the cohorts will be followed in both groups over a specified time period to count the occurrence of disease. Despite the use of a cross-sectional survey to enter the cohorts into the study, the main design remains a prospective or cohort model.

For cohort studies, it is comparatively easy to define the exposure as an intervention, such as nursing care to provide early ambulation in a population of stroke victims. In this circumstance, the control group consists of people without nursing care and, after an allotted time period, the two groups can be compared for several outcomes including client satisfaction, results of nursing education, and illnesses. In fact, all the outcome events recommended by Donabedian in Chapter 10.

Clinical trials are a variant of the cohort study. The prospective design is the same, but the independent variable, the exposure, is to the therapeutic regimen such as an antineoplastic drug of unknown efficacy compared to a control group who are without exposure to the new therapy. Clinical trials usually apply to smaller groups, but when a clinical trial occurs in large populations, it is called an intervention study (synonymous with cohort studies). An example of a clinical trial that was an intervention study is the lipid study on the effects of low-fat diet on hypertension. This was a population-based clinical trial that was an intervention study and showed that low-fat diets do affect cholesterol levels that are already elevated. Similarly, in a clinical nursing study of a total hospital population, primary care nursing was the therapeutic intervention while the control cohort received team nursing.[3]

The third and last epidemiologic research design is the case-control study. In many ways the case-control model is the exclusive domain of epidemiology. Many behavioral disciplines use prospective and cross-sectional designs, and the biological sciences use the experimental and control-group format. Only epidemiology claims the case-control (also called case-comparison) model. Because of the case-finding responsibilities of community health nurses and the clinical responsibilities of graduate public health nurses, this design is particularly adaptable for nursing. Case-control studies always begin with the identification of a group of people with a defined illness. The study is a retrospective model because the exposure has already occurred and is collected from patients and clients as a recalled event from past experience. The comparison group is chosen because of its similarities to the cases in all but one respect: the group members are not ill—hence the title of this kind of research, the case-control study. The cases in case-control design are sick or have a problem; the controls do not. A group of diseased cases (C) is compared to a similar group of non-diseased "cases" ($\bar{C}$), then each group is asked to recall the same exposure event (E) or lack of it ($\bar{E}$). The results are counted and analyzed through the two by two table (or other tabular forms) which we have already discussed in some detail. We have said that the characteristics of epidemiology are the emphasis on groups, the use of observation rather than manipulation, the use of methods of quantification, and, above all, the focus on the outcome event of illness and health. The case-control model epitomizes these distinguishing features of epidemiologic science. Case identification, as a part of the role of the community health nurse, is linked to the ability of the nurse to view the cases as they surface in the community and to identify an unusual group of cases and their potential hazard to other groups. The advantages of case-control methods (besides identifying epidemiologic characteristics!) is that associations between cases and risk factors can be analyzed cheaply and effectively. One of the main drawbacks to this mode is the problem of selecting the control groups and the sometimes questionable validity of the retrospective approach. This is due to the higher possibility of bias in choosing the group for comparison. These designs are diagrammed in Figure 11-1.[4]

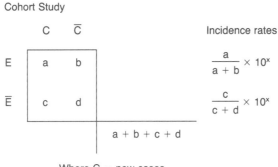

Where C = new cases

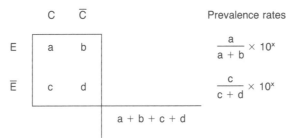

Where C = new and "old" cases

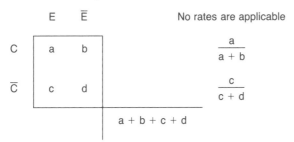

Where C = group of identified problems

FIGURE 11-1 *Epidemiologic research design.*

Only one more fact associated with epidemiologic research will be detailed to complete the vocabulary required for community health nurses to demonstrate the epidemiologic perspective. Risk ratios are generated from epidemiologic studies. They are the single most important and most productive guides to prevention and control of community problems that epidemiology can produce. Risk ratios compare two rates computed from two groups in which one, the propositii, have been exposed to a factor and the other, the control group, is *not* exposed. Risk ratios are called measures of effect because that is their function, that is, they measure the risk of the effects of exposure. Thus, all measures of effect are risk ratios that compare two rates; however, their names differ for each epidemiologic research design. It follows that the study design is indicated by the titles of the risk ratios. Risk ratios are called relative risk (RR) when derived from a cohort study, but are changed to prevalence ratios (PR) when derived from a prevalence model. In case-control studies, rates are not produced in the usual sense; instead, the risk ratio is changed to odds ratio (OR), that is, an estimate of another measure of effect, the RR. The calculations for a risk ratio are summarized as follows: The rate of problems occurring in the exposed group is divided by the rate of problems occurring in the unexposed group. Risk ratios are ratio of rates. Differences between rates can also be calculated and are called attributable risk but are not included in this text.

A moment's thought will reveal that if two rates from two different groups are divided into each other and the rates are equal, the result will be one; therefore, there is *no* risk to the group from the exposure under the investigation. If the rate increases in the exposed group, the result will exceed one (RR > 1) and risk from the exposure will be quantified. If the ratio drops below one, (RR < 1), it means that the exposure *decreases* the risk. For instance, risk of smoking increases the chance of cancer of the lung by 9:1 and the chance of heart disease is doubled and equals 2:1. These numbers are a result of dividing the rates of lung cancer or heart disease in smokers by the rates occurring in the non-smoking population. If there were no risk, the number would be equal or 1:1, usually reported as 1. When an exposure is protective, such as a vaccination or a group experiencing preventive nursing care, the risk ratio will be less than one.

Case-control studies do not produce incidence rates. By a simple mathematical formula, incidence rates can be approximated to form an estimate known as the OR. These important quantifications are also used to identify high-risk profiles for selected diseases and are the basis of the definition of epidemiology as the study of risk in populations. It is obvious that community health nursing benefits from knowledge of epidemiologic risk ratios. These quantifications are applied in practice for the counseling of families and educating the public, for setting priorities for nursing care, and targeting high-risk populations for special services.

■ *Applied Epidemiology as a Problem Solving Method*

Research in epidemiology is a well-defined, painstaking task that respects the rights and privileges of people and strives for validity and reliability through design and statistical analyses. Epidemiologic hypotheses may be described as those postulations that include the community and concentrate on prevention and control as well as quality of services. Hypotheses are carefully reviewed through a thorough search of the literature. Design and methods of collection are supervised with infinite care during the often long and arduous periods of time taken to complete the study. Epidemiologic research is an excellent and time-honored method of establishing risk in populations, of learning causation of disease, and estimating the impact of services for prevention and control of the ills of mankind living together in groups. But in the community, some problems may be so urgent that time for a careful research approach is inadvisable.

Many events occurring in hospitals, nursing homes, or other communities are emergencies requiring prompt intervention. In these compelling circumstances the traditional epidemiologic method is preferred over the new, time-consuming research modalities. When the issue does not easily yield to the quick inductive problem-solving approach, the traditional method may be combined with a case-control study. This research design is the quickest and most economical method of supplementing the problem-solving epidemiologic method for acute problems or emergencies.

Epidemiologic process is comparable to the nursing process explained previously when we aligned and compared the two methods. Now it is necessary to define each step of the acute or traditional problem-solving method for practice and show its application in solving community problems. The steps in the traditional method are as follows.

Traditional Problem-solving Method

1. Establish the existence of an *epidemic*.
2. Verify the *diagnosis*.
3. Make a quick survey of known *cases* and the community situation.
4. Formulate a *tentative hypothesis*.
5. *Plan and conduct* a detailed epidemiologic *investigation*.
6. *Analyze* the data.
7. *Test* the hypothesis.
8. *Formulate* conclusions.
9. Put control measures into operation.
10. Make a report.

These ten steps are necessary to investigate a problem situation. Step one, establishing the existence of a problem or epidemic hazard, is related to step two, the verification of the diagnosis. An epidemic is defined as an unusual outbreak of illnesses or problems, but all problems included in the group must be the same. This may seem obvious, but in practice it may not be easy to be sure that all the cases included in the outbreak are the same, or all complaints relate to the same circumstance. In verifying the number of cases, it is essential to know whether the cases are diagnosed correctly in order to be certain they are the same disease. Sometimes this requires the use of laboratory methods such as microbial cultures and antibiograms. Other times, expensive and time-consuming methods, such as phage typing and DNA probes, may be required. In general, the community health nurse can be of assistance in confirming the medical diagnosis or confirming the nursing diagnosis, as well as in raising the question of whether the cases are new (incidence) or old.

For example, suppose a community health nurse assigned to a school identifies an unusual rate of absenteeism. The nurse will discover that the children have similar symptoms, such as gastrointestinal upset. Familiarity with the school community will enable the nurse to recognize the occurrence of a greater problem relative to what is usual; but to effectively contribute to the epidemiologic investigation, it will be necessary to distinguish illnesses causing gastrointestinal symptoms from food poisoning, and illnesses causing gastrointestinal symptoms from infection such as hepatitis. Initially, the problem may be identified as an epidemic, but an accurate diagnosis is necessary to verify that the cases are the same illness; otherwise, two different diseases manifesting simultaneously may be endemic levels for each disease. These caveats influence the forming of an hypothesis and may be critical in identifying epidemic circumstances.

Of less importance but still relevant is the need to identify old or chronic cases from newly occurring illnesses. Sometimes a chronic carrier state can be the reason for the outbreak, and identifying exposures to old cases can clarify the routes of transmission. Chronic carrier states exist for typhoid and hepatitis B, and many organisms for venereal diseases are shed for many months. Many times it is the community health nurse who is informed about clients' histories and may classify the cases as old rather than new.

Steps three and four are logically connected and relate to the formulation of a tentative hypothesis. The next four steps of the epidemiologic method test and retest the hypothesized association until conclusions concerning the cause of the outbreak can be verified. When the hypothesis is established as reasonable and valid, prevention methods can be put into operation to address the cause and guarantee the effectiveness of control measures. The making of the report is part of the control of the disease because the records may assist in the prevention of future incidents similar to the one under investigation. It is relevant to remember that an initial hypothesis may be discarded and replaced by a more relevant statement of expected association between the frequency of illness and the reason for its occurrence. But more than this, staff nurses in the field may know the community and clients with such detail that the community health nurses' knowledge may be crucial to suggesting the initial and subsequent hypothetical statements. In an outbreak of lead poisoning occurring in a rural commune of about 50 people, it was the public health nurse who had an in-depth knowledge of the health problems existing in the commune. One day she observed an old bathtub, stained and apparently discarded, in a neglected spot in the garden.[5] By recognizing that the abandoned tub may be relevant to the investigation of the epidemic, the nurse drew attention to the tub. She already was aware that the commune made its own wine. It was easy to confirm that the tub was used for winemaking and the alcohol was steadily leaching the lead from the old bathtub. The hypothesis was tested by analyzing the wine for its lead content.

Testing the hypothesis is step seven of the traditional epidemiologic process. Knowing the community situation (step three) is basic to the formulation of the hypothesis and to understanding the relevance of the facts in the epidemiologic process. Hypothesis formulation is obviously a guiding theme of the epidemiologic method just as assessment and nursing diagnosis guide nursing planning and implementation. Three principles govern hypothetical thinking. The first is the knowledge of the community, the second is cluster theory or the grouping of events by what they hold in common, and the third is scientific knowledge about the problem being investigated. Each of these factors influencing hypothesis formulation will be addressed in turn.

Knowledge of the Community

Cases that occur in unusual numbers indicate the need for concern for community safety. The community can be the hospital where the cases of concern may be an increase in fetal loss occurring in nurses staffing the operating room and post-anesthesia rooms. The community may be a nursing home with an unusual outbreak of nosocomal infection. The community may be a neighborhood with unusual groups of childhood malformations near radioactive and chemical waste dumps. When the upsurge of cases occurs, it is putative that the number of cases must be viewed with regard to the geography, the occupation, and the demographics of the community, and other factors in order to form meaningful hypotheses. In conditions of stress that often accompany a threatened or real epidemic, prior knowledge of the community situation is of great advantage in seeking solutions. For the community health nurse, the knowledge of the geography, the occupations, and demographics in the area is basic information for delivering nursing services. This knowledge is already part of the community health nurses' repertoire.

Cluster Theory

Cluster theory, or theory of commonalities, is an applied method of viewing and analyzing the cases provoking the investigation. These cases are grouped according to time, place, and person. This means that time the cases occurred, the places where the cases occurred, and the demographic or personal characteristics of the cases must be examined in detail.

Time

If the cases seem to occur in slowly increasing clusters, it will support a hypothesis of a propagated epidemic or person-to-person spread over time. On the other hand, if the cases seem to cluster in one large group as though they had exploded together at the same time, it is reasonable to assume a common source outbreak or an exposure affecting many people in the same time period. Remember that it is easier to make these kinds of analyses with acute infectious diseases with short incubation periods rather than over long periods of time between the exposures and their sequelae, which happens with long incubation viruses or many environmental exposures. Common source and propagated epidemics are graphed in Figure 11-2 as analyses of time associations.

Place

The cases must be examined for occurrences clustering around a place. When the majority—not necessarily all—of the cases have been in the same place together, such as attending the same function like a picnic or celebration, or if all cases attend the same school or church or have been admitted to the same hospital floor or industry, then the cases share a place in common. The hypothesis would suggest that a singular feature indigenous to the place may be associated with the outbreak.

Person

The cases must be analyzed by person and demographic characteristics they share. In dealing with person, when all the cases share a demographic feature, then the association is reported as age-associated, sex-associated, and so forth. Age association occurs when the cases are mostly in children, ethnic association when cases are mainly in blacks, or sex association when confined to women. The rates increase in these demographic subgroups and can be used to postulate hypotheses as seen in the analysis of the Titanic event (Chapt. 8). In practice, the best hypotheses are made when the increased frequencies can be categorized by time, place, and person.

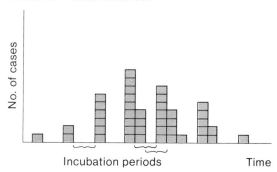

Person-to-Person Outbreak

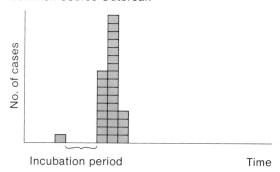

Common-Source Outbreak

*FIGURE
1 1 - 2
Histogram illustrating
propagated (person to
person) distribution
compared with a
common-source
outbreak.*

They are experiences that are held in common. To make one further
point, we have been discussing cases as illnesses. It should be clear
by now that cases can be interpreted in many different ways, especially for nursing concerns. The surge of cases may be instances of client complaints or frequencies of recidivisim in a clinic population of
schizophrenics, or unusual occurrences of missed appointments, or
lack of compliance with nursing education. When these problems
occur with unusual frequency, problem solving may require group solutions for adequate prevention and control through epidemiologic
methods.

Scientific Knowledge of the Problem

Knowing the scientific principles and facts about an event or
case is a crucial factor in the application of epidemiologic methods for
problem solving. Knowledge is associated with the discipline of the
provider involved in the problem-solving process. Thus, knowledge
of nursing, its process and content is essential before epidemiology
can be used and interpreted for nursing care in the community. Spe-

cific knowledge for application to the problem at hand is also essential and involves understanding the familiar categories of acute infectious diseases, chronic diseases, psychosocial illnesses, and delivery of services. The community health nurse requires basic knowledge of nursing care in all these areas: nursing observations then can be used to help solve problems in the community.

It is useful to use the same approach of an event by time, place, and person, when reviewing basic knowledge of the disease or problem entity. In acute communicable diseases, a microbe is involved by definition. Scientific knowledge about pathogens can be analyzed by time, place, and person. Time relates to growth and reproduction of microbes or periods promoting physical changes, for example, in radioactivity. Time is associated with the incubation period—from exposure to disease onset; the place of the microbe refers to the natural habitat of the pathogen microbes where growth can occur. Where a pathogen can live is important: if conditions necessary to support microbial life do not exist, hypotheses for transmission of the organisms are inappropriate. Anaerobic bacteria will not be transmitted through air, and organisms spread by venereal contact fail to have any meaningful survival outside the human body. Many organisms thrive in water and can infect the water supply of populations while other pathogens survive in the rich substrate provided by blood products. Finally, the personal characteristics of the organism are its biochemical and metabolic responses or the knowledge of whether a pathogen is acid or alkaline labile. This information will influence choice of disinfectants for control procedures. The knowledge of all these facts influence hypotheses formulation for the investigation and for identifying prevention and control methods.

There are other exposures besides infectious pathogens. Outbreaks can occur from radioactive or chemical substances. Chemical products can become more toxic or be neutralized depending on where they are situated. Some toxins mimic infections. Metal fume fever presents with the symptoms of influenza but is a result of exposure to chemicals from welding. Knowledge of the chemical and physical properties of substances can assist in promoting policies for prevention and control. For instance, ultraviolet light (UVL) fails to penetrate fluids; therefore, the blood in the surgical field prevents its effective penetration, and UVL is of minimal use in operating rooms to prevent nosocomial infections. Knowledge of where exposures occur influences judgments made for methods of prevention.

Time, place, and person should also be considered in hypothesizing cause. Different exposures have different time periods before they produce problems. Exposure to cotton-laden air, to coal dust, or asbestos will occur many years before the disease develops. Time is a useful variable in applied epidemiology, often requiring special knowledge of the natural history of the disease. The use of time through the application of incubation periods used to be applied in outbreaks of hepatitis. Before our present methods of laboratory testing to confirm cases of hepatitis, the incubation period was a guide to differentiate hepatitis A from hepatitis B. Hepatitis A has an incubation period of 2 to 6 weeks whereas hepatitis B takes 2 to 6 months between exposure and the onset of the disease symptoms. This remains an appropriate quick assessment for identifying epidemics with symptoms of hepatitis.

And finally, the characteristics of the exposure variable or the suspected cause of the illness in the individual often assist in defining new prevention and control methods or identify the violation of control policies. Characteristics of microbes are obviously not demographic; these are reserved for humans. The "person" characteristics associated with exposure to a pathogen may be interpreted as the reaction of the microorganism to acids or alkaline, or whether they are opportunistic or commensal, or whether they are destroyed by excessive cold or heat. The personal characteristics of exposure to toxins are their capacity for aerosolization, or whether they are tasteless or odorless. Cases can be irritating or lethal. These are the characteristics of exposure that must be considered and applied to the problem situation appropriately. A general, broad knowledge of nursing science is a prerequisite for applied epidemiology.

The hypothesis is a fundamental step used to guide the plan and conduct of the investigation. It focuses and directs the collection of information and controls the actions of the multidisciplinary team in planning and conducting a detailed epidemiologic investigation (step five). Analysis will lead to testing the hypothesis (steps seven and eight). To be effective, the hypothesis will also imply, covertly or overtly, the appropriate methods of prevention and control. Control methods are put into operation and will be included in the final report (steps nine and ten). The epidemiologic method can be described as the ability to make scientific observations for prevention and control of community problems through the logical structuring and testing of hypotheses. Methods of hypothesis formulation are summarized in Figure 11-3.

This description of the epidemiologic process has taken each step of the method and discussed fundamental ideas relevant to its application in practice. The process, however, is fluid and continuous with one step depending on its predecessor. It requires a problem to give it life and illustrate the major purpose of the method for prescribing policies for prevention and control. An example of an investigation that required large-scale input from nurses, physicians, and others, and also illustrated the interaction of the public health community when a national threat is recognized is toxic shock syndrome (TSS). The investigation of TSS occurred in this decade. Epidemiologic methods were used exclusively in solving this distressing outbreak, and epidemiologic research methods were used for its final solution.

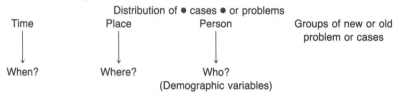

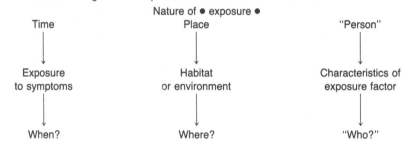

FIGURE
1 1 - 3
Problem solving
hypotheses
formulation.

■ *An Epidemiologic Investigation: Toxic Shock Syndrome*

• *Step 1: Establishing the Existence of an Epidemic*

Before any epidemic can be identified, the endemic or usual number of cases in a community must be established. TSS was considered a new disease until it could be verified that a similar syndrome had occurred prior to the epidemic problem. Unlike AIDS, which is thought to be caused by a newly mutated virus (hence, a new disease), TSS had some history. It did not exist under the diagnostic criteria finally accepted as definitive for a case of TSS, but something very closely allied to toxic shock was identified by Todd, a Denver pediatrician, in 1978.[6,7] This report of seven cases differed from the epidemic because it occurred only in children—three boys and four girls. Todd attributed the cases to the toxin of, perhaps, *Staphylococcus aureus*, which in England was called *Streptococcus pyogenes*, emphasizing its association with purulence. This is the same organism that, when ingested through the gastrointestinal tract in large enough doses, is responsible for intestinal disease (food poisoning). *S. aureus* caused the pandemic of nosocomial wound and skin infections in the 1950s. In TSS, the symptoms were systemic and the patients were severely ill: it was not known if it was caused by the same pathogen.

For the purpose of establishing an epidemic situation, it was thought that if the disease had preexisted, it was very rare. Alternatively it might have been a new variant of an old disease or perhaps a new disease entity. Endemic levels were thought to be about 1/100,000, a rare event; therefore, when over a 100 cases occurred early in 1980, an epidemic situation was identified with 299 cases reported to the Centers for Disease Control (CDC) in the first 9 months of 1980.[8] A review of similar cases for the last 10 years showed fewer than 50 cases for 1978 and even fewer in the years 1970–1977 (Fig. 11-4).[9]

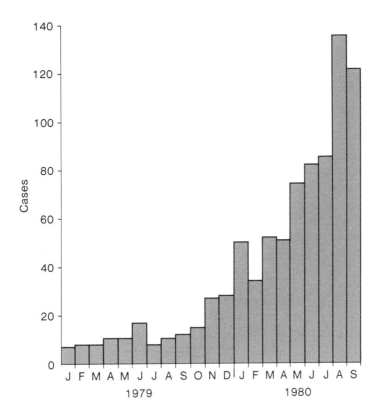

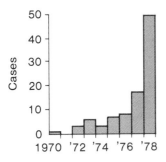

FIGURE 11-4
Number of cases of toxic shock syndrome (TSS) reported from January 1979 through September 1980. (CDC: Toxic shock syndrome, United States 1970–1980. MMWR 30[3]:26, 1981)

- *Step 2: Verifying the Diagnosis*

So few cases had been reported prior to the epidemic that it was difficult to determine whether the cases in the literature were exactly the same as the cases involved in the present problem. Accordingly, all the cases defined as TSS were diagnosed through specific criteria developed to assure similarity of the cases. By stipulating these methods of diagnosis, only the cases meeting the defined set of signs and symptoms were said to be part of the epidemic. The criteria were restrictive; although they were highly sensitive in denoting a real case of toxic shock, the specificity or ability to denote a non-case was comparatively low. The case diagnosis was made when a patient had hypotension, a rash with exfoliation of the skin, hyperemia of the mucous membranes (particularly in the vagina and the oropharynx and conjunctiva), a temperature of 102° F, and finally, renal involvement. Other symptoms could occur in addition to these criteria, such as gastrointestinal symptoms and disseminated intravascular coagulation disease, but the diagnosis was not dependent on the presence of extra symptoms. In short, patients were toxic, were in shock, and were seriously afflicted.

The question of including old cases with the (new) incidence of disease revealed that some cases were recurrences. The problem of a chronic carrier state was unknown, and it was not clear whether *S. aureus* was the culprit. The immediacy of treatment with antibiotics often precluded a successful culture to identify a pathogen. Laboratory tests did not at first assist in defining cases as old and new or carrier states. One other measure of the cases could be analyzed to estimate the virulence of TSS. Among 299 cases in 1980, there were 25 deaths. The case fatality ratio was therefore 25:299 or 9.4%. To put it another way, 1:12 cases died from the disease. This was later adjusted to 5.6% for the entire epidemic period.

- *Step 3:   Make A Quick Survey of Known Cases and the Community Situation*

It can be seen that the analyses of virulence of TSS could be included in step three as easily as it could be included in·defining the problem. The community affected was the United States as cases occurred in 46 states. In Utah, Minnesota, and Minneapolis, the frequency was higher than in the southeastern states, perhaps due to better recording and surveillance. These states started to work with the CDC in Atlanta, Georgia, and the community was mobilized to solve the epidemic. The nursing literature reflected the general concern and, although the role of the bedside nurse in critical care of TSS patients was emphasized, the public health nursing role was seen as keeping the public informed and educated about the latest information on TSS, identifying groups at high risk and informing the public in appropriate prevention and control of the disease.[10] Most of the current information called for interpreting graphs and figures used by epidemiologists involved in the national investigation.

A review of known cases—the cases identified when an epidemic was suspected and subsequently acknowledged—were analyzed using the cluster theory or theory of commonalities. To exemplify this part of the method, we will use the 299 cases reported to the CDC from January to September, 1980. These cases will be reviewed for any clustering by time, place, and person. A distinctive feature of this epidemic was that the majority of cases occurred during the menstrual cycle. Figure 11-5 shows the same histogram used

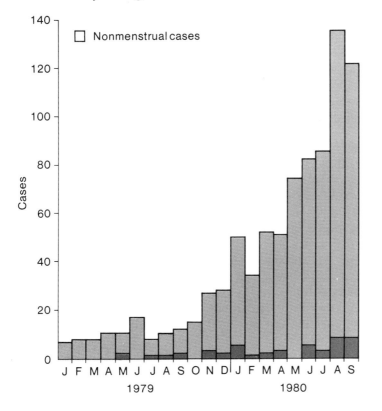

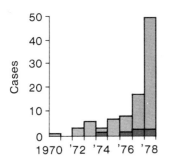

FIGURE 11-5 Confirmed cases of toxic shock syndrome, United States, 1970 through September 1980. (CDC: Toxic shock syndrome, United States 1970–1982. MMWR 31[16]:201, 1982)

to establish the epidemic, but also shows the proportion of non-menstrual cases as shaded areas of the graph.

Demographic variables were analyzed for clustering within the "person" or demographic categories of sex, age, and race for the 299 cases. Cases were predominantly female (95.5%). The average age was 24.5 years with a range of 51 years (6–64 years), and 97% of the cases occurred in Caucasians. These commonalities are summarized in Figure 11-6.

Analyses by time showed that the epidemic had been developing since 1978, slowly at first but increasing rapidly in 1980. Place analyses showed that it was mainly in the northern states, a fact that was only explored later but was consistent with ethnic clustering.

- *Step 4: Formulate a Tentative Hypothesis*

Once more the overlap between steps becomes apparent as the third and fourth parts of the process intermingle. Hypothesis formulation depends on the information gleaned from the quick survey of cases and the analysis of the community situation. In this epidemic, knowledge of the disease was dubious. Todd and others had postulated that TSS was a result of infection by *S. aureus*. Examination of the cases first identified in the epidemic had shed little light on the disease process. No foci of infections by this agent, such as lung abscess, wound infection, or boils, was consistently observed in the cases. The distribution of the cases did not indicate exposure to a common source, and person-to-person spread was not confirmed. The characteristics of *S. aureus* by time, place, and "person(al)" characteristic shows that the disease is dose-related and occurs 4 to 6 hours after entry into the body. The places where the organ can live are plentiful. It resists drying and so can be a contaminant in the environment although it thrives under slightly moist conditions. It is a facultative anaerobe, enabling the pathogen to exist with and without oxygen. It

F I G U R E 1 1 - 6
Commonalities in cases (1980)— demographics, toxic shock syndrome.

- Sex
  ♂ : ♀
  Male : Female
  14 : 285

- Age
  6–64 year of age
  Average ($\bar{X}$) = 24.5 years

- Race
  97% of cases were white
  3% of cases were nonwhite

- Other (among females)
  95% were menstrual cases
  5% were nonmenstrual cases

requires a portal of entry into the body such as ingestion into the intestines or through an abrasion of the skin.

Analysis of the places where the pathogen could form a reservoir showed that it could multiply in contaminated food; however, initially it was not clear if the pathogen existed as a natural commensal in the vagina. The association with menstruation suggested there might be other exposures such as chemical poisoning possibly associated with birth control or type of menstrual protection. At that moment, the hypotheses were formulated around this postulated association between exposure to contraceptives and the methods of protection used for menstrual hygiene. After a review of the cases, the following hypotheses were postulated.

> Hypothesis #1: There is an association between methods of contraception and the occurrence of TSS.
> Hypothesis #2: There is an association between methods of menstrual hygiene and the occurrence of TSS.

• *Step 5: Plan and Conduct a Detailed Epidemiologic Investigation*

The planning and implementation depend directly on the hypotheses formulated in step four. In this study, the hypotheses did not depend on the collection of cultures or other laboratory tests. Also, the places where the cases occurred were scattered across the country with higher frequencies in some states. Interviewing all cases (which is a traditional approach) was time consuming and difficult. Non-cases would consist of half of the population, and random sampling for rare diseases is not a method of choice. The plan, therefore, was to conduct case-control studies. Cases were reported to the CDC and were well documented by dates and diagnoses. Controls could be selected as an appropriate comparison group. States where cases seemed to group together were either asked or volunteered to perform local case-control studies to test the hypotheses. Utah, Wisconsin, and later Minnesota joined the epidemiologic investigation and shared their results with the teams conducting a case-control investigation, the CDC.

In the initial study from the CDC, 50 cases were matched with 50 controls chosen from the healthy roommates and relatives of the cases, matched by sex and approximate age. Cases (C) were asked about contraceptives and types of menstrual protection used within the past year. No brand names were requested. Non-cases ($\bar{C}$) were asked about contraceptives, if any, and type of methods of hygiene used for the last menstrual period.

In Utah, a case-control study was performed, but very few cases were found at first. In Wisconsin, 31 cases were matched with 93 controls, increasing the comparison group threefold—a good research technique that reduces bias. The control group was chosen from clients attending a family planning clinic and matched by age and sex similar to the CDC study. The questions concerning menstrual protection did not include the brand of tampon.

- *Step 6: Analyze the Data*

   The data from CDC was analyzed in tables, and the hypotheses were tested through statistical methods. This was also done for the Utah and Wisconsin studies. Often, testing the hypotheses may consist of culturing the food or culturing an individual suspected of harboring the pathogen. In the Broad Street pump investigation, the hypothesis was tested by establishing that the street drain had direct access to the well water. In the Titanic example, the observations that best fit or explained the hypotheses were used as a test. Because of the case-control format, the hypotheses in this example were tested through analyzing the statistical significance of the associations.

- *Step 7: Test the Hypothesis*

   In Utah, the first analyses showed no statistical significance between cases of TSS and contraceptives or cases of tampon use. This was thought to be due to the very small sample size. As the number of cases increased, Utah's findings confirmed the final CDC results.[11] In Wisconsin, the association between cases and use of contraceptives and tampons were significant. Wisconsin assumed tampons to be a cofactor to the type of contraception. This means that for the contraceptives to cause illness, the tampon must also be used. In their initial study, the CDC found a significant association between disease and tampon use ($p = 0.002$). The results occurred by chance (no true association) only twice in every 1,000 studies. CDC's results are shown in Figure 11-7. CDC reviewed all results and decided to test another more precise hypothesis to detect the brand of tampon. Their third hypothesis follows:

   Hypothesis #3: One brand of tampon is associated with TSS occurrence. Before planning and conducting a study to test Hypothesis #3, they evaluated the previous case-control

F I G U R E
1 1 - 7
First case control study—analysis of hypothesis associating toxic shock syndrome with tampon use, CDC 1980. (Adapted from Shands KN, Schlech WF, Hargrett NJ et al: Toxic shock syndrome: Case control studies at the Centers for Disease Control. Ann Intern Med 96[2]:895–898, 1982)

	Tampons used (E)	Other used (Ē)	
Cases (C)	43	7	50
Controls (C̄)	30	20	50
	73	27	100

Controls matched to cases by age and sex
($p = 0.002$)

study and became concerned that error or bias was distorting the results. The comparison group was faulty. By choosing close friends or relatives of the afflicted women (dependent variable) the choice of menstrual protection could have been shared between the friends or relatives. It is not uncommon that women are influenced by the friend's choice or purchase of sanitary protection. Epidemiologically, this is expressed by saying that the variable was not truly independent of the groups of cases and controls. Other criticisms of the CDC's study were the limited number of controls (they had selected one control for each case, a ratio of 1:1) and the fact that the cases were asked slightly different questions from those asked of the comparison group. The Wisconsin results were also reconsidered. Although the role of contraceptives could not be ruled out, the choice of control group by the Wisconsin investigational team was suspect. It would be reasonable to expect that more clients attending family planning clinics would use contraceptives than would the general population. It was thought that this association might be spurious even though the tampon association, the second hypothesis, verified their own results.

A second study was planned by the CDC. This time the control group was increased to a ratio of 1:3 cases to controls. The new set of 50 cases excluded any case participating in the first study. Each case of TSS identified three friends who were *not* relatives or housemates to form a comparison group matched by sex and approximate age. Lastly, both groups received exactly the same questionnaire, so that type of tampon used was requested for each group in exactly the same terms. Information was gathered through a telephone survey. The new hypothesis was reformulated and retested using steps 4 through 7. The results again showed a significant relationship between TSS and tampon use and an OR of 7.0 in using the Rely brand. This risk ratio means that risk of TSS is increased seven times through the use of Rely tampons. The probability of being wrong or having the results as a chance event was less than 1 in 10,000 ($p < 0.0001$) (Fig. 11-8).

- *Step 8: Formulate Conclusions*

Conclusions about the association of TSS with tampon use, regardless of the first reports of being a cofactor with contraceptive use, were taken seriously. The case fatality ratio was too high not to follow through on merely tentative conclusions. Even though in our example we have taken 299 cases from January to December, the first study for which the hypothesis was formulated occurred earlier and the association, though unconfirmed, was published in June of that same year.

	Tampons used (E)	Other used ($\bar{E}$)	
Cases (C)	50	0	50
Noncases ($\bar{C}$)	124	26	150
	174	26	200

$p = 0.006$
Each case identified 3 friends of same sex and approximate age
(no relatives or housemates).

	Rely used (E)	Other brands ($\bar{E}$)	
Cases (C)	30	12	42
Noncases ($\bar{C}$)	30	84	114
	60	96	156 (Total excludes missing data or multiple brand use)

$p < 0.0001$
or = 7.0

FIGURE 11-8

Second case control study to list the hypotheses that a brand of tampon was associated with TSS, CDC. (Adapted from Shands KN, Schlech WF, Hargrett NJ et al: Toxic shock syndrome: Case control studies at the Centers for Disease Control. Ann Intern Med 96[2]:895–898, 1982)

This action was supported by the fact that several investigators had published their concerns about the same time.[12,13]

- *Step 9: Put Control Measures into Operation*

The report that TSS was tampon-associated was published as a precautionary measure. Media attention and public outcry contributed to voluntary controls by women. After the case-control studies were satisfactorily completed, Rely was recalled in September, 1980. The effectiveness of control measures is a method of final testing of the hypothesis. In the epidemic of kuru, for instance, the decline of the disease coincided with the reduction of the mourning ritual, substantiating the truth of the hypothesized association. In TSS, the use of tampons in general was reduced 21% between June and December, 1980 due to intense media coverage. Cases were already in decline before September, partly as a response to widespread publication of the epidemic. Rely was pulled off the market in September of this same year and consequently cases dropped dramatically after this date. Supporting evidence for the hypothesis was provided from a review of the sales of Rely. In 1974, the tampon was test-marketed as a longer lasting protection compared to other tampons due to a new, nonabsorbent material, carboxymethyl cellulose, that replaced the previous absorbent cotton and other materials in the manufacturing process. In 1978, a major marketing thrust was made on a national basis and by 1980 Rely had captured 17% of the market in sanitary protection. But as sales climbed, so had the cases of TSS until eventually about 71% of the cases were associated with this brand of tampon.

- *Step 10: The Final Report*

Before the report could be finalized, some questions concerning the pathogenesis of TSS required an answer. The most effective prevention and control policies are based on knowledge of the cause of problems and their precursors. Once more the epidemiologic method was put into operation. Cases were reviewed to see if the isloation and identification of an infectious organism had occurred. Of the 50 cases selected for the first case-control study, only 17 were cultured before antibiotic therapy was administered. Of these 17, 16 were positive for *S. aureus.* This and other evidence suggested that there must be a reservoir of this pathogen before a case of TSS could develop. The first hypothesis was that Rely tampons were contaminated with this pathogen during manufacturing. To follow this association, a plan to culture tampons during manufacturing at the Rely factory was implemented. The plan was guided by the knowledge that the characteristics of the pathogen would allow it to survive in a dry environment for a limited amount of time. Also heat destroyed the organism but not its toxin. No source of contamination could be found during the manufacturing process and the hypothesis was discarded.

The second hypothesis was that the organism was harbored in the vagina of women as a natural commensal. Surprisingly it was not known whether all or few women carried *S. aureus* as part of their vaginal flora. A quick survey of clients attending a family planning clinic in Atlanta showed that 7% were colonized with the organism. It was possible to carry the staphylococcus asymptomatically! Testing the hypothesis involved a review of records of TSS cases and showed that of 44 patients who had been cultured vaginally, only one was negative. Additional evidence to test this hypothesis was provided by the fact that recurrent cases always cultured positive for *S. aureus* and also that male and female cases not associated with menstruation had a focal point for sepsis from this same pathogen. Because of the pathogen's ability to survive in aerobic and anaerobic conditions it was thought that tampons left in place for long periods irritate the vaginal wall permitting the resident bacteria to enter the blood stream through tiny abrasions in the vaginal mucosa. Non-absorbent materials such as carboxymethyl cellulose act as a plug in the vagina, preventing leakage and permitting longer periods of retention of the tampon. Unfortunately, the non-absorbent material may be more irritating to the vaginal lining than other tampons made from absorptive cotton. Policies for prevention and control were then identified that would give protection to the public. Women can almost entirely eliminate their risk of TSS by not using tampons. Women who choose to use them can decrease their risk by intermittent use and by replacing tampons at frequent intervals during the menses. Education of the public is still necessary to promote early diagnosis and prevent further outbreaks. There probably will always be an endemic number of cases not associated with menstruation that remain stable and will not respond to these methods of prevention and control.

A final report of the epidemic showed that of the total confirmed cases (941), 99% were in women, 98% of whom had onset during a menstrual period. Eleven cases occurred postpartum. The age range for females was 54 years (6–61 years) with a mean of 23 years. The final graph of the epidemic appears in Figure 11-9.

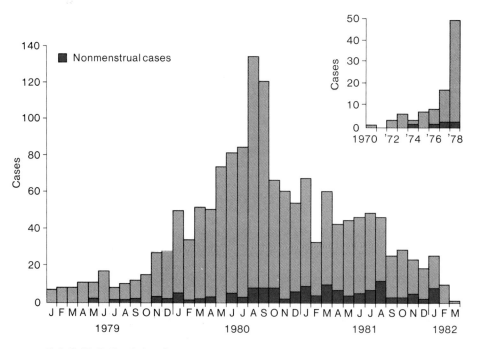

F I G U R E   1 1 - 9
Confirmed cases of toxic shock syndrome, United States, January 1970 through March 1982. (Adapted from Shands KN, Schlech WF, Hargrett NJ et al: Toxic shock syndrome: Case control studies at the Centers for Disease Control. Ann Intern Med 96[2]:895–898, 1982)

*T*his chapter describes and illustrates the two main problem solving methods that epidemiology uses in practice: epidemiologic research method, labelled "new", and the epidemiologic method for solving acute problems in communities, labelled "traditional." The two methods are versions of the same scientific approach inherent in epidemiology. They are presented separately to emphasize epidemiology as a research method as well as a problem-solving process.

Epidemiologic research involves approaches developed for chronic diseases and long-term exposures to environmental hazards. Although these methods are effective for modern epidemics such as accidents and occupational diseases, they are also adaptable to investigation of epidemics of communicable diseases. Cohort, prevalence, and case-control research designs are defined and very briefly, the estimates of effects of exposures (risk ratios) are mentioned to facilitate the community health nurses' understanding of public health vocabulary to enhance multidisciplinary collaboration. The 11 steps of the traditional epidemiologic method are detailed with special emphasis on hypothesis formulation. The ability to postulate an effective hypothesis parallels the assessment and nursing diagnosis process; testing the hypothesis is akin to evaluation in nursing process. The application of research methods and traditional methods is illustrated through analysis of TSS, the epidemic of Toxic Shock Syndrome.

The value of the epidemiologic perspective for the generalist public health nurse is that it facilitates the contribution of nurses to the multidisciplinary team when solving outbreaks in the community. Epidemiology heightens the awareness of the nurse in identifying unusual clusters of cases during nursing practice. The knowledge of the community nurse is indispensable to the facilitation of the epidemiologic process during epidemic stress, regardless of the size and extent of the hazard to the population.

Summary

1. Susser MW, Watson W: Sociology in Medicine, 2nd ed. London, England, Oxford University Press, 1971
2. Miettinen OS: Theoretical Epidemiology, Principles of Occurence. Research in Medicine. New York, John Wiley & Sons, 1985
3. Chavigny KH and Lewis A: Primary care nursing. Nurs Outlook 32:6:322–325 1983
4. Schelesselmann JJ. Case-Control Studies: Design, Conduct, Analysis. New York, Oxford University Press, 1982
5. Osterud HT, Tufts E, Holmes MA: Plumbism at Green Parrot Farm. Clin Toxicology 1–7, 1973
6. McKenna UG, Meadows JA III, Brewer NS, Wilson WR, Perrault J: Toxic shock syndrome, a newly recognized entity: report of 11 cases. Mayo Clin Proc 55:663–72, 1980

References

7. Todd J, Fishaut M, Kapral F, Welch T: Toxic shock syndrome associated with phase-group-I staphylococci. Lancet 2:1116–8, 1978
8. Centers for Disease Control: Toxic Shock Syndrome—United States. MMWR 29:229–30, 1980
9. Centers for Disease Control: Follow-up on Toxic Shock Syndrome. MMWR 29:441–5, 1980
10. Wroblewski SS: Toxic shock syndrome. Am J Nurs 81:1:82–85, 1981
11. Centers for Disease Control: Toxic Shock Syndrome—Utah. MMWR 29:495–6, 1980
12. Shands KN, Schmid GP, Dan BB, Guidotti RJ, Hargrett NT, Anderson RL, Hill DL, Broome CV, Band JD, Fraser DW: Toxic shock syndrome in menstruating women. N Engl J Med 303:25:1436–42, 1980
13. Davis JP, Chesney PJ, Wand PJ, LaVenture M: Toxic shock syndrome. N Engl J Med 303:25:1429–35, 1980

Contemporary Community Health Nursing Roles in Intramural Settings

CHAPTER

12

LEARNING OBJECTIVES

After reading and understanding the contents of this chapter, the student will be able to:

1. *Name the essential role components of the three community health nursing roles that take place in intramural settings.*

2. *Identify five commonalities among all community health nurses, regardless of practice setting.*

3. *Describe the certification process for occupational health nurses, school health nurses, and infection control nurses.*

4. *Discuss leading causes of morbidity and mortality among the working population, the school-aged population, and persons with hospital-acquired or nosocomial infections.*

5. *Compare and contrast occupational health nursing, school health nursing, and infection control nursing as speciality community health nursing practices.*

Introduction

You may remember from Chapter 6 that one of the many ways communities can be categorized is by physical boundaries. When the community is characterized by specified institutional boundaries such as in schools, hospitals, or any number of industrial or agency settings, the community is said to be intramural or contained within walls or limited grounds. While intramural communities certainly interact with and are impacted on by their greater environments such as neighborhoods, cities, or regions, they may be visualized as being contained within common buildings including adjacent structures such as parking lots.

We know these intramural settings qualify as communities because people who interact consistently within these communities form territorial or relational bonds, and because the people have personal or environmental characteristics in common as well as other criteria used in varying definitions of community.

The purpose of this chapter is to familiarize the reader with three community health nursing roles that have evolved over time to meet the specialized needs of populations that live, work, visit, or go to school in intramural settings. Thus, the scope and nature of practice of the occupational health nurse (OHN), the school health nurse (SHN), and the infection control nurse (ICN) will be discussed in this chapter in concert with the major causes of morbidity and mortality of client populations.

Community health nursing roles that have evolved to meet the health needs of populations in extramural communities will be discussed in the next chapter. As discussed in Chapter 6, extramural communities are those that have broader and larger geophysical boundaries such as neighborhoods, cities, or even more universal parameters such as the world.

■ *Commonalities of all Community Health Nursing Roles*

Identifiable if subtle commonalities exist (or should ideally exist) among the speciality roles of OHN, SHN, ICN, home health nurse, hospice nurse and the communicable disease nurse clinician.

Client

The first commonality among all these roles is that all these practices are focused on population aggregates or whole communities of people as opposed to practice which focuses one-on-one (nurse to client). In other words, while these speciality clinicians may center on a single client's health needs whenever that becomes necessary or appropriate, the overall concern is achieving and maintaining well-being for the *entire* population of service.

Education Preparation

Because the community health nursing specialities are concerned with whole populations, a second commonality among them is the fact that educational preparation should include a blending of public health sciences, nursing science, and advanced nursing practice, as would be true for any community health nursing role. Advanced nursing practice includes skills such as individual physical assessment and family and community assessment competencies. In fact, with the possible exception of home health and hospice nursing, experts in the other specialities recommend preparation at the master's level.

These recommendations for graduate preparation may impact on future occupants of these speciality roles, but the reality is that the vast majority of clinicians functioning in these areas are not presently educated at the master's level. In fact, most hold diplomas in nursing. However, as the pool of master's-prepared nurses grows, and as they learn to make their roles cost-effective, it is most likely that they will have the competitive edge over lesser prepared but more experienced nurses.

Practice Goals and Philosophical Foundation

A third commonality that can be identified across these community health nursing speciality practices is the fact that the philosophical set is oriented toward prevention and nursing interventions based on the levels of prevention rather than a disease or medical model. The goal of each of these practice specialities is to promote health and normal development and to prevent injury illness or even emotional duress (primary prevention). When non-health phenomena occur, the goal is to diagnose and treat promptly and prevent disability (secondary prevention). When the health state is irreversibly compromised in some way, such as a traumatic amputation of finger digits in an industrial setting, the goal becomes restoration of maximum functioning (tertiary prevention). Whenever disease or injury occurs, the community health specialist investigates the phenomenon to arrive at safety or preventive measures that will serve to protect the rest of the population against a similar episode.

■ *Practice is Intradisciplinary*

The fourth commonality of all the community health speciality roles is that they are all intradisciplinary in nature. For example, the OHN works with occupational health physicians, toxicologists, industrial hygienists, management, and any number of governmental or regula-

Commonalities within Community Health Nursing Roles

- Client—nursing practice is focused on population aggregates or whole communities of people
- Educational preparation—a blending of public health sciences, nursing science, and advanced nursing practice
- Practice goals and philosophical foundation—nursing intervention based on the levels of prevention rather than a disease or medical model
- Practice is intradisciplinary in nature
- Emphasis on cost-effective practice

tory bodies and their representatives. The ICN works closely with all members of the hospital infection control committee such as physicians, nursing and hospital administration, operating room and central supply personnel, and representatives from purchasing.

Practice is Cost Effective

The fifth commonality among all the community health specialities, and virtually all of health care, is the emphasis on cost effectiveness. The OHN's practice must result in savings and increased productivity for the employer, and further, some mechanisms must be identified that will allow the OHN to document those savings. Similarly, the ICN, and frequently the whole infection control effort, must be demonstrably cost effective. Every time a potential nosocomial infection is prevented, the client and the hospital saves money, but without specific and sometimes sophisticated documentation, these savings are frequently not recognized by hospital administration.

The Occupational Health Nurse

Health hazards associated with work settings were recognized hundreds of years ago. For example, miners in the second century A.D. were reportedly encouraged to protect their respiratory tracts from dust by covering their noses and mouths with fish bladders.[1] Occupational health hazards and exploitation of the work force were accepted facts of life in the United States through and beyond the Industrial Revolution. According to Silberstein (1981), occupational nursing was first recognized as a speciality shortly after the American Industrial Revolution.[1] As mentioned in Chapter 1, Rathbone's district nurses in Liverpool visited industrial settings in the late 1800s, but it is unclear what their specific functions were.

The first educational courses specific to industrial nurses was offered at Boston University in 1917. Attempts of industrial nurses to gain knowledge in their speciality field were accompanied by efforts to organize various local, state, and regional groups. Subsequently, the American Association of Industrial Nurses was founded in 1941; then in 1977, that organization changed its name to the American Association of Occupational Health Nurses, Inc.[1]

Certification of Occupational Health Nurses

Two avenues currently exist whereby practicing OHNs may achieve certification. The first is through the American Nurses' Association (ANA) which offers a generalist in community health nursing. Requirements for the ANA certification include a bachelor's degree in nursing and months of experience. However, the certification examination preferred by many OHNs and their employers is awarded by the American Board for Occupational Health Nurses (ABOHN). The ABOHN offers certification to registered nurses currently employed in occupational health who also have 5 cumulative years experience in OHN and can document 60 hours of formalized continuing education within the previous 5 years. Currently, there is no degree requirement to take the ABOHN certification examination, but that guideline is subject to change.

In 1986, there were ten master's level OHN programs in the United States, and others were in planning phases.

Occupational Health Nursing as a Speciality Practice

The following seven basic principles of occupational health nursing were developed by Brown (1981), and they show the strong interrelationship between the role of the OHN and community health nursing.[2]

1. The occupational health program should be in conformity with the provisions of the Occupational Safety and Health Act of 1970 (PL 91-596).
2. Occupational health care is essentially an interdisciplinary team effort.
3. The occupational health unit must be staffed by qualified, professional personnel, must have administrative stability, and must have the understanding and support of both management and labor.
4. The quality of the work environment is of vital importance and is central to the prevention of disease and injury.
5. The workers themselves must participate in achieving a common goal—a high level of wellness as a measure of the quality of life.

6. Occupational health professionals must understand the dynamics of the American labor movement and work cooperatively with the union leaders in their establishment.
7. Occupational health is an essential component of community health; they are interrelated and interdependent.

The Occupational Safety and Health Act of 1970 was described in Chapter 9, but its essence was to promote safe and healthful employment environments for all working Americans. The OHN should be thoroughly familiar with the provisions of the 1970 Act and subsequent legislation that affects occupational nursing practice.

The OHN's job responsibilities outlined below are adapted from the American Association of Occupational Health Nurses.[3]

1. The OHN plans and develops nursing care that is consistent with the overall objectives of the parent company health program.
2. The OHN plans and submits an annual budget proposal to support nursing services.
3. The OHN participates in research designed to improve delivery of nursing services.

A cursory review of the principles, job responsibilities, and objectives of OHN practice will convince even the novice that specialized education is probably the most systematic and thorough way to prepare for such a role.

Leading Causes of Morbidity Among American Workers

Knowing the major causes of morbidity among worker populations helps the community health nurse understand some of the parameters and concerns of OHN practice. The ten leading work-related diseases and injuries in the United States are as follows.

The Four Major Objectives of Any OHN Program Are To

1. Protect the employee against health hazards in the work environment
2. Facilitate placement and ensure the suitability of the individual according to the individual's ability and physical and emotional makeup
3. Ensure adequate medical care and rehabilitation of the occupationally ill and injured
4. Encourage personal health maintenance among all employees[4]

Ten Leading Work-Related Diseases and Injuries in the United States

1. Occupational lung disease
2. Musculoskeletal injuries
3. Occupational cancers (other than lung)
4. Severe occupational traumatic injuries
5. Cardiovascular disease
6. Disorders of reproduction
7. Neurotoxic disorders
8. Noise-induced loss of hearing
9. Dermatologic conditions
10. Psychological disorders

All ten leading causes of morbidity among workers cost the economy billions of dollars and cause permanent impairment, early disability, and sometimes death for the affected individual. For example, 2.1 million workers experienced disabling injuries in 1981, and 70,000 of those were permanently impaired. In all, the cost for workplace injuries alone is estimated to be $32.5 billion.[5]

Demographic Profile of Occupational Health Nurses in the United States

Considerable attention has been given to cost-effective practice in occupational health nursing. Specifically, one study that contrasted occupational health programs in plants which had OHNs on staff with programs that had no OHN as a part of their program found that inclusion of an OHN in a health program can provide a substantial economic benefit where significant occupational health program in which the environment did not contain numerous occupational hazards was found not to be cost effective by the same researchers.[7] For further guidance in calculating the cost effectiveness of any given OHN practice site, the reader is urged to consult the periodic literature.

■ School Health Nurse

Lillian Wald can be credited with pioneering the concept of the SHN. It was through her experiences with the children in the neighborhood that surrounded the Henry Street Settlement that she became convinced of the need for an organized governmental agency to address the unique needs of children. Not only did Wald start her own brand of school nursing, but partially through her efforts, the United States Children's Bureau was created in 1922.

Educational Preparation and Certification

The ANA and the American Association for School Health (AASH) support bachelor's preparation and certification for entry into SHN practice. However, the American Association for Health, Physical Education, Recreation and Dance recommends graduate-level preparation for SHN practice.[8]

To sit for the ANA certification exam as a school nurse practitioner, the individual must have graduated from a master's program in school health or hold a bachelor's degree in nursing plus a certificate program in school health that was at least 9 months in length. In 1986, there were only three accredited master's programs in school health nursing, but others have been proposed. Additionally, several states require state certification as a requisite to practice.

School Health Nursing Functions as a Speciality Practice

In 1980, there were an estimated 22,000 nurses engaged in school health nursing in the 91,000 schools throughout the country. At that time, there were about 20 programs offering school health nursing in a continuing education format that would serve to qualify participating nurses to sit for the ANA school nurse certification exam.[9]

SHNs perform comprehensive physical, cognitive, and psychosocial evaluations, manage a variety of minor illnesses or injuries, and place special emphasis on teaching students to be responsible for their own health promotion and maintenance. The SHN collaborates with physicians, other health care personnel, educators, and parents in providing health care. Additionally, the SHN uses advanced physical and health assessment skills to identify factors that may place the student at risk of acquiring learning disorders or other physical or emotional problems.[9]

Morbidity in School Populations

The health status of the nation's 46 million school children has improved in the last few decades, largely as a result of prevention and control of infectious and communicable diseases. Still, the health status of children is affected by environmental, economic, and technologic changes in society and within the family unit.[10] Sometimes there is a limited enthusiasm for school health programs because "school children are the healthiest group in the population."[11] However, while the incidence of prevalence of many diseases is lower in school-aged children, a significant volume of illness is experienced by this group. Many children aged 5 to 17 have reading or other learning disabilities, and an estimated 20% have potentially correctable vision problems that, without intervention, can serve to impair learning. Further, it is likely that as more women join the labor force, need for comprehensive school-based health programs will increase.[12]

Communicable diseases ranging from chickenpox to sexually transmitted diseases still impact on children as do nutritional and dental disorders. But there are also more recently described health problems such as behavioral disturbances, accidents, injuries, adolescent pregnancy, substance abuse, and family violence including homicide and suicide. There are also increasing numbers of handicapped and chronically ill children who are full- or part-time students in the school system.

It should also be noted that multiple social and family factors impact on the physical and psychological health of school-aged children. Fifty percent of school-aged children currently have mothers who work outside the home and by 1990, it is estimated that 25% of all children will live in single-parent families.[12,13]

Low family income is another factor that impacts on school health since children from low income families are more likely to be in poor health, to lose more school days, and even to be hospitalized longer than children from higher income families. As an example of the relationship between income and health maintenance, in 1980, 50% of all American families reported that they cut back on one or more health-related items: that figure was 60% among minority families and 72% among single-parent families. Leading causes of mortality among school-aged children is shown in Table 12-1.

Cost Considerations in School Health Nursing

Several studies have been done in the past 10 years to ascertain the costs of comprehensive school health nursing programs. One researcher estimated the cost of a complete school health program to be $96 to $128 per student per year.[9] Another group reported a similar cost of $120 per student annually. Unfortunately, these costs are generally in excess of that which could be totally supported by either local health departments or individual school districts. Therefore, financing of comprehensive school health programs will require innovative sources or pooling of financial resources from federal, local, and private funding agencies.

■ The Infection Control Nurse

Of all three intramural nursing specialities in community health, the ICN is the most recently evolved. In 1959, an "infection control sister" (nurse) was appointed in a Great Britain hospital and was assigned the following responsibilities: (1) documenting nosocomial infections; (2) recommending specific measurements to prevent the

TABLE 12-1
Cause of Childhood Deaths in the United States (1981) by Number of Deaths per 10,000 Population and Percent Due to Specific Causes

Number of Deaths Per 10,000 Population

		Age			
Cause of death	1–5	6–11	12–17	12–15	16–17
All causes	6.4	3.1	6.0	4.4	9.1
Accidents and violence	2.9	6.1	4.2	2.7	7.0
Diseases and conditions	3.4	1.5	1.8	1.6	2.1

Percent of Deaths Due to Specific Causes

	1–17	1–5	6–11	12–17	12–15	16–17
All causes	100.0	100.0	100.0	100.0	100.0	100.0
Accidents and violence	58.4	46.1	51.3	69.9	62.5	76.8
Accidents	50.0	41.1	49.7	56.5	52.5	60.4
Suicide	2.6	—	0.3	5.4	4.0	6.7
Homicide	4.6	3.4	2.4	6.5	4.5	8.3
Diseases and conditions	41.6	53.9	48.7	30.1	37.5	23.2
Neoplasms	10.8	9.2	17.2	8.9	11.2	6.8
Malignant neoplasms	10.2	8.8	16.3	8.4	10.5	6.5
Leukemia	4.3	3.5	8.0	3.2	4.3	2.1
Congenital anomalies	6.5	12.2	6.6	2.5	3.4	1.6
Heart	3.4	6.7	3.2	1.3	1.7	0.8
Nervous system	5.1	7.3	5.6	3.3	4.1	2.6
Respiratory system	4.8	8.0	4.3	2.9	3.8	2.1
Circulatory system	4.2	3.9	4.0	4.5	5.4	3.7
Infective and parasitic	2.6	4.4	2.6	1.4	1.9	0.9

(National Center for Health Statistics, Division of Vital Statistics: Unpublished data from the national vital registration system. In Select Panel for the Promotion of Child Health. Better Health for Our Children: A National Strategy, Vol IV p 326. Washington, DC., DHHS, 1981)

occurrence of nosocomial infections; and (3) assessing the effectiveness of interventions. It was not until 1963 that the role was implemented in the United States, and by 1977 the great majority of hospitals with over 250 beds had an ICN and some kind of hospital-wide infection control program. Although health professionals other than nurses filled positions of infection control practitioners (ICPs), a national survey between 1976 and 1977 showed that 94% of those positions were filled by a registered nurse.[15]

Educational Preparation and Certification

Currently, ICPs are certified by the Association of Practitioners in Infection Control (APIC). Prerequisites include 2 years of experience in infection control practice, but there are no formal educational requirements. In fact, registered nurses, microbiologists, or practitioners prepared in other disciplines such as public health and medicine sit for the same exam. ICPs are expected to demonstrate knowledge in the following areas: education, epidemiology and statistics, patient care practices, employee health, microbiology, infectious diseases, management and communications, and sterilization and disinfection sanitation. Upon successful completion, the individual becomes certified in infection control and can use the C.I.C. designation after his or her name.

As of early 1987, there was only one master's program in infection control nursing in the United States. Several other continuing education programs were offered by federal, state, and private agencies. Additionally, the APIC organization has prepared a starter package of information for newly appointed practitioners who have had little or no formal training in infection control. That packet can be obtained by calling the National APIC headquarters at (312) 949-6052.

Infection Control Nursing Functions as a Speciality Practice

The ICN is responsible for surveillance, prevention, and control of nosocomial infections. To accomplish this broad role function, the ICN acts as an educator, a consultant, a researcher, a manager, a clinician, a role model and so on. To achieve maximum infection control program effectiveness, there should be one ICN per 250 hospital beds. When there are multiple ICNs, one is typically designated as coordinator and assumes additional administrative responsibilities.

ICNs usually work Monday through Friday during the daytime, but may rotate to other shifts or weekends when program responsibilities such as staff development programs mandate a variation in work hours. Even though ICNs typically work daytime hours through the week, they assume 24-hour responsibility for all of their job parameters.

Demographic Profile of Infection Control Nurses in the United States

As pointed out before, prior to 1970, only a few hospitals employed an ICN, but by 1977, over 80% had employed at least one ICN. That change was at least partially implemented as a response to the Joint Commission for Accreditation of Hospitals' guidelines that mandated the existence of an infection control program.

The ICN in smaller hospitals (those under 300 beds) generally works part time in infection control and spends the rest of the work week doing supervision or quality assurance, whereas the ICN in larger hospitals works in infection control full-time.

A nationwide survey conducted by the Centers for Disease Control (CDC) revealed that ICNs in larger hospitals had generally completed a higher level of nursing education and had attended more continuing education infection control courses than their cohorts in smaller hospitals. Of all the registered nurses in ICN positions, almost 25% had baccalaureate degrees, and a very small percent (0.7%) had master's degrees. Thus, the majority of ICNs had diplomas or associate degrees.

Morbidity and Mortality Associated with Nosocomial Infections

Overall morbidity and mortality of nosocomial infections will be addressed in detail in Chapter 16, but their general distribution and impact on ICN practice will be discussed briefly here. First of all, even though the national incidence of nosocomial infections is 6%, that rate is usually higher in more complex care settings such as teaching hospitals or inpatient settings where clients stay for prolonged periods of time, as in an extended care facility.

Nosocomial infections are highest on surgery service, followed by medicine and gynecology. The urinary tract is the body site most frequently infected (usually in conjunction with the placement of indwelling Foley catheters), followed by the lower respiratory tract (as in pneumonia) and surgical wounds. In fact, infection in these three sites accounts for almost three fourths of all reported nosocomial infections.[17]

In 1984, 1% of all nosocomial infections caused death while 3% contributed to death. These figures show that the percentage of infections reported to have caused or contributed to death has not changed significantly over a 3- or 4-year period. Also for a 3-year time period, infection rates have been highest on the surgery and medicine services, probably because of their high-risk patient population.[17]

Cost Consideration in Infection Control Nursing Practice

According to Haley (1986), a sound program in infection control can reduce the incidence of nosocomial infections by 32%, and that program for each group of 250 beds would cost about $60,000 annually. If a 250-bed hospital reduced nosocomial infections by 32%, it could thereby prevent over 150 nosocomial infections and three to five avoidable deaths a year. That prevention would result in avoiding 600 extra days of hospitalization and would reduce hospital costs by approximately $360,000 a year. The net savings for that institution would be $21,000 a month.[18]

> Nationwide, establishment of the most effective infection control programs in all hospitals would prevent 750,000 nosocomial infections, 10,000 deaths, and 2.5 million extra hospital days, and would save more than $1.3 billion annually. Inasmuch as the programs would cost only approximately $200 million, the net savings would be just over $1 billion per year.[18] (p 32)

Summary

*T*he community health nursing speciality roles in occupational and school health and infection control are joined by the fact that they are based on a combination of public health and nursing science, and by the commonality that their practice settings are intramural in nature. They are different in that they care for different client populations with different health problems and have different methods of resolution.

Nursing as an entity is competing with individuals prepared in other disciplines such as health education, industrial hygiene, or laboratory technology (to name three). These professionals are willing to displace nursing and to largely discredit the unique contribution that nursing makes to these speciality practices. In fact, in limited numbers and in some settings, they have succeeded. For example, there is a tendency in some areas to hire non-nurse health educators instead of registered nurses to fulfill the needs of school health programs or to hire microbiologists instead of nurses for infection control programs. If professional nursing is to retain and enrich its legitimate place in these and other specialities, nurses must be educationally prepared, politically astute, and nursing practice will have to be fiscally sound.

References

1. Silberstein CA: Nursing role in occupational health. In Jarvis LL (ed): Community Health Nursing: Keeping the Public Healthy, pp 123–140. Philadelphia, FA Davis, 1981
2. Brown ML: Occupational Health Nursing: Principles and Practice. New York, Springer-Verlag, 1981
3. A Guide for Establishing an Occupational Health Nursing Service. New York, American Association of Occupational Health Nurses, 1977
4. Coryn JM: The occupational health nurse. In Olishifski, JB (ed): Fundamentals of Industrial Hygiene. Chicago, National Safety Council, 1979
5. Centers for Disease Control: Annual Summary 1984. MMWR 33(54):97, 1986
6. Cox AR: Profile of the occupational health nurse. AAOHN J 33(12):591–593, 1986

7. Little AD: Costs and Benefits of Occupational Health Nursing, DHHS (NIOSH) Pub No 80-140. Cincinnati, National Institute for Occupational Safety and Health, 1980

8. Withrow C: School health. In Stanhope M, Lancaster J (eds): Community Health Nursing: Process and Practice for Promoting Health, pp 718–743. St Louis, CV Mosby, 1984

9. Igoe JB: Changing Patterns in School Health and School Nurses. Nurs Outlook 28:486–492, 1980

10. Gephart J, Egan MC, Hutchins VL: Perspectives on health of school-age children: Expectations for the future. J Sch Health 54(1):11–17, 1984

11. Meyerstein AN: The value of periodic school health examinations. Am J Public Health, 59:1910–1926, 1969

12. Meeker RJ, DeAngelis C, Berman B, Freeman HE, Oda D: A comprehensive school health initiative. Image 18(3):86–91, 1986

13. Select Panel on the Promotion of Child Health: Better Health for Our Children: A National Strategy, Vol III: A Statistical Profile, DHHS Pub No 79-55071. Washington DC, 1981. (Cited in Edgil A: A Grant Proposal for School Health Nurse Clinicians. University of Alabama at Birmingham, 1986)

14. Yankelovich, Skelly & White, Inc: Family Health in an Era of Stress. The General Mills American Family Report, 1978–1979. 1980

15. Axnick, KJ: A historical perspective. In Axnick KJ, Yarbrough M (eds): Infection Control: An Integrated Approach, pp 1–5. St Louis, CV Mosby, 1984

16. Emori TG, Haley RW, Stanley RC: The infection control nurse in U.S. hospitals, 1976–1977: Characteristics of the position and its occupant. Am J Epidemiol 111:592–607, 1980

17. Centers for Disease Control: Nosocomial Infection Surveillance, 1984. MMWR 35(1SS):17SS–29SS, 1986

18. Haley RW: Managing Hospital Infection Control for Cost-Effectiveness. Chicago, American Hospital Publishing, 1986

Contemporary Community Health Nursing Roles Within Extramural Settings

CHAPTER

13

LEARNING OBJECTIVES

After reading and understanding the contents of this chapter, the student will be able to:

1. Discuss the differences and similarities between community health nursing roles in intramural versus extramural settings.

2. Describe the major role functions of the home health and hospice nurse.

3. Explain the overall goals of home health and hospice nursing.

4. Summarize how the notion of cost effectiveness has influenced the practice of all community health nursing specialities.

5. List the criteria a client must meet in order to qualify for hospice care.

6. Cite differences in requirements for accreditation and licensure for home health care agencies.

7. Name the advantages of hospice care compared to care of the terminally ill in a hospital or without hospice support in the home.

Introduction   *A*s discussed in the preceding chapter, nurses who function within home health and hospice agencies are examples of community health nursing specialists whose practice is focused on extramural communities. Like all community health nursing roles, the knowledge base for these specialties is a combination of nursing and public health sciences. The client population in extramural communities is less confined geographically and is not generally contained within institutional walls. For example, the home health nurse travels throughout a designated area to visit clients and deliver nursing care. Because the population is more scattered, caseloads are likely to be heterogeneous demographically, that is, clients within any given caseload are likely to be different in age, sociocultural background, and health beliefs or behaviors.

Unlike nurses who specialize in intramural populations, the only certification available to nurses who work in extramural community health nursing settings is currently offered by the American Nurses' Association. That certification program is entitled the Generalist in Community Health Nursing and is available to bachelor's level nurses who have had a certain amount of experience in any one of a number of distributive settings. Currently, there are very few graduate programs offering nursing specialties in home health or hospice nursing, partly because these roles can be effectively implemented by bachelor's level nurses. As master's level programs are offered, it is likely that the curricula will emphasize either the administrator or practitioner role. Hopefully, bachelor's level curricula will offer courses and clinical experiences to help prepare entry-level nurses for roles in these distributive settings.

In this chapter, the notion of home health and hospice agencies will be introduced as will the clinical nursing practices that have paralleled the growth of these facilities. Additionally, a new speciality role in communicable disease control will be proposed.

∎ *Home Health Nurse*

Historically, people were cared for in the home, usually by family members or occasionally by a skilled person such as the midwife. Skilled or systematic nursing in the home is a much newer phenomenon. Even the early Visiting Nurse Associations in Boston and other American cities in the late 1800s did not initially offer skilled nursing care at the bedside. In fact those "nurses" were more often than not lay people whose religious convictions directed them to minister to the sick and disabled in the home. The modern era in home health nursing began when Lillian Wald recruited and specially trained nurses of the era to deliver state-of-the-art care in the home.

Despite her visionary approach to family and community-oriented nursing care, there is little doubt that Wald would be astonished by the degree of technology and controversy that characterizes the environment of home health care at the dawn of the twenty-first century. Although the home health care setting lacks some of the advanced life support features available in the hospital, the home health nurse of today can expect to encounter clients who are being treated with a variety of high-tech equipment such as renal dialysis and parenteral fluid replacement. Although it initially seems a dichotomy, today's home health nurse is truly a specialized generalist.

Even though an integral part of an interdisciplinary team, the home health nurse typically visits clients at home armed only with professional expertise, sound clinical judgment, a few portable supplies, and an ability to innovate. On any given day, caseloads may range from a 29-year-old male paraplegic with multiple decubiti who must be taught self-catheterization to an elderly schizophrenic woman with complex cardiopulmonary pathology, or a 15-year-old unwed mother who is also a drug abuser.

Given the complex social, emotional, and physical health problems, and the fact that case is delivered in a comparatively uncontrolled community environment, it is clear that the home health nurse must possess a diverse knowledge base as well as access to all types of community resources. These are some of the reasons that the home health nurse is considered a specialist in generalized nursing care. Aided by this discussion, it also becomes clear why home health agencies typically prefer to hire nurses with one or more years of experience before attempting to orient them to the specifics of the nursing role.

In general, home health care is directed toward developing and enhancing the health capabilities of clients, their families, and the greater community. Direct professional nursing care in the home setting may actually last an hour or less a week, yet that care must positively influence the client's well-being for all those other hours when the nurse's care plan is implemented by home health aids or family members.

When in a client's home, the home health nurse enters an environment that is controlled by the client and the family. Other nursing environments, such as clinics or hospitals, are largely controlled by health care personnel. Because the setting is different and the focus is more universal, that is, on family well-being, the nurse must have a unique set of skills including an understanding of the interaction between individual health and that of the family and the community.

The primary reason a home visit is made is to perform some kind of nursing activity that will ultimately facilitate client system growth toward a higher level of well-being. But before these therapeutic nurse–client interactions can happen, the nurse must gain the family's trust and, in essence, become a nonjudgmental part of the home environment. At that point, effective and meaningful communications can be established.[1]

Because each home or apartment reflects innumerable personal and cultural values, the home health nurse should be familiar with beliefs and behaviors that impact on the health of individual clients and families. Additionally, it is helpful for the nurse to develop working definitions of key terms like health or well-being, illness, family, community, and nursing that are congruent with the overall philosophy of the employing agency. Likewise, the home health nurse should be skilled in family and community assessment techniques so that application of the nursing process will include crucial human and environmental variables that affect the individual's potential for health realization.

One of the primary responsibilities of the home nurse is to conduct skilled nursing assessments of the physical, emotional, and social status of the client. Such assessments provide the data necessary to make critical decisions about the client's response to various medical treatment strategies. It is the home health nurse who is frequently the one responsible for communicating to the individual physician how the client is responding to ongoing treatment between visits to the doctor.

Doses of medication such as insulin, anticoagulants or antiarrhythmics are increased, decreased, or stopped on the basis of physical findings of the home health nurse or the symptomatology related by the client. Likewise, through systematic physical assessment, the presence of new or different signs and symptoms are assessed and reported to the physician if necessary. As in all care settings, the physician manages aspects of medical treatment, but it is the nurse who is responsible for all nursing aspects of care, including consulting with the physician when appropriate. In essence, the home health nurse is the link between the family, the greater community, and the physician.

Another vital function of the home health nurse is that of teacher. Individuals and their families or ongoing caregivers must be taught how to care for the client safely and effectively. Not only must individual clients and their families understand how to perform caregiver tasks, they should also understand why any given procedure is important. To be an effective client educator, the home health nurse must incorporate some basic teaching–learning principles such as identifying signs of readiness to learn, communicating in language

Primary Responsibilities of the Home Health Nurse

> - To conduct skilled nursing assessments of the physical, emotional, and social status of the client, family, and community
> - To communicate to the individual physician the progress and on-going treatment of the client
> - To be an effective client educator
> - To employ professional expertise, sound clinical judgment, the ability to innovate and understand the interaction between individual health and that of the family and community
> - To provide nursing care directed toward developing and enhancing the health capabilities of clients, their families, and the community

which can be understood, allowing ample time for questions and return demonstration, and avoiding the tendency to overwhelm the client by giving more information in a given teaching session than the client can absorb. Periodic assessment of the client's retention is advised, and reteaching should be performed based on the findings of that assessment.

Varying personal and professional qualities of the home health nurse have been identified in the literature. For example, a home health nurse should be able to function as a family counselor and a family advocate relative to health matters. Personally, the home health nurse has also been described as a person who is comfortable in nonstructured environments and possesses a high degree of tolerance for different lifestyles and habits.[1]

■ Licensure and Accreditation of Home Health Care Agencies

The federal government has mandated that all home health care agencies be licensed by the state in which it is located with the exception of some rural agencies. Licensure is defined as "the granting of a specific privilege by a government authority or agency, permitting acts that would be unlawful in the absence of such permission."[2] A home health care license may be denied by the state for any number of reasons including failure to show that standards of care and services are adequate. In most states, licenses must be renewed annually.

Although accreditation is available to home health care agencies, as of late 1984, only 76 home health agencies had applied for and met accreditation standards. Designed to assist agencies in evaluating and improving the quality of care, the National League for Nursing initiated accreditation services for home health care agencies in 1975.

■ *Cost Considerations in Home Health Care Nursing*

The last two decades have seen a tremendous proliferation in home health care agencies. In Chapter 19, considerable discussion will be directed at that growth as well as the political, social, and economic repercussions that have followed, therefore, related discussion is limited here.

In 1977, Medicare and Medicaid programs spent $13.2 billion dollars on home health. By 1983, the yearly expenditure was $28.8 billion. Everyday, Americans spend nearly $1 billion for health care, with 42% going to hospitals, 19% to physicians, 24% for other professional services, 8% to nursing homes, and less than 7% on programs whose emphasis and concerns is with health promotion. While hospital employment of nurses had increased 35% by 1984, the percentage of nurses employed in all community settings had increased by only 5%.[3]

The push for cost containment in illness care has resulted in re-imbursement programs that encourage shorter stays in hospitals. In fact, between 1981 and 1984, the average length of stay in the acute care hospital decreased from 9 days to 7.5 days while the average length of stay in home health care decreased from 3 months to 2 months for the acute level of client care. At the same time, the complexity of home health nurses ". . . are under increasing pressure to justify the need for their services."[3 (p 46)]

One of the major forces affecting the growth of home health care markets is the renewed and strong pressures by government and big business to contain total health care costs. The idea behind this push to home care is that if home care can reduce the incidence and duration of hospitalization, it will be essentially cost effective. But one of the keys to cost-accountable home health is delivery of services that are reimbursable by various forms of health care insurances like Medicare, Medicaid, and private companies. When clients who need home health care have no insurance, little or no income, or insurance that does not reimburse for home health care, the agency is caught in the middle between providing free services and providing no service at all. Needless to say, voluntary agencies that have a large proportion of indigent clients experience great difficulty balancing an already strained budget.

The other aspect relative to cost benefits is that some of nursing's contributions, especially illness prevention, health promotion, and health maintenance (primary prevention), have traditionally been hard to measure or quantify in dollars and cents.[4] For example, how does one price health education that ultimately prevents a disease episode such as a heart attack or stroke? Even though one can say that for every heart attack averted, dollars, disability, suffering, and lives are saved, one cannot accurately differentiate between those times when primary prevention strategies are effective and those incidences when disease would or would not occur regardless of nursing activities such as health education.

Even though home care may be more cost effective than institutional care, some would say that no care at all is still cheaper in the short run. So home health nurses must simultaneously deal with more acutely ill clients as well as justify and document why skilled nursing services are required.

■ *The Hospice Nurse*

The notion of hospice was actually conceived in medieval Europe. Early hospices were established and maintained by various religious orders that offered nourishment and protection to the sick, the dying, and the poor. The first modern hospice was established in England in 1950, and it focused on caring for the terminally ill.[5] Since the adoption of the hospice concept in this country approximately 15 years ago, the number of persons choosing to die at home has increased steadily. In 1984, one survey identified some 1,429 hospice organizations in the United States alone that provided a wide range of services in which the hospice nurse played a major part.[3]

When an individual becomes incurably ill, client and family may experience a series of crises as they face health care costs, loss of work and recreation, deterioration in appearance, loss of function, and the ultimate threat that is represented by loss of life. Incurable illnesses that are accompanied by prolonged disability and discomfort can destroy the client's self-concept as well as damage family relationships.[5]

According to a statement by the National Hospice Organization in a 1984 pamphlet entitled, "The Basics of Hospice," hospice philosophy affirms life and ". . . exists to provide support and care for a person in the last month of incurable illness, so that life can be lived as fully and comfortably as possible". Rather than seeking to prolong life, hospice care is directed toward promoting optimal qualify of life and death with dignity. The hospice nurse helps the family to function as normally as possible and helps to reduce the number of outside influences.

Five types of organizational patterns have been identified that characterize hospice agencies across the country. First, a hospice may be a department within any given home health care agency. Second, hospices may be freestanding facilities with or without hospital affiliation, but with a contractual agreement with some home health care agency for services if needed. Third, some hospices are volunteer organizations with no physical facilities. Fourth, some hospice agencies exist in parts of an existing facility such as a nursing home that pro-

The Advantages of Hospice Home Care

1. Homecare generally costs less than institutional care and partial reimbursement for services is available under various insurance plans.
2. The family is treated as a unit and basically retains some control over the environment.
3. Lifestyles of clients can be carried out as usual and clients can exercise preferences for diet and activity.
4. The hospice nurse is available to teach comfort and support measures and to monitor the physical and psychological status of client and family. The hospice nurse also counsels and helps the family to resolve conflicts and promotes positive communication patterns.[6]

The Disadvantages or Problems Associated with Hospice Care

1. Family caregivers may become exhausted by the demands of 24-hour care.
2. Cost-reimbursement for professional services and supplies may not be provided by some insurance plans.
3. Emergency situations as perceived by caregivers may create anxiety and decrease coping behaviors.
4. The bulk of the care may be shouldered disproportionately on a single care provider unless there is adequate planning and preparation for spreading the tasks among others.[6]

vides skilled nursing services. While most hospice operations offer home-centered care, a fifth organizational configuration is the hospice that is hospital-based. Just as hospice services are not necessarily right for all clients, some people prefer to die in a controlled environment and so opt for a hospice located in a nursing home or hospital setting.[6]

To qualify for hospice services in the home, the following five qualifications must be met by the client:

1. Control of symptoms such as pain must be possible in the home setting.
2. At least one person must be able and willing to care for the client at home.
3. Professional staff, such as hospice nurses, must visit the home at some stated interval to complement the service of the home care provider.
4. Suitable equipment and supplies such as a hospital-type bed and other comfort and convenience devices must be made available in the home.

5. Immediate inpatient back-up availability must be guaranteed should the client and/or family desire hospitalization.[7]

Accreditation and Licensure of Hospices

The nursing role within the hospice agency is one in which holistic care is given to the client and family. The hospice nurse cares for the family unit as physical, psychosocial, and emotional support services are rendered. Some of the functional roles that hospice nurses assume include caregiver, teacher, support person, counselor, and client advocate. Primary care is continuous and individualized. As in any home setting, the hospice nurse uses nursing knowledge to make decisions about the care regimen. The hospice nurse is accountable to the client system and to the interdisciplinary hospice team.[8]

The major nursing goals for hospice clients are: (1) the promotion of an optimal level of physical comfort; and (2) the promotion of family participation in the physical and emotional care of the client. The hospice nurse must exercise judgment as to the appropriateness of care measures such as turning and back care depending on how the client tolerates such activity.[8] Hospice nurses must understand that if the client's condition is not curable, preventive efforts such as range of motion and scrupulous back care assume little importance if these procedures are perceived as painful or intrusive. The client should be kept as clean as possible, and bladder and bowel functions should be maintained. All care interventions are based on allowing the client to experience as high a level of well-being as possible. Additionally, the hospice nurse works with the client, the family, and the physician to achieve a level of analgesia which is acceptable to the client without imposing unnecessary sedation.[9]

The two major nursing goals related to the psychosocial and emotional needs of the client system are "to promote open honest communication among family members and to promote coping with the grief and sense of loss experienced by the patient and family throughout the period of involvement."[8] One of the most effective things a hospice nurse can do is to take time to listen to what the client and family have to say. Emphasizing family strengths and helping the family to use their own problem-solving skills assists them in dealing constructively with the realities of the situation. Because care of the terminally ill homebound is continuous, caregivers and/or family members should be encouraged to provide coverage for periods of time when they want to be free to attend to other matters.

The relationship between the hospice nurse and dying clients and their family is a special one. When clients die, the nurse will probably experience some degree of grief. If that grief as well as other job stresses are not adequately handled, the nurse can become emotionally impaired or "burned out." No one should enter hospice nursing until they have first dealt with their own beliefs and attitudes about death. Some also advise that hospice nurses should learn how to effectively use emotional support offered by others on the hospice team.

Cost Considerations Relative to Hospice

One of the major problems with talking about costs related to hospice care is that there are several different types of hospice organizations and, therefore, costs vary. In one study conducted in 1977, the cost of a home-based hospice program was compared to costs associated with a nursing home and an acute care hospital. The researchers found that acute hospital care was four times more expensive than nursing home care, and ten times greater than care in a home-based hospice.[10]

In 1980, another group of researchers compared the cost of caring for terminally ill patients between those cared for by a home-based hospice program and those cared for in the hospital. The mean cost per day for hospice care was $42 compared to $441 for hospital care. Actual cost differences for 2 weeks of care ranged from 4.0 to 74.0 times greater in the hospital. Interestingly, nursing care accounted for 56% of the bill for home-care clients, whereas only 3% of the charges were for physician care. For hospital care, nursing care was included in the per diem room rate, accounting for 44% of the total cost, while physician charges were 15 times greater than in home or hospice settings.

■ Communicable Disease Prevention and Control: A New Nursing Role?

The prevention, surveillance, and control of communicable diseases in the community is handled differently by various official health departments at state and local levels. In some instances, there is a department of infectious or communicable diseases that may be headed by a public health physician who may or may not utilize professional nurses on staff. Duties of such departments include compiling incidence data on communicable diseases ranging from sexually transmitted diseases to tuberculosis and food-borne outbreaks. This departmet would also have responsibility for reporting certain "reportable diseases" to central authorities such as the Centers for Disease Control. It would also have case finding, treatment, and contact-tracing for sexually transmitted diseases.

Such a communicable or infectious disease branch would also assume responsibility for investigating any outbreak or epidemic phenomena within its geographic jurisdiction. At the state level, peripheral responsibilities that might be addressed are licensure and inspection of agencies such as day-care centers and nursing homes.

A bachelor's- or master's-prepared nurse with the appropriate background in public health sciences, such as sanitation and epidemiology, and nursing preparation in infection control competencies could function to coordinate all the activities that are usually assigned to health department personnel responsible for prevention and control of infections in the community. Additionally, this nurse could assume responsibility for prevention and control of infectious phenomena in home health care clients. This communicable disease nurse specialist could also be expected to participate in continuing education of nursing personnel relative to prevention and control of infection in all client population segments.

Some health department-affiliated nurses across the country have historically had some responsibilities for prevention and control of infectious diseases, but the role proposed here would be much broader than some in existence now. This communicable disease nurse specialist would also have to be a skilled consumer and producer of research so that a scientific base for practice could be established.

In short, this role would parallel the role of the infection control nurse in the hospital, except the client population would be extramural, and the infections of interest would not be limited to those that were hospital-acquired. And while there may not be a very large pool of infection control nurses prepared at the post-bachelor's or master's level, there is a sufficient cadre of prepared persons to test the feasibility of such a position.

Summary

*H*ospice and home health nursing have much deeper historical roots than the community health specialties that nurse intramural populations. Infection control is easily the newest specialty role and yet, some of public health nursing's earliest efforts were directed at prevention and control of infections like tuberculosis. As society and health care needs evolve, community health nursing will continue to refine existent roles and give birth to new ones.

References

1. Cherryholmes LG: The qualities of a home health care nurse. In Stuart–Siddall S (ed): Home Health Care Nursing: Administrative and Clinical Perspectives, pp 155–161. Rockville, Md, Aspen Systems, 1986
2. Torrens PR (ed): Hospice Programs and Public Health Policy p 84. Chicago: American Hospital Publishing Co, 1984
3. Caserta JE, Addiss S: The economics of community health: Dealing with realities. In Sorensen GE (ed): The Economics of Health Care and Nursing, p 43–63. American Academy of Nursing Presidential Papers and Addresses for the 1984 Annual Meeting & Scientific Session, Kansas City, Mo, 1985

4. Mundinger MO: Home Care Controversy: Too Little, Too Late, Too Costly. Rockville, Md, Aspen Publications, 1983
5. Waters PS: Hospice nursing. In Stuart–Siddall S (ed): Home Health Care Nursing: Administrative and Clinical Perspectives, p 215–222. Rockville, Md, Aspen Systems, 1986
6. Spiegel AD: Home Health Care: Home Birthing to Hospice Care. Owings Mills, MD, National Health Publishing, 1983
7. Zimmerman JM: Hospice–Complete Care for the Terminally Ill. Baltimore, Urban and Schwarzenberb, 1981
8. Waters PS: Hospice nursing. In Stuart–Siddall S (ed): Home Health Care Nursing: Administrative and Clinical Perspectives, p 215–222. Rockville, MD, Aspen Systems, 1986
9. Elkins CP: Community Health Nursing: Skills and Strategies. Bowie, MD, Robert J. Brady, 1984
10. Ward BJ: Hospice Home Care: Expansion of a hospital based home health agency. Paper at the annual meeting of the American Public Health Association, Washington, DC, 1977

Clinical Health Problems in Contemporary Populations

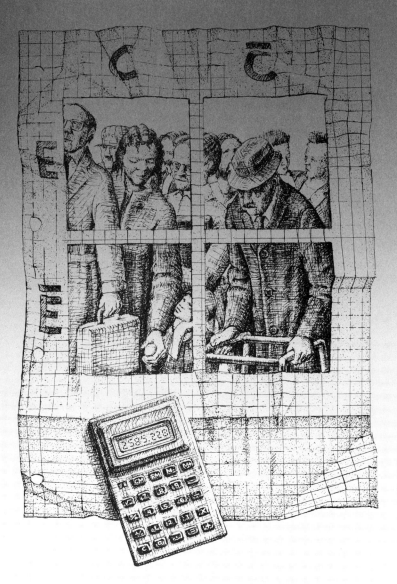

Epidemiologic tables contain frequencies that describe groups and associate events with the rise and fall of disease, tragedy, and accomplishment through community services. Tables show patterns; they evaluate the progress of community activities; and they are warning signals of hazards. Tables tell the story of people, of human beings who form a community.

Family Violence

LEARNING OBJECTIVES

After reading and understanding the contents of this chapter, the student will be able to:

1. State the nature and effect of Public Law 93-247.

2. Cite the prevalence, morbidity, and mortality associated with family abuse.

3. List the factors associated with an increased rate of spouse abuse.

4. Compose your own definition of family violence based on the one given in this chapter.

5. Relate the signs and symptoms of child abuse according to the National Center for Child Abuse and Neglect.

6. Elaborate host and geographic (person and place) variables associated with family violence.

7. Define "incestuous behavior" and cite its estimated rate in the United States.

8. Compare and contrast the relationship between alcohol abuse and family violence.

Introduction

*A*cts of family violence range from negligence to physical battering and sexual molestation. Any family member, whether infant or grandparent, may be a victim of violence, and any child or adult may be the perpetrator. As will be seen, family violence is seen in virtually all geographic settings, among all ethnic and racial groups, among all religions and all occupational and socioeconomic levels. For purposes of this discussion, violence is the use of physical force with the intent of causing injury or death.[1]

Unlike their adult cohorts, children are ostensibly protected by individual states' adaptations of the Child Abuse Prevention and Training Act of 1974 (PL 93-247). That Act directed the creation of a National Center for Child Abuse and Neglect within the Department of Health and Human Services, which serves as a clearing-house for information and resource material on child abuse. Although it is essentially illegal to batter anyone, there is less legal authority and much less societal concern with wife or husband beating than with child abuse.

Regardless of legal statutes, any type of family abuse is grossly underreported. Because these phenomena are underreported, official statistics such as those shown in Table 14-1 should be interpreted with caution. Examination of these official statistics shows that blacks and racial minorities are overreported as child abusers, but in reality, it is probably much more accurate to say that instances of physical injury among minorities with low annual incomes are more often reported to officials.

■ *Incidence of Child and Woman Abuse*

The National Center for Child Abuse and Neglect estimates that between 1 million and 6 million children are abused or neglected in the United States each year.[2] One conservative estimate of mortality associated with child abuse is that 5,000 children die each year in this country as a result of abuse.[3]

Each year in the United States, 3 to 4 million women are assaulted in their homes by their husbands, former husbands, boyfriends, or lovers. This particular estimate includes 1.8 million women who are living with a man, and another 1.8 million who are single, legally separated, or divorced.[1] In a Texas survey, it was estimated that some 358,595 women had required medical treatment sometime in their lives because of abuse.[4] It should also be noted that a significant number of rape victims, suicide attempters, mothers of abused chil-

TABLE 14-1

No. 295. Reported Child Neglect and Abuse Cases, by Division: 1978 to 1983

Year	U.S., total	New England	Middle Atlantic	East North Central	West North Central	South Atlantic	East South Central	West South Central	Moun- tain	Pacific
Total number of reports (1,000):										
1978......	606.6	33.4	76.3	69.1	68.8	96.3	59.5	52.9	38.6	111.7
1979......	707.4	41.3	85.5	104.8	66.6	126.2	61.5	61.7	31.9	127.8
1980......	785.1	48.3	91.8	105.3	77.7	154.5	58.2	69.7	37.7	141.8
1981......	846.2	39.0	101.9	110.5	85.7	174.8	66.1	88.4	37.3	142.5
1982......	924.1	49.9	105.5	126.0	96.8	182.1	75.4	95.8	41.5	151.0
1983......	1,001.4	58.5	101.0	141.6	93.8	228.5	62.3	103.0	49.5	163.3
Percent change:										
1980–1981	7.8	−19.3	11.0	4.9	10.3	13.1	13.6	26.8	−1.1	.5
1980–1982	9.2	27.9	3.5	14.0	13.0	4.2	14.1	8.4	11.3	6.0
1982–1983	8.4	17.2	−4.3	12.4	−3.1	25.5	−17.4	7.5	19.3	8.2
Reports per 1,000 population:										
1978......	2.7	2.7	2.1	1.7	4.0	2.7	4.1	2.3	3.6	3.7
1980......	3.5	3.9	2.5	2.5	4.5	4.2	4.0	2.9	3.3	4.4
1981......	3.7	3.1	2.8	2.7	5.0	4.6	4.5	3.6	3.2	4.4
1982......	4.0	4.0	2.9	3.0	5.6	4.8	5.1	3.8	3.6	4.6
1983......	4.3	4.7	2.7	3.4	5.4	5.9	4.2	4.0	4.0	4.9

[1]Based on Bureau of the Census estimated resident population as of July 1.

Source: American Humane Association, Denver, CO. *National Analysis of Official Child Neglect and Abuse Reporting*, annual and unpublished data.

(U.S. Bureau of the Census; Statistical Abstract of the United States; (106th edition). Washington, D.C., 1985–1986)

(Derived from data provided by state child protective services personnel to the National Study on Child Neglect and Abuse Reporting, conducted by The American Association for Protecting Children, a division of The American Humane Association, and funded through the National Center on Child Abuse and Neglect, OHDS, DHHS. Represents total number of child maltreatment reports documented within the states, including substantiated and unsubstantiated reports. Also, the figures embody the variation among states with respect to whether they use individual child reports or reports which indicate all involved children in the family. Minus sign (−) indicates decline.)

dren, alcoholics, psychiatric patients, and women who miscarry or abort also have a personal history of being battered.[1]

Much of the following discussion on family violence was adapted from research conducted by Straus, Gelles and Steinmetz that was subsequently published in book form in 1981. Findings were based on a national survey using a random sample of the 46 million families in the United States in 1976. Family was defined as any couple who indicated that they were married or living together. One adult member of each of the sample families was interviewed, and an attempt was made to interview equal numbers of adult males and females. The total sample consisted of 2,143 families. A major limitation of the study was that the couple had to be living together at the time of the interview and, therefore, no information was obtained on single-parent families.

▌ *Spouse Violence*

Every year, in approximately one out of six couples in the United States, one partner commits at least one violent act against the other partner. Over the entire span of a relationship, the chances are almost one out of three that your spouse will hit you.[5] When violence occurs, it tends to be a recurrent feature of the marriage. Even though married men and women are roughly equally apt to become violent, men have higher rates for the most dangerous and injurious forms of violence. Men tend to do more physical damage, and a large number of attacks seem to occur when the wife is pregnant. Whereas men who are subjects of physical abuse tend to get out of a marriage, women are statistically more apt to remain in the marriage. Interestingly, the same is true with alcoholism. Ninety percent of men leave an alcoholic wife, but a lower proportion of women leave an alcoholic husband. Although there are no absolute measures that accurately predict spouse abuse, characteristics that seem statistically related to both wife- and husband-beating are as follows[5]:

- Husband employed part time or unemployed
- Family income at or below poverty level
- Husband is a manual worker
- Husband is very concerned about economic security
- Wife is very dissatisfied with her family's standard of living
- The couple has two or more children
- The couple disagrees over how to raise or discipline children
- Either or both spouses grew up in a home where the father hit the mother
- The couple has been married less than 10 years
- The couple is aged 30 or under
- The family is non-white and part of a racial minority
- Both parents score very high on stress index tests
- The wife is dominant in family decisions
- Husband or wife is verbally aggressive to the other
- The family does not participate in any organized religion

▌ *Violence Toward Children*

In general, research has found that men tend to be slightly more inclined to approve of the use of physical force on children than women. Additionally, younger Americans (under 50 years of age) were found to be much more likely to view slaps and spankings as "necessary, normal and good."[5] Although there are some parents who never use physical force or violence on their children, the majority of parents reported that they used some form of violence sometime in their child's life. Some portion of children are kicked, bitten, or punched; a few are threatened with a gun or knife; and one in 1000 children had a parent who either shot (or tried to shoot) or stabbed (or tried to stab) them in 1975.[5]

In general, younger children are more likely to be struck by their parents and struck more frequently than are older children, but violence toward children occurs at all ages. Also, evidence suggests that violent behavior is learned, or at the very least, violent behavior begets violent behavior. Not only does it appear that children who are abused grow up to become abusive parents, but studies on other types of adult violence show a similar history. For example, studies on violent inmates in San Quentin prison found that 100% of these individuals experienced extreme violence between the ages of 1 and 10 years of age.[5] Arthur Bremer, the would-be assassin of George Wallace, wrote in his diary "My mother must have thought I was a canoe, she paddled me so much." Additionally, some of the darkest figures in the 1960s and 1970s, such as Lee Harvey Oswald, Sirhan Sirhan, and Charles Manson, all reportedly experienced violent childhoods.[6]

The National Center for Child Abuse and Neglect has identified the following as signs of abuse in children:

1. Any injury in an infant under 12 months of age
2. Gross or multiple injuries in a child of any age
3. Repeated injuries or fractures in various stages of healing
4. Intracranial injuries
5. Unexpected weight loss
6. Severe malnutrition or failure to thrive, especially in very young children
7. Venereal disease or signs of genital trauma[7]

Furthermore, when the caregiver relates an inadequate or conflicting history about a child's injuries or when medical care is not sought promptly, child abuse may be a possibility. In interactions between the abuser and the child, inappropriate demands and expectations may be communicated as well as displays of unreasonable and inappropriate discipline. Living situations that include unusual stress, isolation, or inadequate social support systems are often associated with an increased incidence of child abuse.[7]

▪ *Violence Between Brothers and Sisters*

Even families who are reluctant to talk about wife beating or child abuse readily admit that sibling violence is a part of most family lives. In Straus and associates' study, it was found that sibling violence occurs more frequently than parent–child or husband–wife violence: the older the child, the lower the rate of sibling violence, but boys in every age group were generally more violent toward their siblings than their girl cohorts. The highest level of violence among siblings occurred when a boy had only one brother.[5]

Each year three out of every hundred children are kicked, bitten, or punched by a parent, and two out of every hundred spouses kick, bite, or punch each other. But a whopping forty-two out of every hundred children aged three to seventeen kicks, bites, or punches a brother or sister each year.[5]

■ *Some Host and Geographic Variables in Family Abuse*

Experts and lay people alike have traditionally viewed family violence as a problem particular to the lower socioeconomic class. The research on the subject in the 1960s and 1970s was based primarily on instances of family violence identified by police or medical records. But because poor, powerless people are more likely to get caught and labeled for their illegal acts, it was instances of violence among the lower class that were most often recorded. In contrast, middle and upper class families tend to be somewhat physically insulated in separate homes, and they tend to rely on private medical and legal agencies, which are much less likely to report instances of violence.[5]

Southern states have always had higher rates of lethal violence, including homicide, than other regions of the country. In spite of that and the fact that southerners are more apt to own guns than people in other parts of the country, southerners were not found to be more prone to engage in domestic violence. The southern region of the United States had the lowest rate of abusive violence toward children, but the midwestern region had a rate of child abuse that was 100% higher than the rate in the South.[5]

As for the effect of urban versus rural settings for violence, it was found that while sibling and wife abuse were similar between the settings, families that lived in cities with a population of 1 million or greater had higher rates of abusiveness toward children and between husband and wife.[5]

As for the effect of race on family violence, it has been found that parental violence is highest among American Indians, Orientals, and other racial minorities, but little difference exists between blacks and whites. Wife abuse is several times more common among black families than among white families, but husband abuse is highest among minorities. Sibling violence was highest in families composed of racial minorities, but lowest in black families.[5]

In 1981, Straus and associates reported the following data relative to the relationship between violence and religious backgrounds:

(1) sibling abuse was lowest among families where the mother was Jewish and highest in families of minority religions (not Catholic, Protestant and Jewish); (2) child abuse was lowest among Jews; (3) wife abuse was lowest among Jewish families; (4) the rate of husband abuse was lowest among Protestants. Jewish women, who lived in the least violent homes, had a rate of abusing their husbands that was more than double the rate for Protestants; and (5) in families where both husband and wife were of the same religion.[5]

Family violence evidently occurs at all ages, just as it does in all social classes, but younger couples tend to be more violent than older ones. The most violent fathers and husbands were those who had graduated from school, whereas the least violent were grammar school dropouts and men with some college education. College-educated women were the least likely to be abused by their husbands or to stay in abusive marriages, whereas women who had not completed high school were the most likely to be physically abused.[5]

Families earning more than $20,000 in 1975 had half the reported rate of violence that occurred in families at or below the poverty level. Families living at or below the poverty level had a rate of violence between husbands and wives that was about 500% greater than the rate of violence in families with moderate or high incomes. Men and women who held blue-collar jobs had higher rates of all types of family violence than people who had white-collar occupations. Further, when a man was employed part time or was unemployed, there was more severe violence in the home than when the father or husband was employed full time.[5]

■ *Incestuous Behavior in the Family*

Even though incestuous behavior may occur between any two or more members of a given family, father–daughter incest is thought to be one of the most common manifestations of the problem. Like instances of family abuse, there are no reliable counts of the incidence and/or prevalence of incest, but it is conservatively estimated that over 1 million American women have been sexually victimized by their fathers or other male relatives.[9] For purposes of this discussion, incest is defined as any sexual activity or intimate physical contact that is sexually arousing between nonmarried members of a family.[10]

> In the physically abusive family, the parent tries to beat the child into meeting his or her needs. In the incestuous family, the parent or other relative uses sex and seduction.[10]

The daughter who is victimized by paternal incest is approximately 11 years old at the onset and is typically the oldest daughter at home.[13] Sexual contact is initiated through the use of bribes, rewards, intimidation, or exploitation of her need to trust the father-figure as well as her desire for affection.[14,15] Further, according to one researcher, physical force is rarely required. The incestuous relationship is typically progressive and the frequency of contact ranges from incidental to as often as more than once a week, and this relationship typically lasts from 1 to 3 years or more.[13] Viewing the incestuous encounters from a family dynamics standpoint, de Chesnay reported the following:

> . . . the mother in homes where exploitative sexual abuse occurs tends to be emotionally distant and aloof toward the children. In such homes, it is no exaggeration that vulnerable family members typically view the father as the parent who loves them. The father interacts more with the children and provides significant amounts of caretaking, despite deviant episodes.[16]

Fathers who engage in incestual relationships with their daughters are not purely after sex, but rather power and control. These are essentially self-indulgent men who feel justified in using their children to meet their own sexual needs.[16]

Research to date reveals that daughters who are victims of incest are affected in varying ways. Immediate or short-term effects include guilt, depression, learning difficulties, sexual promiscuity, running away, somatic complaints, confusion over sexual identification, and fear of sexuality.[17]

Long-term effects, or those that occur 6 months or more after the incestuous relationship is terminated include sexual promiscuity, illegitimate pregnancies, homosexual tendencies, alcohol and drug abuse, frigidity, and neurotic symptoms.[18] Other long-term effects on the victim include difficulty forming trusting relationships, impaired sexual relationships, idealization of men, hostility toward women, depressive symptoms, and even suicide attempts.[19]

It is difficult to predict how these relationships between father and daughter might affect the structure and functioning of the family, but it has been suggested that for the problem to persist, each family member must assume and continue "a role that encourages incest and discourages behavior that could disrupt the cycle."[20]

■ *Alcohol Abuse and Family Violence*

Although there is a statistical relationship between alcoholism and family violence, family violence does not result from alcoholism any more than alcoholism results from family violence. Even so, the community health nurse must be alert for signs of family violence and incest when working with families who have alcoholic members. Research has shown that many alcoholics were themselves abused as children and/or have physical abuse and incest as a part of their family history.

Alcohol abuse does not cause marital violence, but the two behaviors seem to occur in family systems that look similar. These
families are closed systems, isolated from the community, and
have many family secrets.[21]

In fact, alcoholism and child abuse have the following characteristics in common: (1) low frustration tolerance; (2) low self-esteem;
(3) compulsivity; (4) dependency; (5) immaturity; (6) severe depression; (7) problems with role reversals; (8) difficulty experiencing pleasure; and (9) lack of understanding of the needs and abilities of infants and children.[22]

▪ *Application to Community Health Nursing Practice*

In some instances, primary prevention in the form of educational
strategies aimed at enhancing understanding of different developmental levels or at opening lines of communication within the family can
act to prevent instances of abuse or violence. For example, the family
needs to understand why aging members or adolescents behave as
they do. Other times, anticipatory guidance and recognition of individual needs for privacy or recreation by the home health nurse can
act to disarm potentially violent episodes within the family. As an example, when the whole family or even one or two members are consistently homebound caring for a dependent member, it is important
for the community health nurse to encourage the family to arrange
breaks or periods of time when they can attend to other tasks or leisure activities. In other instances, violence or abuse is emotionally or
culturally ingrained, and thus primary prevention strategies may be
ineffective.

When family violence does occur, the signs, symptoms, and
manifestations are highly variable from one population or family to
another. Often family members may feel guilty, fearful, or threatened
by exposure, and they may make deliberate attempts to conceal or
even ignore the problem. Because violence among family members
constitutes a significant threat to a realization of individual and family
well-being, the community health nurse must be alert to the fact that
violence symptomatology may range from subtle to overt. The first
community health nursing responsibility according to secondary prevention strategies is to be a competent case finder. In order to detect
instances of possible family abuse, the community health nurse must
be a sensitive and knowledgeable case finder. In other words, it is important to know the risk factors associated with family violence, to be
aware of cultural attitudes toward violence in the home, and to establish a rapport with family members that is amenable to open and honest communications.

Once a problem related to family violence is suspected, whether it is confirmed by family members or not, a second vital community health nursing role is to objectively document observations and/or verbal confirmations in written form. For many legal and ethical reasons, the community health nurse should not attempt to intervene other than to provide family members with information about where they may obtain temporary shelter or other protective arrangements. Instead, the community health nurse should take written documentation back to the employing agency according to established protocol.

The great majority of health agencies that employ community health nurses will have written protocols or established referral experts who will assume responsibility for further investigation and intervention on behalf of abused family members. In some cases, community health nurses with advance preparation may be specially educated and trained to intervene beyond case finding and initial documentation of the problem. However, at the entry level, the nurse's practice responsibilities are generally limited to epidemiologic case finding, meticulous and objective documentation, and referral to a social or law enforcement agency. Finally, it should be noted that as a tertiary prevention modality, most victims of physical and/or sexual abuse will benefit from professional counseling. Accordingly, the community health nurse should assure that such counseling is made accessible for the client or the whole family when possible.

Summary

*T*he United States Public Health Service in its Health Objectives for the nation estimated that 2,000 to 5,000 deaths and up to 4 million injuries are inflicted on children by parents each year. The goal is that by 1990, injuries and deaths of children inflicted by abusing parents should be reduced by at least 25%. A second goal is to greatly increase the reliability of data on the incidence and prevalence of child abuse and other forms of family violence.[8] Although there are many forms of family violence, such as homicide, suicide, and even elderly abuse, our discussion has been limited to physical abuse between and among members of the nuclear family. Even though we have focused on interpersonal violence, there are also greater consequences of assaultive behavior and spouse abuse. When violence occurs, it diminishes the quality of life for the victims, their families, and their communities. Violent behavior can result in fear, distress, depression, alcoholism, and even suicide or homicide. Suffice it to say that bruises and contusions are probably the most innocuous results of violence in the American family. Community health nursing roles based on the levels of prevention include education strategies, anticipatory guidance, epidemiologic case finding, accurate and objective documentation, and referral.

References

1. Rosenberg ML, Stark E, Zahn MA: Interpersonal violence: Homicide and spouse abuse. In Last JM (ed): Maxcy–Rosenau Public Health and Preventive Medicine, 12th ed, pp 1399–1426. Norwalk, CT, Appleton-Century-Crofts, 1986

2. National Center for Child Abuse and Neglect: Study Findings: National Study of Incidence and Severity of Child Abuse and Neglect, U.S. Department of Health and Human Services Pub No 81-30325. Washington, DC, Government Printing Office, 1981

3. Fontana VJ: Somewhere a Child is Crying: Maltreatment—Cause and Prevention. New York, Macmillan, 1973

4. Teske RH, Parker ML: Spouse Abuse in Texas: A Study of Women's Attitudes and Experience. Huntsville, TX, Criminal Justice Center, Sam Houston State University, 1983 (Cited in Rosenberg)

5. Straus MA, Gelles RJ, Steinmetz SK: Behind Closed Doors: Violence in the American Family. Garden City, NY, Anchor Books, 1981

6. Button A: Some antecedents of felonies and delinquent behavior. J Child Psychol 2:35–38, 1973

7. Public Health Service: Child abuse/neglect: A Guide for Detection, Prevention and Treatment, Pub No (HSA) 75-5220, pp 5–6. Washington DC, Government Printing Office, 1979

8. Public Health Service, Office of Disease Prevention and Health Promotion: Public Health Service implementation plans for attaining the objectives for the nation. Public Health Rep 98(5)Suppl:167–168, 1983

9. Finkehor D: Sexually Victimized Children. New York, Free Press, 1979

10. Justice B, Justice R: The Broken Taboo: Sex in the Family, p 25. New York, Human Sciences Press, 1979

11. Gagnon J: Female child victims of sex offenses. Soc Probl 13:176–192, 1965

12. Landis JT: Experiences of 500 children with adult sexual deviation. Psychiatr Q (Suppl) 30:91–109, 1956

13. Brunngraber LS: Father–daughter incest: Immediate and long-term effects of sexual abuse. ANS 8(4):17, 1986

14. Burgess AW, Holmstrom LL: Sexual trauma of children and adolescents. Nurs Clin North AM 10:551–563, 1975

15. Herman JL: Father–daughter Incest. Cambridge, Harvard University Press, 1981

16. What families won't tell: Insights into the incest taboo. Medical Center Magazine—The University of Alabama at Birmingham 30(2):19, 1986

17. Kaufman I, Peck AL, Taguiri CK: The family constellation and overt incestuous relations between father and daughter. Am J Orthopsychiatry 24:266–279, 1954

18. Lukianowicz N: Incest I: Paternal incest II: Other types of incest. Br J Psychiatry 120:301–313, 1972

19. Herman JL, Hirschman L: Families at risk for father–daughter incest. Am J Psychiatry 138:967–970, 1981

20. de Chesnay M: Father–daughter incest: Issues in treatment and research. J Psychosoc Nurs Ment Health Serv 22(9):15, 1984

21. Lawson F, Peterson JS, Lawson A: Alcoholism and the Family, p 153. Rockville, MD, Aspen Systems Corp, 1983

22. Spinetta JJ, Rigler D: The child abusing parent: A psychological review. Psychol Bull 77:296–304, 1972

Substance Abuse

LEARNING OBJECTIVES

After reading and understanding the contents of this chapter, the student will be able to:

1. *Cite the overall rate of alcohol and tobacco use in the United States, and do the same for marijuana and other illicit substances.*

2. *Describe known racial/ethnic characteristics among minority drug abusers.*

3. *Cite the rates and types of substance use/abuse among high school populations in the United States.*

4. *Compare and contrast various preventive strategies for drug abuse and discuss some of the known barriers to healing or educating the abusers.*

5. *Discuss the rate of drug abuse among youths, young adults, and adults over time.*

Introduction

*U*se and abuse of all kinds of drugs, including tobacco and alcohol, is a worldwide public health problem. In the United States, nearly one third of all deaths (between 450,000 and 600,000 premature deaths annually) are attributed to drug abuse of some sort. Some of these substances have been used throughout history in virtually every culture and civilization. We will review some of the host variables associated with substance abuse, look at associated morbidity and mortality, and examine overall preventive strategies.

■ *Tobacco Use*

Aside from being the largest single preventable cause of illness and premature death in the United States, cigarette smoking is the major single cause of cancer mortality in the United States. Smoking is also a causal factor for coronary heart disease and arteriosclerotic peripheral vascular disease as well as the most important cause of chronic obstructive lung disease. Smoking is also associated with an increased risk of bladder, pancreatic, and renal cancer as well as peptic ulcer disease. Besides its harm to the unborn fetus, cigarette smoking acts synergistically with oral contraceptives to increase the risk of coronary heart disease and some forms of cerebrovascular disease; with alcohol to increase the risk of cancer of the larynx, oral cavity, and esophagus; and with asbestos and some other occupationally related substances to increase the likelihood of cancer of the lung and larynx. Smoking is also the major identifiable cause of residential fire deaths and injuries as well as a contributor to accidental injuries.[1]

More than 30 million smokers have quit since 1964, and the proportion of adult smokers has declined from about 42% in 1965 to approximately one third today. Even so, as many as 50,000,000 Americans smoked in 1981, and more than 4,000 cigarettes were consumed per capita in the United States.[2]

In 1984, about 70% of all high school seniors had tried cigarettes at some time, and 30% had smoked regularly during the preceding month. Fourteen percent of seniors reported smoking half a pack or more per day, and the prevalence of smoking was higher in adolescent females than in their male cohorts.[3] The use of drugs is interrelated in that young people who smoke are also reportedly much more apt to have used alcohol and/or marijuana than nonsmokers.[4] Overall, daily smoking among high school students dropped from 29% to 20% between 1977 and 1981, and daily use of a half of a pack a day or more fell from 19.4% to 13.5%. Since that time, however, it is believed that smoking rates have remained constant.[5]

The prevalence of cigarette smoking among black males has consistently exceeded that of white males, but only small differences exist between black and white females. The differences observed between black and white males are not explained by occupational, educational, or income differences, although the percentage of blacks who never started smoking is lower than whites. Once started, blacks are less likely to attempt to quit or to quit successfully. Also, in general, whites are heavier smokers than blacks, but blacks tend to smoke cigarettes higher in tar. The effect of these differences between races on morbidity and mortality are not always clear, but it does appear that smoking-related cancers are particularly high among blacks.[6]

On the average, Native Americans have lower smoking-related lung cancer rates than whites, but the relative frequency of lung cancer differs among Native American tribes. For example, Native Americans of the Southwest, who seldom smoke, have low rates of smoking-related lung cancer.[6]

Although the prevalence rates of smoking for Asian/Pacific Islanders are unknown, people from that area do exhibit an excess incidence and mortality for some smoking-related cancers. For example, Hawaiians have an excessive mortality rate for cancer of the lung, and the incidence of esophageal cancer is higher for Japanese and Chinese persons than for whites. Also, Chinese individuals seem to have a high rate of pancreatic cancer, which is associated with cigarette smoking.[6]

It has been estimated that at least 12 million people in the United States used smokeless tobacco (*e.g.*, snuff and chewing tobacco) in 1985. Use of these substances is increasing, especially among adolescent and young adult males. It is also known that experimentation with and adoption of the tobacco habit usually occur during adolescence; therefore, prevention programs must frequently focus on this age group.[7]

■ *Alcohol*

The use of alcohol is of major public health importance because of its relationship to many acute and chronic physical, psychological, and behavioral problems. The important health problems related to alcohol use are alcohol dependence, injury, accident, violence, and medical complications such as gastrointestinal, nervous, cardiovascular, and respiratory system debilitation. Also of importance is the association between alcohol intake and a range of adverse pregnancy outcomes and fetal abnormalities caused by the embryotoxic and teratogenic effects.[8]

Currently, average consumption of alcohol for all persons older than 14 years of age is 10% higher than 10 years ago, and is equivalent to about 2.75 gallons of ethanol per person per year. Approximately 10 million adult Americans (*i.e.*, 7% of those 18 years of age or older) can be considered problem drinkers. Moreover, there are an estimated 3 million youthful problem drinkers aged 14 to 17.[1]

In addition to the social costs to family and community, the economic costs as a result of alcohol misuse are substantial: an estimated $440.4 billion in 1977. Overall, 10% of all deaths in the United States are alcohol-related. Cirrhosis, which is strongly linked to alcohol intake, ranks among the ten leading causes of death in this country. Table 15-1 is a summary of alcohol-related problems.

Data exists that indicate that alcohol abuse has a major impact on the health of blacks. For example, the cirrhosis mortality for blacks is twice that of nonminorities. Few studies exist on the subject of alcohol and blacks, but survey results have shown that black males begin to report high rates of heavy drinking and social problems due to drinking after the age of 30, compared to white males where heavy and problem drinking is concentrated in the age group of 18 to 25 years.[6]

The Indian Health Service reports that five of the top ten causes of death among Native Americans are directly related to alcohol. These are accidents (21%), cirrhosis of the liver (6%), alcoholism (3.2%), suicide (2.9%), and homicide (2%). In fact, the age-adjusted mortality rates from alcohol-related causes of death are three times higher among Native Americans than among other groups. For example, it is estimated that 80% of all deaths by suicide and 90% of homicides are alcohol-related.[6]

The overall impression that Asian/Pacific Islanders do not consume as much alcohol as the general population is generally supported by research studies. Research on the so-called "flushing reaction" shows that approximately 50% of persons of Asian background metabolize alcohol much more quickly than do Caucasians, causing a "flushing reflex," and a high degree of discomfort, which may provide some protection against heavy drinking and related problems.

The frequency of alcohol consumption for all Americans is shown in Table 15-2.

■ *Cocaine*

Cocaine comes from a plant, Erythroxylon coca, which grows on the moist eastern slopes of Peruvian and Bolivian mountains. The natives in those regions have chewed the leaves for their stimulating effect for 5000 years. Shortly after 1850, scientists isolated an alkaloid from the plant and dubbed it cocaine. Sigmund Freud worked with the substance, reported on its local anesthetic effects, but also became de-

TABLE 15-1

A Summary of Alcohol-Related Physical, Psychological, and Behavioral Problems

Psychological and behavioral	Hypertension
Acute alcohol intoxication	Death from ischemic heart disease
Acute alcohol poisoning	
Hangover	***Respiratory***
Blackouts	Obstructive sleep apnea
Alcohol dependence	Chronic obstructive lung disease
	Pneumonia
Acute alcohol withdrawal and alcoholic	Lung abscess
psychoses	Pulmonary tuberculosis
Acute alcohol withdrawal syndrome	Laryngeal carcinoma
Delirium tremens	Carcinoma of the lung
Acute auditory hallucinosis	
Depression	***Endocrine/metabolic***
Attempted suicide	Hypoglycemia
Suicide	Hyperglycemia
	Diabetes
Neurological	Gout
Subclinical neuropsychological	Lactic acidosis
impairment	Derangements of mineral metabolism
Epilepsy	
Peripheral neuropathy	***Reproductive***
Cerebral atrophy	Depressed testicular function
Cerebellar atrophy	Depressed ovarian function
Wernicke-Korsakoff syndrome	Carcinoma of the breast
Traumatic head injury	
Death from cerebrovascular disease	***Musculoskeletal***
	Acute and chronic myopathy
Gastrointestinal	Ischemic necrosis of the head of femur
Oropharyngeal carcinoma	Osteoporosis
Acute esophageal dysfunction	
Mallory–Weiss syndrome	***Hematological***
Esophageal varices	Anemia
Esophageal carcinoma	Impaired leucocyte response to infection
Erosive gastritis	Thrombocytopenia
Acute gastroduodenal ulceration	
Atrophic gastritis	***Traumatic injuries***
Gastric carcinoma	
Disturbed small bowel motility	***Ethanol-drug interactions***
Intestinal malabsorption	
Large bowel carcinoma	***Nutritional deficiencies***
Subclinical pancreatic dysfunction	
Chronic pancreatitis	***Pregnancy outcome and developmental***
Pancreatic carcinoma	***disorders***
Fatty liver	Spontaneous abortion
Alcoholic hepatitis	Perinatal mortality
Cirrhosis	Low birth weight
Hepatocellular carcinoma	Impaired development (physical, behavioral,
	intellectual)
Cardiovascular	Congenital birth defects
	Fetal alcohol syndrome
Cardiac arrhythmias	Pseudo-Cushing's syndrome in breast-fed
Alcoholic cardiomyopathy	infants
Cardiac beriberi	Alcohol withdrawal in newborn

(Reprinted with permission from Rankin JG and Ashley MJ: Alcohol-related health problems and their prevention. In Last JM (ed): *Maxcy–Rosenau Public Health and Preventive Medicine*, p 1941. Norwalk, Ct, Appleton-Century-Crofts, 1986)

pendent on the drug. An American surgeon, Dr. William Halsted, also worked with cocaine and like Freud, became dependent on it.[9]

By late 1986 it was estimated that some 22 million Americans had used cocaine, and over four million were either dependent on or in the process of becoming addicted to it. Though not as popular as marijuana, cocaine usage is thought to be rising, and the price is low enough to attract youngsters. In one survey, 50% of college students said that cocaine was easy to get and that they didn't see much risk in using it.[9]

Although initial purchases of cocaine may be inexpensive, addiction is unbelievably expensive. Calls to the nation's cocaine hotline established the fact that steady users spent anywhere from $635 to $3150 a week for the drug. The large majority of users experienced sleep problems, chronic fatigue, severe headaches, and sore nasal passages. Psychologically, most complained of depression, anxiety, irritability, apathy, paranoia, and difficulty concentrating. Such symptomatology has created what is called the cocaine paradox: what starts out as elation euphoria ends up as depression and fatigue.[9]

Cocaine is a versatile drug in that it can be eaten, drunk, injected, smoked, or sniffed. It provides a short-acting euphoria, but its

T A B L E 1 5 - 2
Frequency of Alcohol Consumption by Sex, Age, and Family Income: 1984*

Frequency of Alcohol Consumption	Total[1]	Sex	
		Male	Female
Never or less often than once a year	30	24	36
More often than once a year, less often than once a week	34	27	39
Once or twice a week	14	17	12
Three or more times a week	22	32	13
Percent who drink 5 or more drinks, at one sitting[2]	17	23	12

*In percent. Covers persons 18 years old and over living in households in the 48 contiguous States. Based on a sample survey of approximately 2,100 persons conducted in the last months of 1984. Data are subject to sampling variability. Survey responses are based on self-reported consumption of beer, wine, and distilled spirits.

[1]Includes persons 18 and 19 years old not shown separately.   [2]Based on number of persons who drink alcohol.

ability to kill even infrequent or first-time users by initiating cardiar-rhythmias is well known. Distributors of cocaine and other designer drugs like Ectasy and Rhapsody advertise these substances as "nectors of the gods of filmdom, rockdom and sportsdom along with the promise of excitement and sexual proclivity."[9]

Use of Other Drugs

Drug misuse seems generally to be increasing in America. For example, there are an estimated 16 million current marijuana users, and cocaine is enjoying a renewed popularity. Misuse of barbiturates also remains a significant problem with at least one million persons believed to be misusing these drugs, and with an estimated 30,000 persons physically addicted. Heroin addiction is one of the most serious problems, and its addiction rate has "stabilized at an estimated one-half million persons in this country."[1]

The misuse of drugs leads to a number of social and health problems. For example, the toll from heroin includes premature death

Age			Family Income			
20–34 years	35–54 years	55 yr. and over	Less than $6,000	$6,000–$15,000	$15,001–$30,000	$30,001 and over
22	28	45	46	38	27	19
36	35	28	29	32	38	32
18	14	9	13	14	13	17
24	23	18	13	16	21	32
22	15	8	10	21	34	35

Source: Medical Research Institute of San Francisco, Alcohol Research Group, Berkeley, CA, unpublished data.

(U.S. Bureau of the Census. Statistical Abstract of the U.S.: 1986, 106th ed. Washington, D.C., 1985)

and severe disability, family disruption, and crime committed to maintain the habit. A special problem is the relationship of marijuana to automobile accidents, especially when used in combination with alcohol.[1] Drug use by type and age group is shown in Table 15-3.

■ *Marijuana*

Approximately 25% of the population has used marijuana at least once. Its use is believed to be most prevalent between the ages of 18 and 25, but it must be remembered that reliable data on illicit drugs is virtually nonexistent.[2] Marijuana is the most commonly used illegal drug in America. An estimated 16 million Americans have used marijuana during the previous month.[10] The daily use of marijuana by high school students decreased from 21% in 1982 to 17% in 1983.[5]

T A B L E   1 5 - 3
Estimates of Drug Use, by Type of Drug and Age Group: 1974 and 1982*

Type of Drug	Percent of Youths			
	Ever used		Current user	
	1974	1982	1974	1982
Marijuana	23.0	26.7	12.0	11.5
Inhalants...........................	8.5	(NA)	.7	(NA)
Hallucinogens	6.0	5.2	1.3	1.4
Cocaine...........................	3.6	6.5	1.0	1.6
Heroin.............................	1.0	(Z)	(Z)	(Z)
Analgesics	(NA)	4.2	(NA)	.7
Stimulants[1].......................	5.0	6.7	1.0	2.6
Sedatives[1]........................	5.0	5.8	1.0	1.3
Tranquilizers	3.0	4.9	1.0	.9
Alcohol	54.0	65.2	34.0	26.9
Cigarettes	52.0	49.5	25.0	14.7

NA Not available.   Z Less than .5 percent.   [1]Prescription drugs.

(Current users are those who used drugs at least once within month prior to the study. For 1982, based on national samples of 1,581 youths (12–17 yrs. old), 1,283 young adults (18–25 yrs. old), and 2,760 older adults (26 yrs. old and over). Subject to sampling variability; see source)

(U.S. Bureau of the Census, Statistical Abstract of the U.S.: 1986, 106th ed. Washington, D.C., 1985)

Although tolerance and withdrawal symptoms are not associated with marijuana use, there is some evidence that alcohol potentiates and produces a form of cross tolerance to cannabis. Certainly the combination of alcohol and cannabis is more dangerous than either alone, and there is increasing data that indicate that marijuana-intoxicated drivers are over-represented in fatal accidents. It is definitively known that complex reaction time is impaired with marijuana intake, and these factors plus the visual and time distortion make driving a vehicle a hazard.[10]

Other effects of marijuana are as follows: free recall is invariably impaired and short-term memory is worsened; speech, thought, attention, and the integration of sensory information is compromised; and the desire and energy to work productively are impaired not only during the intoxicated period, but for chronic users, during the sober interval too. In fact, ". . . serious skills impairment can be measured for more than 10 hours after a single marijuana cigarette."[10]

Percent of Young Adults				Percent of Adults			
Ever used		Current user		Ever used		Current user	
1974	1982	1974	1982	1974	1982	1974	1982
52.7	64.1	25.2	27.4	9.9	23.0	2.0	6.6
9.2	(NA)	(Z)	(NA)	1.2	(NA)	(Z)	(NA)
16.6	21.1	2.5	1.7	1.3	6.4	(Z)	(Z)
12.7	28.3	3.1	6.8	.9	8.5	(Z)	1.2
4.5	1.2	(Z)	(Z)	.5	1.1	(Z)	(Z)
(NA)	12.1	(NA)	1.0	(NA)	3.2	(NA)	(Z)
17.0	18.0	3.7	4.7	3.0	6.2	(Z)	.6
15.0	18.7	1.6	2.6	2.0	4.8	(Z)	(Z)
10.0	15.1	1.2	1.6	2.0	3.6	(Z)	(Z)
81.6	94.6	69.3	67.9	73.2	88.2	54.5	56.7
68.8	76.9	48.8	39.5	65.4	78.7	39.1	34.6

■ *Solvent and Aerosol Intoxication*

Commercial solvents and propellants such as model airplane glue, paint thinner, and gasoline can be inhaled to produce a temporary period of stimulation before depression of the central nervous system occurs. These substances are poured onto a rag, balloon, or plastic bag and sniffed or deeply inhaled.

Abusers of solvents and propellants are primarily school-aged boys. In fact, in one survey, elementary students ranked solvents second to alcohol as most frequently used substances. Junior high school students rated solvents the sixth favorite or frequently used substance, and high school students ranked these substances as seventh in frequency, ahead of heroin, which ranked last.[2]

Inebriation produced by inhalation of solvents is over in minutes, or one can inhale and "stay stoned" all day. Symptoms include delirium, mental confusion, psychomotor clumsiness, emotional instability and impairment of thinking, dizziness, slurred speech, and unsteady gait. Sometimes these symptoms are mixed with impulsiveness, excitement, and overactivity that gives way to physical injury. About 100 deaths are reported every year from intentional inhalation of volatile hydrocarbons.[2]

■ *Phencyclidine*

Phencyclidine (PCP), or angel dust, can be inhaled, smoked, or sprinkled on parsley or marijuana, swallowed or injected. It is readily manufactured by "kitchen chemists" and comes to the consumer in a variety of colors, shapes, and sizes. Effects of PCP ingestion include tachycardia, hypertension, sweating, flushing, drooling, pupillary constriction, a decrease in pain and touch perception, disorientation in time, place, and even person, acute schizophrenic syndrome, psychomotor agitation, and unpredictable destructiveness or violent action. Repetitive intake appears to result in chronic impairment of mental functioning, and during sober periods, the person may demonstrate memory gaps, some disorientation, and difficulty with speech.[2]

■ *Codeine*

Prescription use of codeine is widespread since it is an excellent analgesic and cough suppressant. As an analgesic, it is used in combination with either aspirin or Tylenol because these peripheral analgesics add to the effect of the central action of codeine. Codeine dependence is a rarity—primarily because it has a low binding affinity for the opiate receptor sites, and the euphoria is of low-grade equality. Secondary codeine dependence occurs when heroin and other opiates become unavailable since codeine can partially suppress the heroin abstinence syndrome. It should also be noted that 10% of codeine is secreted as morphine, and thus a positive urine screen for both codeine and morphine may indicate codeine use alone, codeine and morphine sulfate use, or codeine and heroin use.[2]

■ *Over-the-Counter Drugs and Household Hallucinogens*

Many over-the-counter (OTC) drugs used for inducing sleep contain scopolamine among other things. Over use or purposeful overdose of substances like Sominex, Sleep-Eze, and Compoz produce signs of anticholinergic toxicity such as dilated, fixed pupils, dry mouth, flushed dry skin, and rapid pulse.[10]

Other OTC substances containing aspirin or Tylenol can also be dangerous. For example, ingestion of a high dose of salicylates can induce metabolic acidosis resulting in hyperventilation and tinnitus or hearing loss. Acetaminophen toxicity can occur when higher than recommended doses are taken, and heavy use of alcohol and acetaminophen are particularly apt to cause liver damage. Some relatively innocuous substances found in most homes can also be dangerous. For example, nutmeg is a powerful hallucinogen if taken in large doses, and most flavoring extracts like vanilla contain 35% ethanol. Cough syrups may not only contain codeine, but may also contain relatively high amounts of ethanol.

■ *Drug Use Among Minorities*

Although it is difficult to obtain reliable data on drug abuse in any population segment, studies have been done that suggest that drug-related morbidity and mortality in blacks, Hispanics, and Native Americans are greater than among whites. For example, survey results have revealed that drug use within households is generally higher in urban areas than in suburban or rural areas. Since minorities are more likely to reside in inner-city areas, they may be at greater risk for drug abuse as well as for the negative social and health consequences associated with drug abuse. Blacks constitute 11.5% of the total population, but they constitute 22.5% of the population of the inner cities.[6]

Recent data indicates that blacks have higher rates of drug use than whites for marijuana, cocaine, heroin, and illicit methadone. Minorities also seem more likely than nonminorities to be involved with more dangerous drugs and with more dangerous combinations of drugs. For example, 31% of black clients in drug treatment programs reported problems with heroin, cocaine, or PCP. That percentage means that blacks outnumber whites 3:1 in addiction to heroin, cocaine, and PCP.

Between 1982 and 1984, medical examination data showed that cocaine-related deaths among blacks tripled, while they doubled among whites. The percentage of drug-related deaths due to PCP alone or in combination with other drugs increased in blacks from 50% in 1983 to 58% in 1984. Other data sources indicated that blacks were somewhat more likely than whites to have used more dangerous routes of cocaine administration, such as injection, smoking, or free-basing.[6]

Hispanics constitute a greater proportion of inner-city dwellers than do blacks, and they also have an increased risk of drug abuse and its consequences. In addition to heroin, cocaine and PCP, Hispanics reported widespread use of inhalants. Between 1982 and 1984, cocaine-related deaths among Hispanics tripled while they doubled for whites. A 1981–1982 New York Police Department study of drug-related homicides found that 34.2% involved Hispanic victims.[6]

Data on drug abuse by Native Americans is scarce, but it appears that they are twice as likely to be in treatment for a drug-abuse related problem than are whites. Use of inhalation drugs such as solvents is reported to be significantly higher for Native Americans than for their white cohorts.[6]

■ *Drug Abuse Among High School Students*

Survey findings conducted in the last few years suggest that the overall illicit drug use among high school students is declining slowly from the peak levels attained in the 1970s, but the United States still has the highest reported drug abuse rates in the industrialized world.[3] Use of illicit drugs was down to 32% in 1983 from 39% in 1979. Much of this decline is attributed to a drop in the most popular of illicit drugs, marijuana. Among the other drugs that showed the greatest declines in use were amphetamines, methaqualone, and lysergic acid diethylamide (LSD). Additionally, the annual prevalence of barbiturate use in 1983 was 5%, which was less than half of what it was in 1975 (11%).[5]

But not all drugs showed a decline in 1983. Inhalant use has remained fairly stable since the 1970s, and heroin, of which the annual prevalence among high school students stands at 0.6%, has not changed appreciably. Nearly all young people have at least tried alcohol by the end of their senior year in high school, and the great majority have used it in the previous month. The rate of occasional binge drinking rose from 37% in 1975 to 41% in 1979 and has risen in years since.[5]

The use of cocaine more than doubled between 1975 and 1979 and then leveled off in 1980 and 1981 at 12%. The prevalence rates in both 1982 and 1983 were 11% among high school students, suggesting that the period of dramatic increase is over. However, it has also been found that cocaine use continues to rise sharply in the years after high school. From a descriptive epidemiologic standpoint, it is interesting to note that the western and northwestern regions of the United States have cocaine use rates that are roughly twice those of the south and north central regions.[5]

Thus, although it appears that overall drug usage rates are declining for high school students, the following is still true:

1. Roughly two thirds of all American young people try an illicit drug before they finish high school.
2. Fully 40% of high school students have illicitly used drugs other than marijuana.
3. At least one out of 18 high school seniors is actively smoking marijuana on a daily basis, and fully 17% have done so for at least a month at some time in their lives.
4. About one out of 18 high school students is drinking alcohol daily, and 41% have had five or more drinks in a row at least once in the past 2 weeks.
5. Some 30% of high school students have smoked cigarettes in the prior month, a substantial proportion of whom are daily smokers, or soon will be.[5]

▮ *Prevention Strategies*

Multiple primary prevention strategies have been planned and implemented in an effort to lessen the chance that young persons would be willing to try licit and illicit drugs. One of these strategies was a media campaign staged in the 1960s and 1970s that attempted to impress upon the populace the harmful effects of drugs, but because some of these campaigns unrealistically exaggerated the effects of drugs, they actually created a credibility gap. As a result, a moratorium was imposed and special guidelines were established by the White House (Special Action Office for Abuse Prevention), which would guide the development of related campaigns and materials.[11]

A second primary prevention strategy aimed at reducing the incidence and prevalence of drug abuse was the development of drug information and education programs in the schools. These programs varied in quality, and in some instances, students actually seemed to have experienced an increased likelihood of drug usage after exposure to the drug education programs. It was subsequently suggested that "exposing children who have high anxiety levels regarding drugs to drug education programs may alleviate this anxiety and unwittingly promote drug abuse."[11]

A third approach to prevention was developed in the 1970s and evolved from humanistic educational techniques, which was also called the generic approach to abuse prevention. The idea behind the generic approach was to address the fact that students who tended to develop drug-related problems also tended to have low self-esteem, greater evidence of alienation from their parents and society, deficits in interpersonal skills, and negative attitudes toward authority. Thus, the generic prevention programs were designed to overcome some of the general problems of youth without focusing directly on drug use per se. Overall, research has shown that these programs have not been very effective in preventing drug-related behavior.[11]

Currently, there are some preventive approaches that show some promise of reducing the incidence of drug abuse. One of them, the macro approach, emphasizes a focus on the entire environment in which a child is living. One technique is a public information campaign that not only communicates the adverse effects of drugs in a straightforward way, but also utilizes what is known about the motivation for drug use. An example of this factual and straightforward information is shown in Figure 15-1.

Another promising approach to primary prevention involves positive peer pressure strategies. In this technique, youths are trained to resist the subtle or explicitly persuasive arguments that emanate from their peers or the media. With the use of positive peer role models, both in the classroom and on videotape, they have been able to promote the idea that saying "no" to a cigarette or any other drug is a socially acceptable and desirable thing to do. The results of this method of primary prevention have been promising and the National Institute on Drug Abuse has devoted a large portion of its research program and resources to determining both the efficacy and cost effectiveness of this approach. Of particular promise has been a method that combines school-based peer interventions with media programs targeted at prevention of substance abuse.[11]

Although at first one may not think so, there is a lot of evidence that indicates increasing prices for liquor (as in the instance of increasing taxes) results in a lower per capita consumption. One researcher in the area says that ". . . a doubling of U.S. federal liquor tax would reduce the nation's cirrhosis mortality rate by at least 20%."[12] In fact, research data have shown that even alcohol-dependent persons reduce their alcohol consumption when costs rise.[13] Likewise, a lack of physical accessibility and legal accessibility seemed to decrease consumption of alcohol.[8]

■ *Acquired Immune Deficiency Syndrome: The Drug Connection*

The transmission of the acquired immune deficiency syndrome (AIDS) virus is highly correlated with substance abuse and a history of sexual intercourse with multiple partners. In fact, intravenous (IV) drug abusers, both habitual and recreational, form the second largest risk

FIGURE 15-1
Symptoms of drug abuse. (Used with permission, Birmingham News, Sunday, November 16, 1986, p 5)

Symptoms of drug abuse

Legend:
- [•] Symptoms of abuse
- [*] Symptoms of withdrawal
- [•] Dangers of abuse
- [#] How taken

Drug	Drowsiness	Excitation & hyperactivity	Irritability & restlessness	Belligerence	Increased sweating	Euphoria	Depression	Hallucinations	Panic	Irrational behavior	Confusion	Talkativeness	Rambling speech	Slurred speech	Laughter	Tremor	Staggering	Impairment of coordination	Hyperactive reflexes	Depressed reflexes	Dizziness	Anxiety	Constricted pupils	Dilated pupils	Unusually bright shiny eyes	Inflamed eyes	Runny eyes and nose	Loss of appetite	Increased appetite	Insomnia	Distortion of space or time	Nausea and vomiting	Abdominal cramps	Diarrhea	Constipation	Physical dependence	Psychological dependence	Tolerance	Convulsions	Unconsciousness	Hepatitis	Psychosis	Death from withdrawal	Death from overdose	Possible chromosome damage	Orally	Injections	Sniffed	Smoked
Methamphetamine		•	•		•	•		•	•			•				•						•		•	•			•									•	•			•	•		•		#	#		
Other stimulants	•	•	•			•	•	•				•				•			•					•				•									•	•			•			•		#	#		
Barbiturates			*	•		•	•	*		•	•			•		*	•	•		•		*	•							*		*	*			•	•	•	•	•	•		•	•		#	#		
Other depressants			*	•		•	•	*		•	•		•	•	•	*	•	•		•		*		•						*		*	*			•	•	•			•			•		#	#		
Lysergic acid diethylamide (LSD)		•				•	•	•		•	•		•			•		•						•							•						•	•				•			•	#			
STP						•		•			•		•					•						•							•						•									#	#		
Phencyclidine (PCP)							•	•	•	•					•	•																					•				•					#	#		
Peyote		•	•			•	•	•					•							•	•	•		•													•	•			•					#	#		
Psilocybin		•				•	•						•								•	•		•							•						•	•			•					#	#		
Dimethyltryptamine (DMT)							•			•														•							•						•									#	#		
Morphine	•				*	•	•		•		•			•		*				•		*‡	•	*			*	•		*		*	*	*		•	•	•		•	•			•		#	#		
Heroin	•		*		*	•	•		•		•			•		*				•		*‡	•	*			*	•		*		*	*	*		•	•	•		•	•			•		#	#	#	
Codeine	•		*		*	•	•		•		•			•		*				•		*‡	•	*			*	•		*		*	*	*		•	•	•		•	•			•		#	#		
Hydromorphone	•		*		*	•	•		•		•			•		*				•		*‡	•	*			*	•		*		*	*	*		•	•	•		•	•			•		#	#		
Meperidine	•		*		*	•	•		•		•			•		*				•		*‡	•	*			*	•		*		*	*	*		•	•	•		•	•			•		#	#		
Methadone	•		*		*	•	•		•		•			•		*				•		*‡	•	•			*	•		*		*	*	*		•	•	•		•	•			•		#	#		
Exempt Preparations	•		•		•	•	•				•					*				•		*	•	•			*	•		*						•	•				•			•		#	#		
Cocaine	•	•	•			•	•					•			•				•					•				•									•							•		#	#	#	
Marijuana	•					•																				•			•		•						•									#			#
Amphetamines	•	•	•		•	•		•	•							•					•			•				•									•	•			•	•		•		#	#		

This chart indicates the most common symptoms of drug abuse. However, all of the signs are not always evident, nor are they the only ones that may occur. Any drug's reaction will usually depend on the person, his mood, the dosage of the drug and how the drug interacts with other drugs the abuser has taken and contaminants within the drug.

group for AIDS; and IV drug abusers form a direct link to two other increasing risk groups, heterosexual partners and subsequent off-spring.[14]

Because of the subculture to which many IV substance abusers belong and the many risks involved in obtaining drugs, drug users are frequently distrustful of outsiders. This distrust compounds the difficulties in delivering health education. Yet, in the absence of an effective vaccine or treatment for AIDS, health education remains the most effective means for halting the spread of the disease to uninfected individuals.

Intravenous drug users need to know how AIDS is transmitted, and they need some conception of their own vulnerability and how their behavior can be modified to prevent transmission of the virus. If individuals are already antibody-positive, they need to know how they can modify their behavior to decrease the chances that the virus will be transmitted to others, and they need to know how they can care for themselves to reduce the chances that their infected but asymptomatic state can be managed to lower the chance that they will develop the clinical disease. Finally, they need information on treatment or prevention breakthroughs and information on how and where they can be tested for the presence of the virus.

The research to date indicates that communication among IV drug users is oral rather than written or printed. Not only do many addicts have difficulties in reading and writing, they are weary of written documents since much of what they do is illegal. Additionally, the drug subculture often develops folklore belief systems that tend to downplay disruption of the IV drug users' activities and values.[14] Finally, it is important to realize that the risk of death was present in the life of the IV drug abuser long before the risk of AIDS. Dubious drug quality, informers, incarceration, and illness from malnutrition or disease are a few of the risks assumed by users, and for this reason, AIDS may not be particularly feared and motivation to change behaviors to prevent infection may be low.

Even though the occasional or recreational IV drug users may have little identity or membership in the drug subculture and may not share many of the characteristics of drug addicts, they are still at risk for AIDS and other communicable diseases since not only are many of the drugs immunosuppressive, but their use impairs judgment and perception. For example, individuals who are well-versed in techniques of safe sex may fail to practice these techniques when drug or alcohol impaired. It is also important to realize that drug subcultures and drug behaviors, even drug choices, vary from location to location. Even within any given city, drug behaviors may vary among different races or ethnic groups.

The point was made earlier that IV drug abusers are believed to constitute the greatest source of AIDS transmission to heterosexuals and unborn children. To reinforce that point, one group of researchers found that almost 80% of one large group of IV abusers reported that their primary sexual relationships were with people who did not inject drugs themselves. Additionally, each addict had an average of two children each, and a quarter of the patients indicated that they expected to have additional children.[14] For this reason, health education should include how IV drug users can protect their sexual partners and their potential children.

Guidelines for teaching risk reduction for AIDS and other communicable diseases are listed in Chapter 16. The comments that follow relate to specific techniques for educating IV drug addicts. First, in order to educate IV drug users, one must locate them. Some IV drug users can be reached through programs at drug treatment centers, jails, or prisons. However, in such environments, distrust of staff or even outsiders may be so great that any information given is suspect.[14] One method that has shown some success is having a rehabilitated ex-addict approach individuals within the "street culture." Although IV drug users do not usually invest time or energy in organized activities, one group has recently emerged that was set up by ex-users in New York City. The Association for Drug Abuse Prevention and Treatment has been organized to provide support services to both prevent AIDS and to provide support services to AIDS victims who are current or past IV drug users.

■ *Application to Community Health Nursing Practice*

The problem of substance abuse necessitates that the community health nurse base intervention strategies on all three levels of prevention. First, the community health nurse should be a visible part of a community-wide program to prevent and monitor substance abuse. Although adolescents are most often the target population for community and school-wide educational campaigns, some effort should be directed toward the adult and aging in the population. As people age and acquire chronic conditions that are partly managed by medicinal, diet, and exercise regimens, they need to be taught how to maximize the therapeutic effect of prescribed drugs while minimizing unwanted side effects.

Primary prevention modalities relative to substance abuse are of paramount importance because avoiding intake of drugs is the only way to effectively avoid associated physiologic and psychologic effects. Yet, as pointed out earlier in this chapter, various educational strategies aimed at preventing substance abuse have not proven to be as effective as one might hope. More research is needed to enable health professionals to understand more clearly the numerous factors that initiate and sustain substance abuse behaviors. Further, existing and proposed educational programs must be carefully planned and evaluated as to cost benefit and overall effectiveness.

Secondary prevention activities related to substance abuse involve early diagnosis and treatment and disability limitation or case finding and referral within the context of the community health nursing practice. For purposes of referral for treatment of substance abuse, whether the substance is tobacco, alcohol, prescription drugs, or street drugs, it is imperative that the community health nurse have a working knowledge of community resources that include drug treatment programs and support groups like Alcoholic's Anonymous. Treatment programs vary in length, cost, philosophy and treatment modalities, so what may be right for one client may not be appropriate for another.

Tertiary prevention for the substance abusers equates with efforts to keep the clients free of drugs and efforts aimed at helping them to mobilize personal and social support resources to live life to their maximum potential. Often there is a need for individual and/or family counseling or psychotherapy, as well as vocational counseling. Familial and friendship relations that may have been disrupted during the period of substance abuse must be reestablished or resolved because when needs for acceptance, support and love are met, the rehabilitation process is apt to be more successful.

Summary

Whatever the reason, contemporary Americans seek detachment from reality and physical or emotional solace in drugs ranging from tobacco to heroin. This behavior is not particular to one age range, social class or race. Although the rate of drug abuse, especially of illicit substances, is higher in some parts of the country, drug use is a problem that affects people to some degree wherever they live. The physiologic effects of most drugs in use are known, and their effects on individuals, families, and communities can be roughly quantified. Even the human motivations that prompt people to try any drug for the first or subsequent time are beginning to be revealed. We are even beginning to evaluate various public educational programs in realistic terms by asking, how well do they work?

There is no question that hundreds of millions of dollars could be saved every year in human productivity, health care costs, crime, and other social deficits if the drug problem could be diminished or eradicated. Now it is a challenge to people in public health to realize this miracle without negating anybody's constitutional rights.

Some progress has been made. In 1961, it was "cool" to smoke cigarettes. In the 1970s, it was "hip" to experiment with other drugs. Now, heading into the 1990s, the word is that it is "OK to say no."

1. Public Health Service, Office of Disease Prevention and Health Promotion: Public Health Service Implementation Plans for Attaining the Objectives for the Nation. Public Health Rep 98(5)Suppl, 1983
2. Cohen S: The Substance Abuse Problems. New York, Haworth Press, 1981
3. Alcohol and Other Drug Abuse Among Adolescents. Stat Bull Metrop Insur Co, 65(1):4–13, 1984
4. Levison PK, Gerstein DR, Maloff DR: Commonalities in Substance Abuse and Habitual Behavior, p 9. Lexington, MA, Lexington Books, 1983
5. Johnston LD, O'Malley PM, Bachman JG: Drugs and American High School Students 1975–1983, U.S. Department of Health and Human Services Pub No (ADM) 85-1372. Rockville, MD, National Institute on Drug Abuse, 1984
6. U.S. Department of Health and Human Services: Report of the Secretary's Task Force on Black and Minority Health, Vol I, 1985
7. Centers for Disease Control: Cigarette Smoking Among Public High School Students—Rhode Island. MMWR 35(32):505–507, 1986
8. Ranking JG, Ashley MJ: Alcohol-related health problems and their prevention. In Last JM (ed): Maxcy–Rosenau Public Health and Preventive Medicine, 12th ed, pp 1039–1073. Norwalk, CT, Appleton-Century-Crofts, 1986
9. Barbour JA: Price of Drugs Low Compared to High Cost of User Dependency. The Birmingham News, p 2J, November 16, 1986
10. Cohen S: The Substance Abuse Problems, Vol II: New Issues for the 1980s. New York, Haworth Press, 1985
11. Durell J, Bukoski W: Preventing substance abuse: The state of the art. Public Health Rep 99(1):23–31, 1984
12. Cook PJ: Alcohol taxes as a public health measure. Br J Addict 77:245–250, 1982
13. Mello N: Behavioral studies of alcoholism. In Kissin B, Begeiter H (eds): The Biology of Alcoholism, Vol II: Physiology and Behavior, pp 219–291. New York, Plenum Publishers, 1972
14. Friedman SR, Des Javlais DC, Southeran JL: AIDS health education for intravenous drug users. Health Educ Q 13(4):383–393, 1986

Current Communicable Disease Problems

LEARNING OBJECTIVES

After reading and understanding the contents of this chapter, the student will be able to:

1. *Explain why communicable and infectious diseases are of major concern in contemporary community health nursing practice.*

2. *Describe the morbidity and mortality associated with infectious disease phenomena in the United States.*

3. *Rank the incidence of reportable and non-reportable communicable diseases in the United States.*

4. *Critique the guidelines for home care guidelines for persons with AIDS.*

5. *Elaborate public education strategies aimed at preventing transmission of the AIDS virus.*

6. *Assess the role of the community health nurse in prevention, control, and surveillance of infectious diseases.*

7. *Discuss the public health education guidelines relative to risk reduction for AIDS.*

Introduction

*T*here are at least three reasons why communicable and infectious diseases continue to be a major concern for community health nurses as well as the larger health care community. First, new diseases like acquired immune deficiency syndrome (AIDS) and new disease agents like cytomegalovirus (CMV) continue to emerge periodically. Second, nosocomial or hospital-acquired infections and the related phenomena of antibiotic abuse and drug resistant organisms will continue to be a problem in the 1990s and beyond. Third, vaccine-preventable diseases still cause significant morbidity and mortality in the United States and worldwide.

In addition, communicable diseases affect our economy in terms of lost productivity and health care expenditures. For example, the cost of treating persons with AIDS was estimated at $45.6 billion by the end of 1986.[1] Additionally, acute respiratory syndromes, such as the common cold, are the most common human illnesses and one of the most frequent reasons for seeing a physician. In 1979, it was estimated that approximately 156 million workdays were lost annually at a cost of $24 billion as a result of infectious diseases.[2]

Even though pneumonia and influenza are the only infectious diseases cited among the ten leading causes of death in this country, more than 290 million infectious illnesses occur annually—and that means more than one illness per person per year. It has already been pointed out that these diseases are costly. They also compromise the quality of life for Americans.[3]

As noted before, the only communicable diseases that ranked among the top five causes of death in 1978 were pneumonia and influenza. In 1979, chronic obstructive pulmonary disease replaced pneumonia as the fifth leading cause of death in the United States. Depending on how the data are viewed and how inclusive the topic is, a different picture can be obtained.

> Three million people in the United States, and over 150 million people in the world are still admitted to hospitals each year with infections. In the United States, the death rate from all infectious diseases is 123 per 100,000 persons, making them the number 3 killer after heart disease and cancer.[4]

In the preceding excerpt, Lappe is counting not only the deaths that occur from infectious or communicable diseases in the community, but also the deaths that occur during the course of hospitalization. These nosocomial or hospital-acquired infections may be occurring at a rate of as many as 4 million per year in the United States. Studies have shown that about 1% of all nosocomial infections, or about

30,000, contribute directly to the death of the host (Table 16-1). Another 3.6%, or 90,000 nosocomial infections, contribute to the death of
the host each year.[5]

As can be seen in Table 16-1, the total number of deaths attributed to infectious diseases in the representative year of 1983 was
92,549. That figure makes infectious and communicable phenomena
the fourth leading killer in the United States for 1983 since the third
leading cause was accidents, which accounted for 105,718 deaths.[6]
Additionally, it should be noted that the data in Table 16-1 are under-
counts in that the total figure for infectious diseases would be 152,549
if nosocomial infections that *contributed* to death were counted. One
can also understand that deaths attributable to AIDS would certainly
inflate annual counts of deaths due to infectious diseases since 1981.

Tables 16-1 through 16-3 help to visualize the impact of communicable diseases in this country. It should be noted that the seven
communicable diseases with the highest incidence are those diseases
for which there is no active immunization, except hepatitis B and tuberculosis. However, tuberculosis vaccine is rarely used in the United
States.

■ *The New Communicable Diseases*

Some of today's most prevalent communicable diseases are ones that
have not been recognized until the past few decades. Diseases such
as sexually transmitted chlamydial infections, genital herpes, legionnaires' disease, Reye's syndrome, toxic shock syndrome, Delta Hepa-

T A B L E   1 6 - 1
Number of Deaths in the United States Attributable to
Infectious/Communicable Diseases, 1983

Cause of Death	Number of Deaths
Specific notifiable communicable disease	3,592
Fungal infections	892
Respiratory infections	56,771
Miscellaneous infectious processes*	1,394
Nosocomial infections	30,000–90,000†
Total	92,549–152,549

*Miscellaneous infectious processes include herpes, meningitis (excluding meningococcal
and tuberculosis), mononucleosis, streptococcal sore throat, scarlet fever, and toxoplasmosis.

†Nosocomial infections *contributed* to 90,000 deaths. Nosocomial infection was the direct
cause of 30,000 deaths.

(Data compiled from Centers for Disease Control, Annual Summary, MMWR, 1984)

T A B L E   1 6 - 2
Incidence of Notifiable Communicable Disease: United States, 1984*

Disease	Number of Cases Reported
Gonorrhea	878,556
Chickenpox	190,894
Syphilis (all stages)	69,888
Hepatitis (all types)	52,026
Salmonellosis (excluding typhoid fever)	40,861
Tuberculosis	22,255
Shigellosis	17,371
Measles (rubeola)	2,587
Mumps	3,021
Aseptic meningitis	8,326
Total	1,283,950

*These data do not include estimates of the common cold nor do they include pneumonia and influenza, which are not mandatorily reportable diseases.

(Data compiled from Centers for Disease Control, MMWA, September 17, 1985)

T A B L E   1 6 - 3
Deaths from Specified Notifiable Diseases: United States, 1983

Cause of Death	Number of Deaths Reported in 1983
Tuberculosis (all forms)	1,937
Hepatitis (all forms)	862
Meningococcal infections	459
Encephalitis	164
Syphilis	136
Total	3,558

titis, and AIDS may have been present in the world for an unknown period of time, but it is only in recent years that they have impacted on the population of the United States.

■ *Chlamydia Infections*

Infections caused by *Chlamydia trachomatis* are currently recognized as the most prevalent of all the sexually transmitted diseases (STDs). An estimated 3 to 4 million Americans of both sexes contract Chlamydia infections each year, and the disease may be transmitted to adults and to newborns. In newborns, the infant is infected by way of the birth canal, and the disease is manifested by either conjunctivitis or pneumonia. In adult males, Chlamydia presents as urethritis and in females as mucopurulent cervicitis, or the disease may be relatively asymptomatic. But even when Chlamydia is asymptomatic in females, the scarring of the fallopian tubes can result in ectopic pregnancy or involuntary infertility.[7]

The Centers for Disease Control (CDC) reported that *C. trachomatis* causes approximately 50% of all the reported cases of nongonococcal urethritis (NGU) among men as well as 50% the cases of acute epididmyitis seen each year in the United States. In women, it causes mucopurulent cervicitis, acute pelvic inflammatory disease, and maternal and infant infections during and following pregnancy. In fact, Chlamydia accounts for one quarter to one half of the million recognized cases of pelvic inflammatory disease in this country each year. Additionally, every year in the United States, an estimated 155,000 infants are born to Chlamydia-infected mothers. These newborns are at high risk of developing inclusion conjunctivitis and pneumonia, and are at slightly elevated risk of developing otitis media and bronchiolitis.[7]

Each year, more than $1 billion in direct and indirect costs are expended on these infections in the United States alone, and that cost does not reflect the human suffering. Because there are hundreds of thousands of persons who are either asymptomatic or go untreated, transmission of Chlamydia infections is expected to accelerate in the short run.[7]

The host variables associated with *C. trachomatis* infection are age, number of sex partners, socioeconomic status, and sexual preference. Genital infection is inversely related to age and positively correlated with the number of sex partners. For example, sexually active women less than 29 years of age have chlamydial infection rates 2 to 3 times higher than for those over 30 years of age. Similarly, the rates of urethral infection among teenage males are higher than those for adults. Risk of infection increases with the number of sex partners, and in some studies, lower socioeconomic status and ethnicity have been correlated with an increased risk of chlamydial infections. The prevalence of urethral chlamydial infections among homosexual men is approximately one third of that among heterosexual men, but 4% to 8% of homosexual men seen in STD clinics have had rectal chlamydial infections.[7]

Not only are a large number of chlamydial infections asymptomatic, but they often coexist with other STDs such as gonorrhea. Women who have STDs, such as trichomoniasis and bacterial vaginosis, are also at increased risk of having a coexistent chlamydial infection. Although it is not currently known whether intrauterine devices influence the rate of *C. trachomatis* infection, it is known that people who use barrier forms of contraception, such as condoms or diaphragms, are at decreased risk of chlamydial infection. In contrast, women who use oral contraceptives have been reported to have higher prevalence rates of cervical infections than those who do not use oral contraceptives.[7]

Progress has been made relative to antigen and antibody formation tests for Chlamydia, and cultures and serologic diagnostic tests have improved, but are not yet highly reliable and cost effective. Publications like CDC's Weekly Morbidity and Mortality Report should be consulted for advancements in this area. A review of the other communicable diseases shown in Table 16-4 will follow.

■ *Genital Herpes*

Herpes simplex virus type II (HSV-2) usually produces genital herpes, but herpes simplex virus type 1 (HSV-1) has also been implicated in genital infections too. It is believed that the increase in oral–genital sex is presumed responsible for changing this etiology. In fact, epidemiologists are speculating that HSV-1 and HSV-2 may someday be isolated with about the same frequency from genital lesions.[8]

Genital herpes occurs primarily in adults and is sexually transmitted. Both primary and recurrent infections occur, with or without symptoms. Primary genital herpes infection is more common in adolescents and young adults of lower socioeconomic groups. Recurrent infections may occur at any age as a response to ultraviolet light, x-ray, heat, cold, hormonal imbalance, immunosuppressed status, or emotional disturbances.[8]

Vaginal delivery of pregnant women with active genital infections carries with it a risk of infection to the newborn, causing disseminated visceral infection, encephalitis, and even death. It is also

T A B L E   1 6 - 4
The Incidence of Selected Communicable Diseases in the United States, 1984

Disease	Number of Cases Reported
Chlamydia	3–4 million*
Genital herpes	500,000*
Legionnaires' disease	750
Reye's syndrome	190
Toxic shock syndrome	482
Delta hepatitis	7,834
Kawasaki's disease	†
AIDS	4,445

*Estimates, exact figures not stated in Annual Summary
†Unavailable

thought that genital infection with HSV-2 in adult women may be a risk factor in cancer of the cervix.[9]

The community health nurse should know that direct contact with lesions produced by HSV-1 or HSV-2 can cause a herpetic paronychia (Herpetic Whitlow) which can be painful and can be complicated by systemic symptoms such as acute membranous pharyngitis.[9] Secretion of the virus in the saliva of infected persons may last as long as 7 weeks after recovery from stomatitis. Persons with primary lesions are infective for about 7 to 12 days. "Asymptomatic oral as well as genital infections, with transient viral shedding, are probably common."[9] Reactivation of genital herpes may occur repeatedly in up to 50% or more of women following primary infection, and reactivation of the disease may be asymptomatic, but will nonetheless result in more viral shedding. Whenever there is viral shedding, transmission is possible.

■ *Legionellosis and Pontiac Fever*

Legionellosis is not really new at all since an earlier documented case occurred in 1947, and an earlier outbreak was in 1957 in Minnesota. But it was the outbreak in 1976 in Philadelphia that led to the initial identification of the causative organism, *Legionella pneumophila.* The two clinical syndromes associated with this organism are legionnaire's disease and Pontiac fever. Both of these diseases are initially characterized by anorexia, malaise, myalgia, and headache followed by rising fever associated with chills and nonproductive cough. In legionnaires' disease, patchy lung consolidation may progress to bilateral involvement and ultimately to respiratory failure. The overall case fatality rate has approached 15% in hospitalized cases and can even be higher in persons with compromised immunity. Pontiac fever is not associated with pneumonia or death, and clients usually recover spontaneously in 2 to 5 days without treatment.[9]

Legionellosis occurs in other countries as well as in the United States, and although sporadic cases are distributed throughout the year, both sporadic cases and outbreak clusters are recognized more commonly in the summer and autumn. The disease is rarely seen in persons under 20 years of age, in individuals who smoke, and in the immunocompromised. No person-to-person transmission has been documented, and the infected client apparently poses no risk to those in the immediate environment.[8]

■ *Reye's Syndrome*

Reye's syndrome was first described in Australia in 1963 as a type of acute encephalopathy of children. In the ensuing years, it was found that the syndrome is actually a multiorgan system disease that can also occur in older persons. The onset of the syndrome is usually preceded by a respiratory viral syndrome. Interest in Reye's syndrome has been generally heightened by the recognition that use of salicylates has been associated with the sometime rapidly fulminating course of the disorder.[8]

In reality, Reye's syndrome may not be an infectious disease per se, but it occurs universally after viral infections ranging from upper respiratory infection to varicella and gastroenteritis. In this respect, an infectious agent may be synergistic rather than causal.[8]

Even though this disease has been temporally associated with salicylates, it is important to educate clients that acetaminophen can be more toxic to infants and young children when recommended doses are exceeded. It may also be that salicylates are degraded more slowly in young children than in adults. Whatever the case, it is interesting to note that Reye's syndrome has been reported in the absence of salicylate ingestion. Besides salicylates, numerous environmental factors including insecticides and other chemicals have been suspected of playing a role in disease causation.[8]

Reye's syndrome appears to be worldwide and occurs with equal frequencies in both sexes. Even though most cases occur during times of increased influenza activity, sporadic and family outbreaks also occur. The syndrome occurs most often in Caucasians and individuals from urban, lower socioeconomic groups. Although Reye's syndrome had a mortality rate of 80% in 1963, early diagnosis and treatment have reduced that rate to approximately 20% to 40%. Even with aggressive and appropriate therapy, some survivors sustain permanent neurologic damage as evidenced by mental retardation, spasticity, or epileptic-type seizures.[8]

■ *Toxic Shock Syndrome*

First recognized as a distinct entity in 1977, toxic shock syndrome (TSS) became more prevalent in 1980 when almost 900 cases were reported in the United States. Caused by *Staphylococcus aureus* possessing the TSS antigen, TSS has been reported in children with focal staphylococcal skin infections, but it primarily occurs in young women during menstruation or postpartum. Menstrual TSS can be almost entirely avoided by not using vaginal tampons, and the risk can be reduced by using tampons intermittently during the menstrual cycle. Women who experience high fever and vomiting or diarrhea during menses should discontinue tampon use and consult a health care provider.[9] (See previous discussion of this epidemic in Chapter 11.)

■ *Delta Hepatitis*

Delta hepatitis occurs worldwide epidemically or endemically in populations at risk of acquiring hepatitis B infection, including hemophiliacs, drug addicts, others who come into frequent contact with blood, and to some extent, homosexuals. Prevention of hepatitis B virus infection will prevent infection with the delta agent, but among hepatitis B carriers, avoidance of exposure to any potential source of the delta agent is the only effective measure. None of the passive or active vaccines used to prevent hepatitis B is useful in protecting hepatitis B carriers from exposure to the delta agent.[9] At present, there are no products available that would prevent delta infection after infection with hepatitis B.

The delta virus, also known as hepatitis D virus or HDV, is a defective virus that causes infection only in the presence of active hepatitis B infection. Infection may occur as either coinfection with hepatitis B or as a super infection of a hepatitis B carrier. The subsequent disease may be self-limiting or it may progress to chronic hepatitis or fulminant hepatitis.[10]

Delta hepatitis has been found to be present in 20% to 30% of cases of chronic hepatitis B and in acute exacerbation of chronic hepatitis B.[11] Delta hepatitis is endemic to the Mediterranean basin and on the East and West coasts of the United States. On both coasts of the United States, there has been a reported 3% to 12% prevalence of delta hepatitis antigen in prospective blood donors with the serum hepatitis B surface antigen, and that is the highest percentage recorded to date in any population.[12]

■ Kawasaki Syndrome

Kawasaki syndrome was first recognized as a clinical entity in 1967 among 50 Japanese children. Sometimes called mucocutaneous lymph node syndrome, the disease was initially thought to be rare, benign, and self-limiting. However, cases have been reported with increasing frequency both in Japan and in other countries. It was first recognized in the United States in 1971, and more than 25,000 cases have been seen in this country since that time. Overall, there is a 1% to 2% case fatality rate, which is most often associated with sudden death or coronary artery aneurysms.[8] Like Reye's syndrome, the causative agent is unknown, but antecedent viral respiratory illnesses and exposure to mites have both been noted. The mode of transmission is also unknown, but the extant epidemiologic data shows little evidence of person-to-person transmission.[9]

■ Acquired Immunodeficiency Syndrome

AIDS, more than other new disease, is a complex and deadly phenomenon that has already demonstrated variability in its natural history. In fact, it is extremely challenging to make statements about AIDS that will be accurate or even relevant 1 or more years hence. Currently, it is believed that cases of AIDS in the Western world are caused by a new retrovirus, human immunodeficiency virus (HIV) and that the incidence of the disease is doubling roughly every 6 months.

The following questions remained unanswered as of late 1986. What is the absolute range of the incubation period? What variables predict which antibody-positive persons will actually develop the clinical disease? What role does the AIDS-related syndrome, lymphadenopathy, play in the natural history of AIDS? Why do some victims develop Kaposi's sarcoma and other malignancies while others do not? And exactly what role does HIV play in disease causation, and what role (if any) do excretions/secretions like saliva and tears play in the transmission of the disease?

Among the things that are known for certain about AIDS is the way in which it affects the immune system and the fact that is has a very high case fatality rate. We are told that for now, AIDS is a public health problem whose incidence must be slowed by educational campaigns that will serve to disrupt or modify what are believed to be the two primary practices that allow transmission of the virus: intravenous drug abuse and sexual contact. Drug addicts are not only being bombarded with the message that sharing needles is extremely hazardous, but they are also being given sterile needle and syringe units on request in many parts of the country.

Sexual abstinence is not a marketable notion, and thus various guidelines for safe sexual practices have been compiled and are being distributed whenever and wherever local social and political systems allow. An example of such guidelines designed for a universal audience—that is, homosexuals, heterosexuals, men, and women—may be found in Appendix B.

Because the lives of persons with AIDS will potentially be extended through the use of various pharmacotherapeutic substances, it is anticipated that the course of the disease will necessitate periodic hospitalizations as well as long periods of home health care. The CDC has already issued infection control guidelines for the hospitalized person with AIDS, but in the absence of similar directives for home care, infection control guidelines for home care of infected individuals are shown in Appendix C.

As noted in Chapter 15, in the absence of an effective vaccine or specific treatment for AIDS, public health education is the only means by which spread of infection can be prevented. In essence, public health education should be focused on the following points:[13]

Time has proven that some behaviors are harder to modify by any means, including health education, than others. Certainly, it seems reasonable to assume that the two behaviors most closely associated with the transmission of AIDS, sexual behavior and drug abuse behavior, are the hardest of all social behaviors to modify. Because drug and sexual behaviors are ingrained, the following principles for AIDS risk reduction are offered.[13]

Focus of Public Health Information

1. Encourage gay or bisexual men to reduce the number of their sex partners and simultaneously adopt safe sex practices.
2. Dissuade intravenous (IV) drug abusers from sharing needles.
3. Encourage women who are at risk, either by virtue of their own behavior or that of their sexual partners, to seek prenatal screening and to consider postponing pregnancy.
4. Provide adequate counseling to those who seek AIDS antibody testing on the meaning of both positive and negative test results and on the methods that prevent the transmission of the virus.
5. Continue to assure the public that AIDS is not transmitted by casual contact.
6. Encourage all sexually active individuals to be mutually monogamous or to adhere to safe sex practices.

Principles for AIDS Risk Reduction

1. Avoid communicating in a moralistic fashion.
2. Realize that the whole AIDS phenomenon evokes tremendous anxiety, and attempt to develop strategies that acknowledge this stress as well as means for coping with the stress.
3. Utilize existing research findings to ensure that messages reflect existing knowledge, values, attitudes, beliefs, and practices of the specific target population.
4. Be explicit about the often complex and obscure relationship between specific behaviors and likely subsequent health or disease outcomes.
5. When possible, emphasize not only what to do, but also the precise circumstances under which the behavior is to be carried out, the benefits of doing so, and the consequences of failing to do so.
6. Realistically acknowledge the obstacles to change, and build in supports and reinforcements for adopting new behaviors.
7. Without whitewashing the difficulties, establish a positive tone in which fear-arousing information is balanced by constructive suggestions for purposeful action.
8. Strive to characterize the desired behavior as socially desirable by modeling appropriate role models and associating the target behavior with other behavior or qualities that are considered desirable by the target audience.
9. Develop strategies that are likely to engender identification between the target audience and the message.
10. Deliver a clear, coordinated, consistent message or cluster of messages through a variety of reinforcing channels of communication.
11. Seek out individuals who can provide access to the audience and who add credibility to the intended message.

In the light of the newly discovered communicable diseases like the ones discussed here, and others like Lassa fever and Lyme arthritis, the following question is posed even though only time and intensive research can hope to provide an answer. Does evolving technology and its effects on lifestyles encourage the development of new dis-

T A B L E   1 6 - 5
Communicable Diseases and Vaccine Availability

Box 1	Box 2
Communicable Diseases for Which Active Immunization is Available	**Communicable Diseases for Which There is Passive Immunization**
Adenovirus (types 4 and 7)	Botulism (but administration carries with it a great danger of sensitivity reaction)
Anthrax	hepatitis type A (ISG)*
Botulism	Measles (rubeola) (ISG)
Cholera (vaccine has only limited value)	Mumps
Cytomegalovirus (experimental attenuated CMV vaccines under evaluation)	Rubella (ISG)
Diphtheria	Smallpox
Haemophilus influenza (Type B)	Tetanus
Hepatitis B	Varicella-zoster virus infection
Influenza	
Measles (rubeola)	
Meningitis (caused by *Neisseria meningitidis*)	
Mumps	
Pertussis	
Plague	
Pneumococcal infections	
Polio	
Rabies	
Rocky Mountain spotted fever	
Rubella	
Salmonellosis (typhoid immunization afford protection in approximately 70% to 90% of subjects)	
Smallpox	
Tetanus	
Trachoma conjunctivitis (temporary and limited protection study)	
Tuberculosis (BCG effectiveness discussed later in this chapter)	
Tularemia	
Typhus	
Yellow fever	

*Immune serum globulin

eases, or are we simply noticing such events because we have the technology with which to detect and evaluate new diseases?

Even though the contemporary arsenal of vaccines that can effectively induce active immunity numbers about 27 (Box 1, Table 16-5), only seven are recommended for routine use (trivalent oral poliovirus

---

Box 3

Communicable Diseases for Which There is No Active or Passive Immunization Available

Actinomycosis
All arboviruses except yellow fever
Amebiasis caused by *Escherichia* history
Ascariasis (roundworm infection)
Aspergillosis
Balantidiasis
Blastomycosis
Brucellosis (undulant fever)
Candidiasis (moniliasis, thrush)
Cat-bite fever
Cat-scratch disease
Chlamydial infections
Coccidioidomycosis
Clostridium perfringens (food poisoning)
Coxsackievirus
Cryptococcosis
Echoviruses
Enterobiasis (pinworm infection)
Erythema infectiosum
Escherichia coli diarrhea
Gas gangrene
Genital herpes
Giardiasis
Gonococcal infections
Hemorrhagic fever
Herpes virus hominis (simplex infections)
HistoplasmosisImpetigo
Larva migrans
Leprosy
Leptospirosis

Lymphocytic choriomeningitis
Listeriosis
Lymphocytosis
Malaria
Molluscum contagiosum
Mononucleosis
Mycoplasma pneumoniae infections
Otitis media
Parainfluenza virus infections
Pediculosis
Psittacosis
Primary amebic meningoencephalitis
Rhinovirus infections
Rickettsialpox
Roseola infantum
Scabies
Schistosomiasis
Shigellosis
Staphylococcal infections
Streptococcal infections (including pharyngitis, scarlet fever, and erysipelas)
Syphilis
Tapeworm disease
Tinea capitis, corporis, cruris, pedis
Toxoplasmosis
Trichinosis
Viral gastroenteritis

vaccine, measles, mumps and rubella vaccine, and diphtheria, pertussis and tetanus vaccine). The remaining vaccines are not recommended for routine use except for high-risk individuals because the diseases are generally rare and therefore the chance of exposure is low in this country (Table 16-5).

Summary

Times of economic prosperity and scientific advancement have long been associated with greater sexual freedom. Starting roughly in the economic prosperity of the 1950s, greater sexual promiscuity resulted in increases of all the STDs. Not only did the rates of gonorrhea and syphilis rise, but HSV-2 mutated form HSV-1 to become the major cause of genital herpes.

Promiscuous heterosexual intercourse has traditionally resulted in two major physical manifestations: conception and transmission of STDs and other communicable infections. The simultaneous development of effective methods of contraception served to minimize conception, and indirectly, to make sex a more acceptable form of recreation. Homosexuality has played a unique role in the transmission of STDs and other communicable infections. The simultaneous development of effective methods of contraception served to minimize conception, and indirectly, to make sex a more acceptable form of recreation. Homosexuality has played a unique role in the transmission of STDs because homosexuals as a group have more sex partners than heterosexuals, and their sex practices, like anal intercourse, provide multiple opportunities to transmit microorganisms such as shigella, hepatitis B, human cytomegalovirus and HIV.[8]

■ *Immunization*

Immunizations against communicable diseases have resulted in a marked reduction the tool of some infectious diseases that were previously responsible for substantial morbidity and mortality. For example, smallpox has been eliminated worldwide. In addition, while 29,000 cases of polio were reported in 1955 in the United States, through the routine administration of polio vaccine, the number was reduced to eight cases by 1975.

On the other hand, failure to enforce (or to comply with) recommended immunizations such as measles has resulted in a seesaw of annual measles incidence. For example, 385,000 cases of measles were reported in 1963 when the vaccine became available, and by 1968, the incidence fell to 22,000 cases. However, only 3 years later, the count was back up to 75,000 cases. Rates fell but began to jump again by 1976 and 1977. Those jumps in measles rates were not the result of the failed vaccine. They were the result of decreasing immunization levels in populations at risk for the disease.[14]

Because new vaccines are occasionally added and others are improved or overall immunization recommendations change, the community health nurse is urged to consult up-to-date publications, such as the American Academy of Pediatric's *Red Book* before administering routine or special immunizations. Additionally, the package literature should be consulted to ascertain the recommended route of administration, nature and extent of side effects, and information on the proper storage of the vaccine. Although most vaccines for adult use are given either subcutaneously or intramuscularly, the intradermal route may be used for some like typhoid boosters.[15]

Judicious use of smallpox vaccine (vaccinia virus) has eradicated smallpox as of May, 1980. Smallpox inoculation is now only indicated for either certain civilian laboratory workers or members of the military service. The exact reason that some military personnel are vaccinated every 5 years for smallpox is unknown, but it is possibly related to the thought that some opposing force at some point in the future may decide to include the smallpox virus in their arsenal of biologic agents used for germ warfare. In 1986, new guidelines were formulated for military personnel that should act to decrease the incidence of vaccinia.

Misuse or use of smallpox vaccine has been associated with sporadic instances of contact spread of vaccinia. For example, one instance was reported early in 1985 in which a 15-year-old female was referred to a dermatologist in Wisconsin for evaluation of an ulcerated lesion on her left upper lip. The client reportedly appeared mildly ill, had a low-grade fever, complained of fatigue, and had mildly enlarged and tender cervical lymphadenopathy. She was otherwise in good health, with no history of eczema, malignancy, or immunologic deficiency. By history, the client had a friend who had received a smallpox vaccination the last of December as a part of his tour of duty at a United States Army facility. Earlier in January, she had applied compresses to her friend's arm to ease the discomfort of the area surrounding his smallpox inoculation. She was subsequently treated with vaccinia immune globulin (VIG) intramuscularly over 2 days as well as topical antibiotic ointments. Her lesion ultimately healed without scarring.[16]

Fortunately, instances such as the one described above are rare, but the potential for additional cases exists as long as military personnel continue to be immunized. The preferred treatment is VIG, and this can be obtained by calling (404) 329-3145 during the day and (404) 329-2887 evenings and weekends. The community health nurse should understand that such person-to-person spread can be extremely dangerous if the person infected has eczema or is immunocompromised.

There is no evidence that smallpox vaccination has any value in the treatment or prevention of herpes infections, warts, or any other disease. Therefore, the CDC recommends that this vaccine never be used and, in fact, it is no longer available for civilian use for any reason.[17]

■ *Immunization Under Special Circumstances*

Recommendations for immunization under special circumstances are shown in Tables 16-6 and 16-7.

■ *Some Words About Passive Immunization*

In passive immunity, protection is given to the host by inoculation with antibodies derived from another host. The immunity is effective almost immediately and persists for a few weeks before it disappears. There are three types of passive immunity: transplacental immunity,

T A B L E 1 6 - 6
*Vaccines and Toxoids Indicated or Specifically Contraindicated for Special Health Status Situations**

Health Situations	Vaccines or Toxoids	
	Indicated	*Contraindicated*
Pregnancy	Diphtheria and tetanus toxoids (TD)	Live-virus vaccines
Immunocompromised	Influenza Pneumococcal polysaccharide	Live-virus vaccines
Splenic dysfunction, anatomic asplenia	Influenza Pneumococcal polysaccharide	
Hemodialysis	Hepatitis B (double dose) Influenza Pneumococcal polysaccharide	
Deficiencies of factors VIII or IX	Hepatitis B	
Chronic alcoholism	Pneumococcal polysaccharide	
Diabetes and other high-risk diseases	Influenza Pneumococcal polysaccharide	

NOTE: Refer to CDC recommendations on specific vaccines or toxoids for details on indications, contraindications, precautions, dosages, side effects and adverse reactions, and special considerations.

*Unless specifically contraindicated, the vaccines and toxoids generally recommended for adults are indicated.

(Center for Disease Control: Adult Immunization: Recommendations of the Immunization Practices Advisory Committee (ACIP). MMWR 33(18)Supplement:September 28, 1984)

natural passive immunity, and artificial passive immunity. In transplacental immunity, IgG antibodies are transferred from the mother. Since the baby plays no active part in the process, its range of immunity is dependent on the variety of antibodies in the mother's blood.

T A B L E   1 6 - 7
*Immunobiologics Recommended for Special Occupations, Lifestyles, Environmental Circumstances, Travel, Foreign Students, Immigrants, and Refugees**

Indication	Immunobiologic(s)
Occupation	
Hospital, laboratory, and other health care personnel	Hepatitis B Polio Influenza
Staff of institutions for the mentally retarded	Hepatitis B
Veterinarians and animal handlers	Rabies
Selected field workers	Plague
Lifestyles	
Homosexual males	Hepatitis B
Illicit drug users	Hepatitis B
Environmental situation	
Inmates of long-term correctional facilities	Hepatitis B
Residents of institutions for the mentally retarded	Hepatitis B
Travel	Measles Rubella Polio Yellow fever Hepatitis B Rabies Meningococcal polysaccharide Typhoid Cholera Plague Immune globulin
Foreign students, immigrants and refugees	Measles Rubella Diphtheria Tetanus

NOTE: Refer to CDC recommendations on specific vaccines or toxoids for use by specific risk groups, details on indicahions, contraindications, precautions, dosages, side effects and adverse reactions, and special considerations.

*Unless specifically contraindicated, the vaccine or toxoids generally recommended for adults are indicated. (Centers for Disease Control. September 28, 1984)

This is an important point because even though there is transplacental immunity against measles, the child will be born susceptible. To carry the point further, there are still instances of congenital tetanus in infants who are born to mothers not immunized against tetanus. Such phenomena occur with some frequency in underdeveloped nations.

Communicable diseases to which infants often receive natural passive immunity are mumps and diphtheria. Infants receive questionable amounts of immunity to pertussis regardless of the mother's immunity: 40% of all fatalities in the United States attributable to pertussis occur in the first year of life. Natural passive immunity to chickenpox is not thought to occur at all, in fact, infection with chickenpox virus is frequently devastating during the first year of life.

In addition to acquiring natural passive immunity, infants may also acquire disease at birth through (1) infected amniotic fluid; (2) the maternal bloodstream; or (3) direct contact with infected maternal tissue in the birth canal. Specifically, syphilis, occasionally *Listeria monocytogenes*, and less frequently, tuberculosis are acquired through the placenta.[18]

In artificial passive immunity, protection is prompted by administering antibodies obtained from the same or a different species. Antibodies obtained from an immune member of the same species seldom causes severe reactions. An example of antibodies obtained from the same species is immune serum globulin (human) (ISG).

▋ *Animal Serums*

The risk of serum sickness or severe reaction is increased when human hosts receive antibodies produced by active immunization in a different species. Tetanus and rabies serums, formerly produced in animals, are now produced in humans, making them much safer to administer. In the following four types of immunization, animal serum continues to be used: (1) diphtheria, botulism, and gas gangrene; (2) tetanus and rabies exposure when special human gamma globulin is unavailable; (3) snake and spider bites; and (4) disorders in which immunosuppression with antilymphocyte serum is indicated.[19]

Animal serums are avoided unless definitely indicated. Hence, a careful history must be taken before sensitivity testing takes place relative to asthma, hay fever, urticaria, and previous injections of animal serums. This history is followed by sensitivity tests that are administered with necessary equipment and personnel present to recognize and treat adverse reactions. For further information relative to sensitivity testing for serum reactions, the pharmacological information packaged along with these substances should be checked.

■ *Immune Serum Globulins*

ISG produces passive immunity and is an antibody-rich fraction of pooled plasma from normal donors. The advantages of ISG over plasma administration include (1) freedom from hepatitis viruses; (2) concentration of the antibodies into a small volume for intramuscular use; and (3) stable antibody content if properly stored.[19]

ISG has occasional side effects, and for this reason its use is generally limited to disorders in which its efficacy has been established. Currently, there are only four disorders in which the value of ISG is clearly recommended: (1) measles prophylaxis or modification; (2) viral hepatitis type A, or HAV, prophylaxis or modification; (3) viral hepatitis type B, HBV, prophylaxis when hepatitis B virus immune globulin is indicated but not available; and (4) antibody deficiency disease.[19]

There are several other disorders in which the use of ISG may be helpful, but the benefit is not clearly established. One instance in which the value of ISG is highly debatable is related to its use in preventing rubella in the first trimester of pregnancy. It is important to remember that ISG does not actually prevent the occurrence of disease but rather alters or modifies its clinical course.

Special human ISGs are derived from the blood of individuals hyperimmunized or convalescing from specific infections. Because these preparations contain a higher concentration of antibodies to specific microbial agents than do ordinary ISGs, they are helpful in several disorders in which ISG is of no value.

■ *Antibiotic Resistance*

Simply put, "resistance to an antimicrobial (or antibiotic) means that the bacteria are not inhibited by concentrations of the drug that can be achieved in patients."[20] Although many erroneously believe that the use of antibiotics caused various microorganisms to be drug resistant, antibiotic-resistant genes and plasmids were a part of the physiology of the germ cell before antibiotics were discovered; the antibiotic merely serves to create the conditions which favor the overgrowth of preexisting antibiotic-resistant organisms.

Acquired resistance to antibiotics has one important consequence: the client may not get a drug to which the infecting organism is sensitive resulting in treatment failure. This situation can be avoided by conducting a culture and sensitivity before starting antibiotics.

The first evidence of penicillin resistance by *Neisseria gonorrheae* was demonstrated as early as the 1950s. Such strains have been reported subsequently in all parts of the world, but some still respond to higher doses of penicillin, which is given in combination with probenecid. Resistance to other antibiotics, including erythromycin, streptomycin, tetracycline, and chloramphenicol, has been reported also. By 1976 the same highly resistant strains have been reported in numerous parts of the world.[21]

Another common communicable disease, tuberculosis, has demonstrated a capacity for drug resistance in recent years also. For instance, in 1984, there was a documented outbreak of drug-resistant tuberculosis in a group of homeless individuals in Boston. These infected individuals did not respond to treatment with isoniazid and streptomycin, but did ultimately respond with clinical improvement after rifampin was added to the regimen.[22]

In addition to gonorrhea and tuberculosis, a partial list of organisms known to be antibiotic resistant appears below.

Salmonella
Hemophilus
Neisseria gonorrheae
Enterobacteriaceae
Pseudomonas
Staphylococcus aureus
Serratia marcescens

What can be done to combat these resistant strains? First, it is important to appropriately isolate and effectively treat people known to be infected with resistant strains. It is also important to detect carriers or those with subclinical infections with resistant strains. Meticulous initial case finding and then follow-up are essential when people with infections are located. Unfortunately, in many countries of the world, antibiotics may be obtained without a prescription, and this is believed to account for the high rate of chloramphenicol resistance in populations of such countries. It would be helpful if worldwide agreement could be reached on the principles of antibiotic usage. For instance, antibiotics important for treating human infections should be excluded from animal feeds. Antibiotics are excluded from animal feeds in Great Britain but similar legislation has not yet been passed in the United States. Also, no disease should be treated with antibiotics unless positively indicated by clinical and laboratory data. Even tropical gentamicin should be avoided if possible because pathogens such as *Pseudomonas aeruginosa* may acquire resistance in its presence. In essence, every animal or person taking an antibiotic (therapeutically or subtherapeutically) becomes a factory-producing resistant strain of microorganism.[23]

Finally, the principles of control and spread of resistant organisms, which are similar to those of any communicable disease, must be followed (*i.e.*, good surveillance, rapid detection, isolation of infected patients, good hygiene including handwashing, treatment of carrier, and possibly contacts of cases and carriers). Additionally, someday there may be a worldwide antibiotic policy.

▪ *Nosocomial Infections*

As previously defined, infections that are not present or incubating at the time of admission to a care facility are called nosocomial. They concern community health nurses for two reasons. First, the role of the infection control nurse (ICN) is a specialty role whose knowledge base incorporates nursing and public health sciences. The ICN's role has been discussed in Chapter 13.

The second reason community health nurses should be concerned about nosocomial infections is because these infections can occur in any care setting including long-term care facilities and the client's home. Additionally, the client who succumbs to nosocomial infection while hospitalized may require careful discharge planning and follow-up care after discharge.

About 6% of all hospitalized persons contract nosocomial infections, and the rate is probably greater in long-term or extended care facilities. The actual rate varies with the type of institution, being higher in university-based or teaching hospitals, and slightly lower in smaller community level hospitals.

Every year in this country, over 8 million extra hospital days are required to care for persons with nosocomial infections at a cost of $4 billion. As stated earlier in this chapter, nosocomial infections contribute directly to 30,000 deaths and indirectly to another 90,000 deaths every year.[24]

Effective infection control programs, of which the ICN is an integral part, have the potential to reduce nosocomial infection rates by 32%. In contrast, hospitals with incomplete programs or insufficient numbers of ICNs increase infection rates by 18% in the same time period.[24] Thus, it could be said that infection control has scientifically demonstrated its worth, and new models and principles of cost effectiveness are being tested with promising results. It was the Joint Commission for Accreditation of Hospitals that mandated hospital infection control programs in the mid-1970s. How soon similar programs will be required for other types of care facilities such as home health is difficult to predict. But because acquired infections have significant legal, quality care, and economic ramifications, some of these agencies are already involved in surveillance and documentation efforts.

■ *Application to Community Health Nursing Practice*

Communicable and infectious disease phenomena have been in the past, and will continue to be in the future, a significant component of community health nursing practice. Because practice is often located in a wide range of community settings, unique opportunities for case finding, prevention, control, and surveillance of communicable diseases exist for the community health nurse who is well-versed in a variety of public health sciences and innovative nursing strategies.

The picture of communicable diseases in distributive settings is different from what is seen within the hospital because only the most acute or life-threatening conditions are managed in the hospital. Hospitalized individuals are comparatively passive and captive recipients of care, whereas the community health nurse most often deals with ambulatory individuals who are occupied with the activities of daily living and are neither passive nor captive-care recipients.

Practice geared toward prevention, surveillance, and control of communicable diseases in the community necessarily utilizes strategies based on all three levels of prevention. Primary prevention strategies include enforcement of immunization schedules, teaching responsible and safe sex and personal hygiene practices and aseptic principles, such as those related to self-injection of insulin. Additionally, the community health nurse must realize that these primary prevention strategies can only be effective if they are made accessible to and perceived as valuable by the target population. Another primary prevention consideration of prime public health importance is maintenance of safe food and water supplies as well as effective disposal of waste. The latter is of prime importance during natural disasters like floods, or in the instance of toxic chemical waste.

Secondary prevention strategies include case finding and surveillance that, in turn, foster early diagnosis, treatment, and disability limitation. First, the community health nurse should be familiar with the magnitude of endemic levels of various communicable disease phenomena in the community of service for several reasons. For example, how does the population served rate as to the incidence and prevalence of STDs, communicable diseases of childhood like chickenpox and pediculosis, as well as the rarer and more lethal entities such as botulism, tetanus, and hepatitis? It is only by knowing usual or endemic levels that the clinician is able to identify potential epidemic phenomena.

Other activities related to early diagnosis and treatment of infected clients within the context of primary prevention include the monitoring of persons known to be infected with diseases like tuberculosis, hepatitis, and AIDS. For example, persons with chronic hepatitis must be monitored until they can be determined noninfectious.

Persons who have AIDS or who are infected with the AIDS virus must be followed with the dual purpose of maintaining client health and family well-being while simultaneously taking measures to prevent transmission of the AIDS virus. Additionally, in the course of the practice day, community health nurses should be case finding or identifying persons at high risk of infections like AIDS or tuberculosis so that they may be referred for screening and treatment.

Disability limitation strategies are also utilized in the form of teaching family members how to care for persons who are acutely ill with various viral or bacterial-based illnesses. Especially when symptoms, such as fever and diarrhea, involve the very young or the very old, family members should be taught methods for rehydrating the client and monitoring them for signs of physiologic stress that would require prompt referral to a health care provider. Parents should also be carefully counseled as to the expected and untoward effects of routine and special immunizations. Additionally, families should be encouraged to develop an ongoing relationship with care providers, such as physicians and nurse practitioners, so that when emergencies occur, access to treatment is facilitated.

Although the vast majority of nursing interventions with regard to infectious and communicable diseases relate to primary and secondary prevention strategies, tertiary prevention-based interventions come into play when the illness is terminal or when irreversible physiologic or psychosocial changes occur as a result of the disease process. When caring for persons with a terminal disease such as AIDS, tertiary prevention-based nursing interventions revolve around maximizing individual potential to cope with the interval preceding but culminating in death. When possible, family members and/or significant others should be included in the overall plan of care for the person with AIDS.

Another example of tertiary prevention involves maximal rehabilitation of the client who has sustained irreversible physiological or psychosocial damage during the clinical course of an infectious disease. For example, when deafness or other sensory or intellectual deficit occurs as the result of encephalomyelitis, community health nursing interventions focus on maximizing remaining potential for health realization and successful placement of the client within the family and community.

Summary

*A*s we have seen, communicable diseases contribute significantly to the morbidity and mortality of people all over the world. Community health nurses are in a unique position to prevent the occurrence and spread of these maladies as well as to act as case finders and caregivers whenever they occur. Guidelines for safe sex are found in Appendix B.

References

1. Volberding P, Abrams, D: Clinical care and research in AIDS. Hastings Cent Rep, pp 16–18, August, 1985
2. Public Health Service: Healthy People: The Surgeon General's Report on Health Promotion and Disease Prevention, DHEW Pub No (PHS) 79-55071. Washington, DC, Government Printing Office, 1979
3. Public Health Service, Office of Disease Prevention and Health Promotion: Public Health Service Implementation Plan for Attaining the Objectives for the Nation. Public Health Rep 98(5)Suppl:97, 1983
4. Lappe M: Germs That Won't Die: Medical Consequences of the Misuse of Antibiotics. Garden City, NY, Anchor Press, 1982
5. Haley RW, Culver DH, White JW, Morgan WM, Emeri TG: The nationwide nosocomial infection rate: A need for new vital statistics. Am J Infect Control 121(2):159–167, 1985
6. National Center for Health Statistics: Vital Statistics of the United States, 1983, Vol II: Mortality, Part B, DHHS Pub No (PHS) 85-1102. Washington, DC, Government Printing Office, 1986
7. Centers for Disease Control: *Chlamydia trachomatis* Infections: Policy Guidelines for Prevention and Control. MMWR 34(3S)Suppl:53S–74S, 1985
8. Berquist LM: Changing Patterns of Infectious Disease. Philadelphia, Lea & Febiger, 1984
9. Benenson AS (ed): Control of Communicable Diseases in Man, 14th ed. Washington, DC, American Public Health Association, 1985
10. Centers for Disease Control: Recommendations for Protection Against Viral Hepatitis, 34(22):313–335, 1985
11. Nishioka NS, Dienstag JL: Delta hepatitis: A new scourge? N Engl J Med 312(23):1515–1516, 1985
12. Rosina F, Saracco G, Rizetto M: Risk of post-transfusion infection with the hepatitis delta virus. N Engl J Med 312923):1488–1491, 1985
13. Fettner AG, Check WA: The Truth About AIDS: Evolution of an Epidemic. New York, Henry Holt and Co, 1985
14. Public Health Service, National Center for Health Statistics DHHS Pub No (PHS) 83-1232. Hyattsville, MD, 1982
15. Committee on Immunizations: Guide for Adult Immunization, 1st ed. Philadelphia, American College of Physicians, 1985
16. Centers for Disease Control: Contact Spread of Vaccinia from a National Guard Vacinee—Wisconsin. MMWR 34(13):182–183, 1985
17. Centers for Disease Control: Smallpox Vaccine. MMWR 34(23):341–342, 1985

18. Korones SB, Lancaster J: High-Risk Newborn Infants: The Basis for Intensive Care Nursing. St Louis, CV Mosby, 1976
19. Report of the Committee on Infectious Diseases, 20th ed. Evanston, IL, American Academy of Pediatrics, 1986
20. Guiney DG: Resistance to antimicrobial drugs. In Braude AI, Davis CE, Fierer J (eds): Infectious Diseases and Medical Microbiology, p 210. Philadelphia, WB Saunders, 1986
21. Centers for Disease Control: Tetracycline-Resistant *Neisseria gonorrhoeae*—Georgia, Pennsylvania, New Hampshire. MMWR 34(37):563–564, 569–570, 1985
22. Centers for Disease Control: Drug-Resistant Tuberculosis Among the Homeless in Boston. MMWR 34(28):429–431, 1985
23. Levy SB: Playing antibiotic pool: Time to tally the score. N Engl J Med 310(10):663–664, 1984
24. Haley RW: Managing Hospital Infection Control for Cost-Effectiveness. Chicago, American Hospital Publishing, 1986

Community Health Nursing Services in a Changing Health Care System

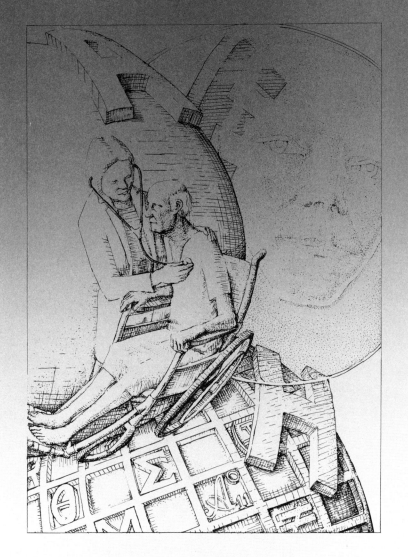

Epidemiology ensures that public health concepts are in full play during delivery of nursing services in the home. These concepts view any family in its community setting and assess the impact of the family's problems on the community at large.

Epidemiology, Health Policy, and Community Health Nursing

LEARNING OBJECTIVES

After reading and understanding the contents of this chapter, the student will be able to:

1. *Define political power, health policy, and politics.*

2. *Understand the influence of government on community health nursing care.*

3. *Apply the public health model to political action for community health.*

4. *Identify the type of epidemiologic research that is used to supply facts to assist health policy decisions.*

5. *Differentiate between health policy research and health services research.*

6. *Differentiate between logical and emotional appeals to groups as part of the political process.*

7. *Apply structure, process, and outcome to health policy analysis.*

8. *Identify the most influential committees in the government structure.*

Introduction

*H*ealth policy is a structured effort of organized groups, such as nursing, to influence government policy for health needs. Political power is defined by Rogge as the ability to influence government officials to use the power of their office to effect a desired outcome.[1] Nurses generally view politics and its associated activities as secondary to patient care; however, community health nursing has always been involved with health policy as part of the nursing process for intervention and planning for aggregates. Understanding the influence of government on community health and access to care is part of public health nursing care.

The public health model, based on Winslow's definition, underscores the reasons for the inevitable involvement and concern of community health nurses with political power, regardless of agency affiliation with the public or private sectors. In order to effect the major mandates of society for maternal and child care to preserve future generations, to control communicable disease, and to promote a safe environment for all, group action is necessary to influence political systems. The implementation of voluntary and government regulations is part of community health nursing. These include nursing home regulation and child and elder abuse affecting health. Government must be influenced to assure that laws and regulations support appropriate community action for health care aimed at prevention and control of disease and disabilities. Families must be protected through outreach programs and constant surveillance of the community, but this is made difficult and sometimes impossible unless it has the force and power of law. Many facets of public health nurses' practice are directly involved in the explanation of state and federal rules and legislation that influence care to the indigent and to the elderly. Home health care is impeded by regulations and policies that apply to an outmoded system of episodic care. Change can only be effective if it is influenced by health professionals and nursing, in particular, so that family needs can be met. Clinical nursing care in the community is directly affected by national and local health policies, which affect access to nursing care. For this reason care of the aged and home health will be discussed in this section as health policy issues.

Vice President Hubert Humphrey is quoted as saying that the moral test of government is how it treats those who are in the dawn of life, its children; those who are in the twilight of life, its aged; and those who are in the shadow of life, its sick, its needy, and its handicapped. A government that can neither educate its children, care and sustain its elderly, nor provide hope and meet the needs of its infirmed sick, its poor, and its disabled, is a government without compassion.[2] In the community, public health nursing has traditionally provided services for the disabled, the indigent, the aged, and the sick at home. Health policy and government decisions affect access to care, funding, and the ability to deliver services, which are part of community health nursing responsibilities.

▌ *Defining Health Policy*

Understanding health policy is as important as understanding research, becoming clinically proficient, and monitoring the quality of nursing care, especially to the community health nurse.[3] Organizing nursing for political action is often effective when it represents groups of nurses such as the National League for Nursing (NLN), the American Organization of Nurse Executives (AONE), the American Association of Colleges of Nursing (AACN), and the American Nursing Association (ANA), the labor union of nursing. These four nursing organizations form a quadriga of political power that seeks to influence the ebb and flow of debate and the outcome in national and state legislatures. The study of health policy is a most important instrument for identifying and prioritizing problems, directing epidemiologic research for nursing, and influencing the decisions which affect the economics of health care in society. Community health nursing is uniquely informed about the way the health care system works, where it fails, and how it can be changed to become more effective for health care delivery. The understanding of how new groups are formed and how they are influenced is basic to effective practice in communities. The epidemiologic perspective, by seeking to quantify and observe group phenomena, provides valuable information concerning political issues.

Definitions of health care policy are myriad. This has much to do with the fact that health policy is procedural and depends on the type of problem for activating its process. Epidemiology, a method-oriented science, is similar in this respect, for it too has multiple definitions. In the same way, health policy has many ways of expressing its character. Some, like Diers, say that health policy is the study of why things happen or health policy is the study of decision making (for health concerns).[4] McGivern says that public policy is the philosophically dictated course of action taken by government.[5] It is easy to add "for health care" to define health policy where "public" is understood to apply to communities. To influence the philosophy that shapes action requires a basic knowledge of community needs and a thorough knowledge of clinical issues.

A policy process has been identified by Sister Donley—one which incorporates the nursing process into its six steps.[6] The steps or methods Donley recommends to effect public policy for health care are extended and adapted to read as follows:

1. The identification of the policy issue
2. The development of the issue, its history, and current status
3. The formulation of goals
4. The involvement of the legislative process
5. The implementation of the legislation process
6. The evaluation of the results

This health policy method follows some of the basic steps of assessment, diagnosis, plan, implementation, and evaluation in the nursing process.

In applying the method, it is important to distinguish between policy and politics. Policy is the goal mentioned in the method; politics is the implementation process. Policy is the objectives that must be clearly understood if the goal is to be achieved: politics is the negotiations required to accomplish the goal. Goals or policy is a function of values and ethics. The goals of health policy are the public good, the prevention and control of disease for the safety of society, and the attainment of quality health services in communities. These goals or policies are compatible with the concepts underlying public health philosophy in the public health model and reflect the values and ethics of community health nursing.

Politics is a quite different matter from policy. Politics is the bargaining process, the arguments pro and con. Politics is the identification of influential allies—all the pull and tug that effects the system to achieve the goals. It is the process incorporated into the public policy methodology and applies to the involvement of the legislature to implement the objectives or policies. Politics is the use of power or influence to achieve identified goals. Success is dependent on considerable political skills, an extensive knowledge of the community, and, importantly, clinical issues, as well as the mobilization of community support.

Knowledge of the community and knowledge of clinical issues is indispensable to the epidemiologic process, and the same knowledge base can be transformed to the political context with ease. The democratic ethos decides on relevant goals through consensus—a variant, if you will, of multidisciplinary approaches guiding epidemiology and public health. Community goals are a way of assuring the safety and protection for the majority of individuals and their families. The ethics and values of public health affect epidemiology as well as political decision making.

Private sector and government agencies are affected by public policies for health. Regulation may be voluntary or may be supported by local statutory laws or may become public laws at the federal level. The influence of accepted policies does not stop at the artificial boundaries of "public or private" domains. Voluntary standards and government laws interact in several ways. Private sector policies compete with federal initiatives. For instance the Diagnostically Related Groups, DRGs, were originally intended to apply only to the elderly population receiving federal reimbursement. This system of prospective payment for hospital and provider services has been adapted by private insurance carriers such as "the Blues," Blue Cross and Blue Shield, where reimbursement applies to all age groups. Another example of private sector initiatives influencing government policy is the Joint Committee on Hospital Accreditation's standards for quality of care, a voluntary program unsupported by tax dollars. This program is a paradigm for government action in this arena and affects policy at all levels.

■ *Epidemiology and Health Policy*

Epidemiology supplies facts to assist health policy decisions. It provides methods of estimating risk to justify the policies of private and government political bodies at several levels of need. Surveys or descriptive studies and prevalence studies help to define issues and prioritize needs. Etiologic studies analyze associations between health policies, costs, and effects on the community. Intervention or experimental epidemiology supplies facts to estimate the effects of regulation and laws on the delivery of care and the risk to health. This area of epidemiology is called health services research. The main focus of health services research is access, quality, and cost of care. In a previous chapter, we discussed an important role of epidemiology in evaluation of quality of care. Evaluation also applies to the effects of implementation of public policies on the health of the group. In short, health services research is important in the formulation of public policy.[7] It is used to strengthen the decision-making processes and to justify funding resources for health manpower and health programs. Health services research focuses on the organization, distribution, and delivery of health care. This includes access to care and the feasibility of delivery of services as well as the financing and cost of comparative systems. Health policy research is a subset or extension of health services research used to address policy issues at local, state, and national levels.

In the government systems, demonstration projects are used to estimate the effects of a delivery of an identified system or specific program before it is adopted to the broader population. Demonstrative projects have special attributes: they afford some feasibility of operation in applying the new program, which is not possible in the controlled conditions of experimental, etiologic, or descriptive epidemiologic design. HCFA, the Health Care Financing Administration, has funded several demonstrations for nursing care including the "channeling" project to maintain the frail elderly in their homes. In this project, costs of care remained the same as in nursing homes but quality of care measured by patient satisfaction increased. Demonstration allows the development of initiatives compatible with the major purpose of the project: adjustments to streamline the delivery of care can be made. When the hospice program was demonstrated at 26 sites to see if it was feasible to cover the services under the Medicare program, adaptations were possible on an ongoing basis. This is similar to the use of pilot research for nursing studies.[8] Government-funded demonstrations now require more effective evaluations: epidemiologic approaches to meet this requirement for scientific evaluation are most appropriate. Retrospective evaluation occurs after the fact and is considerably more difficult than an evaluation method that is part of the original proposal, mainly because of the difficulty in obtaining a control group.

Facts are supplied through epidemiologic research to justify policy. Without facts or with incomplete facts, arguments for change are suspect, and this lack of reliable data is used to discredit efforts to persuade the legislature and community of nursing goals. The role of statistics at local and federal levels contributes to the rational choices that depend on careful interpretation of quantified information.[9] Epidemiologic statistics make many things possible, including the development of logical programming, the planning of procedures, methods of recording data that apply to the administration of the community nursing agency, and evaluation of the results of public health nursing initiatives. In an era of computerization and rapid communication through electronics, statistics can be made accessible to all health departments and community agencies.

But facts alone are not enough. Groups are affected emotionally as well as intellectually. In the courts, plaintiffs suing for malpractice influence juries by showing the injured child and family in the courtroom in an attempt to evoke sympathy. The inclusion of chronic renal failure patients in the Medicare Act is a case in point. During government hearings in Washington, D.C., funds for renal dialysis patients were awarded from legislators who were greatly moved by family case histories reported by parents and spouses, especially when a needy patient entered Congress during the testimony. Other strategies that appeal to the emotions are targeted to altering the perceptions of the public. Influencing group decisions to engage their support is a major part of perceptual change. It demands control of the media to communicate relevant arguments and an understanding of any economic impact that might be used to persuade the group.

Interpretation of the facts is an important consideration when influencing public viewpoints. The evaluation of graphs, figures, ratios, and percentages are important factors affecting the perceptions of the communities, clients, and politicians. Community health nurses are in close contact with families and professional groups. Their interpretations of epidemiologic data must be factual but must also be politically astute. Apropos of meaningful interpretation, it is becoming increasingly necessary to define nursing and, in particular, public health nursing, so that the definitions can be operationalized and quantified not only for reimbursement for nursing care but also for optimal utilization of nursing skills, including epidemiologic approaches. The ANA social statement of what nursing is emphasizes the nursing diagnosis.[10] Implementation and evaluation of care is also needed to define and illustrate the effects of nursing care to legislators and power brokers.

Epidemiology is designed to evaluate services to groups. It gives credibility to community health nursing. Information collected epidemiologically has a database common to all public health workers and improves communication while providing a mutual basis for multidisciplinary actions. Epidemiology is a method of organizing observations in practice and utilizing clinical outcomes of care. Public policy is a process closely allied to ethics and is the ultimate goal of political process: epidemiology helps identify and justify those goals. Politics is the power to achieve goals to make change. Epidemiology provides scientific insights to assist the community health nurse in this process. Ultimately the goal is to protect the public and assure access to high quality, cost-effective community services.

■ *Epidemiologic Approach to Health Policy Analysis*

In order to apply nursing process and methods of analysis for health policy, it is necessary to know the system through which communities are organized and governed. It is essential to have some knowledge of political process and to be able to articulate goals that improve community care. An epidemiologic perspective on health policy uses the Donabedian and Sheps approach by dividing health services into structure, process, and outcome.[11,12] These concepts are equally as applicable to the political system in formulating health policy as they are in evaluating parameters of quality of care. Structure, then, is the organized system of government; process is the political actions undertaken to achieve the goal or outcome. The discussion, therefore, will review structure, process, and outcome in that order.

Structure

Knowing the committee structure of the body politic is essential to defining and prioritizing actions to influence the political process of politics. Government is divided into the executive, judicial, and legislative branches, as any American student learns early in their school experience. The role of government in American life has evolved over time through the interpretation of judges and the response of executive actions and legislative initiatives.[13] In this system, the executive branch has considerable influence that is exerted through its leadership. Chairman of committees and heads of agencies are appointed to positions of influence: the choice is an executive prerogative. It is supported by the highly powerful Office of Management and Budget. Committee assignments are made by seniority in the House and Senate, in the same proportion that makes up the representatives of the party membership in each chamber. While the judicial branch can only be influenced by executive support for the appointment of new members to the Supreme Court, the legislative branch is a committee system with which the executive branch must interact. The legislature writes federal laws, including the tax laws, appropriates money, and can impeach high executives. The veto of the President can be overridden by a two thirds majority in both houses. The President vetoed the formation of an Institute of Nursing, but an alternative plan was put into operation by forming a Center for Nursing Research whose director reports to the appointed head of the Department of Health and Human Services, along with other heads of institutes. The branches of government and their functions are outlined in Figure 17-1.

The committee system in the legislative branch is composed of about 16 committees in the Senate and approximately 32 committees in the House. Most work is completed in subcommittees. Full committees may elect to discuss a controversial issue; otherwise the subcommittees report their recommendations to their parent committee. Only when topics are seriously disputed do they enter the House and Senate for debate.[14] It is useful for community health nurses to know the most powerful committees for all topics including health issues. Their counterparts that exist at the state level and retain similar functions to the committees will be identified. In the Senate, the most influential committees are the Committee on Appropriations and the Committee on Finances. In the House of Representatives, the Committee on Appropriations and the Ways and Means Committee are

FIGURE 17-1
Structure of the U.S. government.

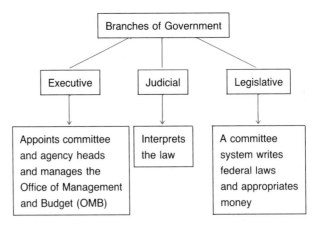

the two most powerful. It is not accidental that the powerful committees in both the House and the Senate control money!

The Appropriations Committee controls the flow of money authorized for programs by other committees. This means that a program for health services may be approved or authorized, but until the money to fund the program is "appropriated" or assigned, the services cannot be activated. The Finance Committee and Ways and Means Committee set the national budget and considers tax legislation—important considerations for public health programs nationwide (Fig. 17-2).

Committees and subcommittees deal with health issues in both Chambers of Congress. Of these influential committees, three in the House and three in the Senate control much of the legislative activities. In the House, the Committee on Appropriations and its subcommittee on labor, health, and human services and education distribute federal funds for individual health programs. The Energy and Commerce Committee and its subcommittee on health and the environment have jurisdiction over public health, health maintenance organizations, food and drugs, clean air, biomedical research, and other health-related responsibilities. The Ways and Means Committee has the power to tax and, in the past, has heavily influenced health financing regulations (Fig. 17-3).

Process

The process of politics is part of democratic government. Efforts of special interest groups like the quadriga in nursing (ANA, NLN, AACN, AONE) or public health are an inherent part of the political process: success depends on political skills. To apply process, the structure of the system must be familiar, and an extensive knowledge of the federal community, the state community, and the local community is imperative. Broad-based community support for a public health issue must be mobilized. Facts, particularly epidemiologic facts, must

Standing Committees

Senate
≙ 16 Committees

House of Representatives
≙ 22 Committees

Most Powerful Committees

Appropriations ......(control assignment ......Appropriations
Committee   of money)   Committee

Finance.........(authorizes expenditure)... Ways and Means
Committee   Committee

FIGURE 17-2 Structure of the committee system in the federal government.

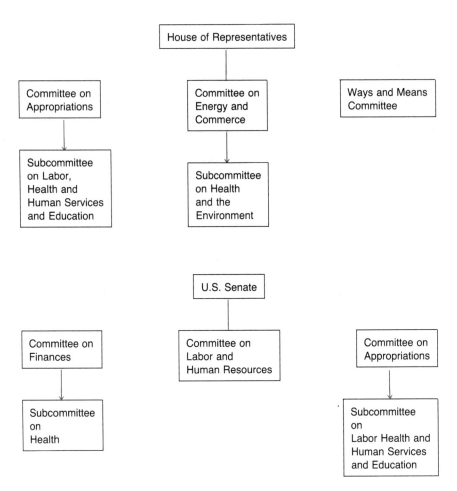

F I G U R E   1 7 - 3
Structure of the Senate and House of Representatives directly concerned with health policy.

be verified and interpreted. The committee structure of the government then can be approached with evidence that is presented clearly: persons of influence may exert their power to accomplish the goal to legislate the policy required. The methodologic steps to advance the identified cause can be applied systematically as part of the process.

Reliance on the rationality of the voters or the persuasiveness of scientific evidence, although appropriate, are seldom sufficient. The prestige of the health professions or the implausibility of the charges of the opposition are also factors that may be inconsequential; these strategies cannot be relied on to turn the tide of opinion towards the wanted objective. A group's power to influence legislation is a function of its finances, the astuteness of its representatives, and its political acumen, rather than the righteousness of its point of view. Political perspicacity includes being informed on the opinion of the health care providers and the opinion of the constituents of the representatives in power positions. It demands establishing working relationships with key committee members and staff and making sure the issues are stated clearly, preferably in written form, to share with relevant groups. This is process. It requires a system of communication between public health workers, lobbyists, and the legislature at all levels.

Outcome

The best justification for any political process for health policy is the public good, increased access to care, and cost-effective, high quality services. Estimates of many of these impeccable outcomes are to be found in effects such as reduction in rates of illness and disability, increased client/patient/community satisfaction, increased independence from the health care system, reduction in rates of recidivism, and so on. These outcomes are, of course, the same as those discussed in Chapter 10 for evaluation of quality of care. But for health policy, the outcomes may be more specific and circumscribed. The goal may be to pass a law to mandate the fluoridation of water. (This issue, by the way, is politically controversial despite scientific facts to support the beneficial effects of fluoride on dental caries.) The outcome may be the formation of an institute of nursing or the provision of "model cities" to fight housing inadequacy. The goal may be defensive; in other words, the aim might be to clarify government positions and/or controls. Whatever the objective, the outcome will be affected by how accurately it can be identified, in the same way that the accuracy of a hypothesis influences the process required to solve an epidemic problem.

The goal must be consistent with current values. The growth of government in health care in the United States has been accelerating, especially since 1935, when the Social Security Act was passed. It has been part of American tradition to value independence, to protect individual rights, and to rule by majority. Established authorities evoke suspicion; these values still affect health policies. In the 1980s, market forces through competition are part of current philosophy and affect all policy making. It is clear that outcomes are tempered by current mores.

■ *Case History in Health Policy*

To illustrate structure, process, and outcome, a well-known case history known as the Baby Doe and Baby Jane Doe legislation will be reviewed. The executive, judicial, and legislative branches of government became involved in the case. The outcome, the "policy", was a defensive goal; that is, health care providers challenged the right of government to determine health care practices in families. The goal included a request for a ruling on the right of government to impose its will in conflict with the individual family's wishes.[15] The Baby Doe case also raised the philosophical questions concerning the prolongation of life in circumstances in which there is suffering from grave illnesses that place a burden on the individual, the family, and society.

The case history began in Bloomington, Indiana where an infant was born with Down's syndrome (Trisomy 21). The baby, unfortunately, also had a detached esophagus. The parents, in consultation with health care providers, decided surgery to sustain life would subject the baby to further hardship and involve the extensive utilization of resources to support a disabled child. These arguments seemed most reasonable to the parents; unfortunately, the Reagan administration took exception.

Prompted by this case, the Department of Health and Human Services (DHHS) issued interim regulations in March, 1983 regarding the care of infants who were handicapped. Section 506 of the Rehabilitation Act of 1973 states that it is unlawful for hospitals receiving federal assistance to withhold life-sustaining treatment from disabled infants. DHHS required that a notice be posted in a conspicuous place in institutions stating that it was against the law to withhold life-sustaining measures. A hotline number for reporting suspected violations of the law was to be included on the poster.

Opposition was registered by numerous professions including the American Medical Association (AMA), the ANA, The American Academy of Pediatrics, the American College of Obstetricians and Gynecologists, and the Nurses' Association of the American College of Obstetrics and Gynecologists. This marked the first time in recent history that medical, nursing, and other professionals were united for a common cause. Together they argued that (1) the rules did not consider the opinions and judgment of the parents; (2) government was interfering with clinical practice; and (3) regulations were issued with only 15 days notice instead of the customary 30-day period. In a legal challenge spearheaded by the American Academy of Pediatrics, the United States District Court for the District of Columbia described the interim rules as "arbitrary and capricious." Margaret Heckler, at that time the Secretary of the DHHS, was criticized for not giving adequate hearing to debate the issue and to listen to the parents' evidence. This is political process.

At this time (November, 1983), a baby was born in Stonybrook, New York with spina bifida and hydrocephalus. This case was called the Baby Jane Doe to differentiate it from the first case. Further questions were raised. Was the withholding of life-sustaining treatment a discriminatory act? Could the government have access to medical records in cases of discrimination? Subsequently the DHHS was denied access to Baby Jane Doe's records on the grounds that the courts

upheld the position that no discrimination had occurred and, therefore, there was no violation.

The final regulations in January, 1984 included the following in-
junctions: notices were to be posted to warn providers of the need to
be alert in the withholding of lifesaving measures for disabled infants
unless death was inevitable; there was to be established a (voluntary)
Infant Care Review Committee (ICRI) and a hotline to be used after
either the ICRI or the State Child Protection Agency had been noti-
fied. The federal government was declared to be "the protector of the
last resort." This was, for the time being, the outcome.

Congress in 1984 amended the Child Abuse Act to include cases
where seriously handicapped infants were denied life-sustaining treatment. The Baby Doe provision included a detailed definition of "withholding medically indicated treatment" and instructed physicians,
nurses, and hospitals on when treatment should be provided. The
Act also required states to participate in child abuse programs and set
up methods to respond to reports of medical neglect.

Final regulations in April, 1985 were revised based on arguments
by the ANA, the AMA, and others that government should not further define "withholding of medically indicated treatment." The definitions were interpreted as "guidelines" without the binding force of
law. This legislation gave doctors and families the right to withhold
care, but their decisions were to be monitored by the government.
The states implemented their own programs. As critical and highly
technical care moves into the home environment, community health
nurses will be affected by these regulations and similar concerns for
quality care. Epidemiologic facts on the risk of death for seriously
handicapped children and costs of care in the family and community
were brought forth in the political arguments, but the case was fought
on the right-to-privacy issue regardless of estimates from group qualifications. The issue continues to be debated.

Summary

*H*ealth policy, or more strictly speaking, public health policy,
is a process of decision making to assure government's use of power
for health care needs. Politics differs from policy in that politics refers
to the negotiation used to persuade groups and alter their perceptions; policy is the goal that is the outcome of the political process.
Policy is a function of values and mores; politics is the skill required
to accomplish that goal. Using an epidemiologic perspective, the political system was analyzed according to structure, process, and outcome. The structure of the government committee system was reviewed with special emphasis on the influential committees for health
policy in both the Senate and the House of Representatives in Congress. Process was described as negotiation—a process heavily dependent on political skills. Outcome was the goal or policy that required

precise identification similar to epidemiologic hypothesis to guide process and planning. Public health nursing is based on a model requiring multidisciplinary efforts and consensus to prevent and control disease for the benefit of the public. Effective public health policy is a method of assuring access to care for communities' needs. Community health nurses have knowledge of clinical issues and familiarity with the community and group needs; hence, they always have been involved with health policy as a means of effecting change. For the communities they service, health policy is the study of political process and the philosophically detailed course of action taken by government. The political process is a method of problem solving akin to the nursing process but focused on the mobilization of the community to affect the legislature. Epidemiology supplies facts to assist health policy decisions. Through health services research, epidemiology assists in the discussion and resolution of political issues and problems. Epidemiology facilitates the development of problem-solving techniques, measuring risk for priority setting and evaluating the impact of new legislation and the withdrawal of old systems, as well as estimating the impact of cost-effective, high quality nursing care. The political process was exemplified through the Baby Doe legislation where the main outcome was to define government role in family/provider decision making. The Baby Doe legislation may heavily influence community health nursing in home care in the future.

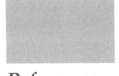

References

1. Rogge, MM: Nursing and Politics: A Forgotten Legacy. #15-1995 NLN. New York, 1986
2. Litman TJ: Robins LS: Health Politics, and Policy. New York, John Wiley & Sons, 1984
3. Maraldo PJ: The Importance of Policy in the Nursing Curriculum: Integrating Public Policy into the Curriculum, #15-1995 NLN. New York, 1986
4. Diers D: Policy and Politics: Implications for Curriculum #15-1995 NLN. New York, 1986
5. McGivern DO: Resources for Teaching Public Policy #15-1995 NLN New York, 1986
6. Donley RS: Teaching Public Policy #15-1995 NLN New York, 1986
7. Merrill JC, Sass MM, Somers SA: Health Services Research and the Formulation of Public Policy. Nurs Res 36(1):26–50, 1987
8. Chavigny KH: A comparison of pilot study and the main thesis on palpation of the pulse in acute cardiac patients. Int J Nurs Stud 10:10:229–238, 1973
9. Balius W Jr: The role of statistics in state health policy decisions: The Massachusetts experience. J Public Health Policy 7:1:12–20, 1986
10. Birkauskas V: Effectiveness of public health nurse visits to primiparous mothers and infants. Am J Public Health 73:5:573–580, 1983

11. Donabedian A: A guide to medical care administration. NY APHA 1965–1969

12. Sheps CG, Taylor EE: Needed Research in Health and Medical Care. University of North Carolina Press, 1954

13. Litman TJ: Government and health: the political aspects of health care—a sociopolitical overview. In Health Politics and Policy, p 3–40. New York, John Wiley & Sons, 1984

14. Grupenhuff JT: The Congress Turnover Rates of Members and Staff. Communications #1, Fall 1982

15. Roe CS: The Case Study Method NLN, New York #15-1995, 1986

Care of the Aged in the Community

LEARNING OBJECTIVES

After reading and understanding the contents of this chapter, the student will be able to:

1. *Define the usual meaning of elderly according to age stratum.*

2. *Understand the role of the community health nurse in allaying anxiety about access to care.*

3. *Apply understanding of Medicare to community health nursing role.*

4. *Define the impact of costs of care to elderly populations.*

5. *Define the areas of content covered by epidemiology research in health services and their role in assisting quality of care in the community.*

6. *Apply the predictors of longevity to nursing care of the elderly.*

Introduction

Nursing has always played a proportionately larger role in care of the elderly than any other discipline. Nursing has become so involved in looking after aged populations that the final intramural setting where aging people are cared for before death is called a nursing home; and yet the challenge of nursing geriatric patients has been, in large part, left to technical nurses rather than professional nurses. Examination of the demographics of aging shows that the population of the elderly is getting increasingly older as more and more people live longer. Nursing has a major responsibility to provide care to the aged that is cost effective and higher in quality than ever before.

As the proportion of elderly (65 years or more) increases, the costs of care for the elderly increases and is a source of anxiety for the aged. Usually this cost is borne by families and by the retired elderly. Eighty percent of all care is given by family members, usually spouses and daughters, and the caregivers in the home require the support and counseling of the community health nurse.[1] Frequently—much too frequently—the elderly are divested of their savings, and many are forced to enter the ranks of the indigent after a lifetime of independence. Many outlive their spouses and live out their lives homeless, lonely, and sick. This situation is not new, and many health care workers have been increasingly concerned as the proportion of aged in the community, estimated at 12%, continues to expand. The task of caring for the aged population has grown. The goals of public health have enabled the professions to promote lifetime wellness, to rehabilitate the stricken, and to provide care for the sick in the community. As the problem of an increasingly older population in the United States has become critical, the role of government in health care has changed the way the system provides for the elderly.

It is the purpose of this discussion to describe nursing care for the elderly in the context of the health policy of the United States. Medicare, a government system for paying for services to the aged, will be discussed so that the responsibilities of the staff nurse in community health care be delineated. Often it is the nurse who counsels the family for placement in nursing homes, who explains the system of health care subsidy, and who guides the family or the elderly person through the morass of bureaucratic paperwork. Epidemiologic perspectives provide insights into meeting elderly needs in the context of community resources and in estimating risk to the elderly. The epidemiology of aging will be outlined to predict future needs for the elderly and to explain the role of community health nurses in meeting these needs. The care of the elderly is also care of the chronically ill, but being chronically ill is not confined to the elderly. Epidemiologic studies have determined that 30% of the chronically ill are below 65 years of age. These problems will be addressed in the next chapter as part of home health care.

■ *Role of Government in Health Care*

In the United States, the role of the government for any reason except national defense has, traditionally, been discouraged. In the early days of the republic, the government had little to contribute to the health care system. As the population increased in America, the government role was highly constrained. In general, government intervention was limited to threats against the common good or the health of the public. In the early days, communicable disease control and environmental sanitation were state responsibilities even though there were no state health departments, and quarantine measures were restricted to controls regulated through port authorities.

It soon became evident that government intervention was necessary to protect society from common risks. Risks shared mutually by communities in the early days of the republic were risks from epidemics of communicable diseases. Thus it became policy to confine government protection of society to hazards perceived as affecting the nation. The care of the destitute was also a government responsibility; therefore, the government role in health care was described as paternalistic, custodial, and most of all, minimal.[2] The first major involvement of the government in health care was the Marine Hospital Service Act in 1798 to provide for sick and disabled seaman.[3] Later this Act was extended to include Indians held on reservations as wards of the state. It was the enactment of delivery of care to Indian populations that gave rise to the Indian Health Service. Regardless of these involvements, health care in America remained a highly personalized matter for most citizens through the 19th century.

In the 1920s, legislation began to be considered for health care services.[4] The Sheppard–Towner Act for Maternity and Infant Care tried, unsuccessfully at first, to establish grants-in-aid or money to assist funds generated at the state level. The target of grants-in-aid was to provide direct services for mothers and infants. This legislation was the forerunner of present-day maternal and child health programs.

When the federal government provides or supplements funds for state health departments, the principle of "state primacy" takes precedence over federal controls.[5] Under the First Amendment of the Constitution, the states have the broad authority to protect the health, safety, and general welfare of the public; however, federal subsidy gives privileges to the national government to make demands and control health care delivery for nursing care and other health care needs through awarding funds conditional upon compliance with federal regulations.[6] Intervention in the private lives of the citizenry for control of communicable diseases has been sustained by the courts in the face of challenge.

In 1935, the Social Security Act was passed. This historic event was a major milestone in health policy in the United States. For the first time, the government had important responsibilities *not* for health care but for income maintenance of the unemployed, the unemployable such as injured workers, the indigent, as well as the retired and the elderly.[7] The Social Security Act was not intended to be a health care measure. Originally its major focus was on maintaining income, not on maintaining the health of the society. The Act set up a public assistance or welfare program for those entirely without resources. A sizable proportion of those without financial support had become needy because poor health had used up their savings and income. Social Security is paid through a tax on all people employed in the workplace. Because of this ongoing replenishment of funds through the working population, the social security funds for retirement benefits remain viable. In fact, the money held to finance retirement is used by government as collateral against which funds can be borrowed.

The part of the Social Security Act that gave federal grants to the states for maternal and child care, crippled children, the blind, and Aid to Families with Dependent Children was based on rehabilitation concepts. Although many humanitarian reasons motivated the Act, the belief that sustained its passage through the legislature was that it returned the injured, the poor, and the needy to the work force. These were the arguments used in the political process to attain the goal (the policy) of increased governmental support and involvement.

In 1950, the Social Security Act was extended to include the permanently disabled and then, in 1960, the Kerr-Mills Act gave medical assistance to the elderly. In 1965, two amendments to the Social Security Act were called Titles XVIII and XIX. Title XVIII was Medicare, government-reimbursement for health care to the elderly. Title XIX was attached almost as an afterthought: this was Medicaid, or care for the poor, an extension of the Kerr-Mills Act. The real problem with Title XIX (Medicaid) was that the determination of eligibility was unclear and was left to the states. As a result, Title XVIII (Medicare) financing of health care to the elderly is a federal program and Medicaid, a welfare program to the indigent, is a state program; hence program administration changes from state to state. It depends on the states to solve broad social problems and invokes state supremacy or the right of the states to autonomy and decision making. The result is a great diversity of benefits and services between rich and poor states.

The cost of Medicaid was not considered at all in the amendment legislation in 1965. In contrast, the Medicare program administered through the Department of Health and Human Services was more explicit about methods of finances and eligibility requirements.

Its application was uniform and used private sector insurance programs as fiscal intermediaries. In other words, reimbursement for care to those 65 years and over was a federal initiative. It was financed through direct reimbursement to hospitals (Part A) and to physicians (Part B) and through insurance carriers. Indirect reimbursement under Part B was used to underwrite educational costs of nurses and physicians especially for those caring for the elderly. Care in the community of the aged was refunded if physicians ordered skilled nursing care for patients in the home. The Visiting Nurses Association, a private-sector initiative in nursing, delivered most public health skilled nursing services prescribed by physicians. A debate about whether Medicaid was income maintenance or a health service program was resolved in favor of income maintenance. The problem is that the elderly are most likely to be sick *and* without funds due to their illnesses. Government assistance is therefore through "mixed" administrations through federal offices and, when the elderly become indigent, through state administrations.

■ *Health Policy for the Elderly Since 1970*

Since 1970, the years have been distinguished by recession and escalating inflation. It soon became evident that the 1965 amendment to the Social Security Act had increased the use of the health system by the aged as well as the rest of the population based on direct reimbursement of fee-for-service. Fees were governed by the policy of reasonable cost. By 1970, claimants had escalated with explosive force. In a period of higher interest rates, third-party reimbursers such as insurance companies attempted to recoup their losses from investment of capital; nevertheless, decompensation occurred, and insurance premiums started to rise as hospital costs soared. Total health care expenditures rose to 12.6% of the gross national product in 1986 (Table 18-1).[8,9]

In 1972, a further amendment to the Social Security Act mandated a professional services review through peer organizations to determine the medical necessity of services to Medicare recipients a utilization review. States who failed to implement utilization reviews were subject to the withholding of federal funds; however, costs continued to rise in spite of these efforts.

In 1971, health maintenance organizations (HMOs), prepaid health care plans, became a national centerpiece.[10] An HMO provides a specific set of health care benefits to an enrolled group for a predetermined periodic payment without regard to actual services provided. No legislation was passed regarding HMOs until 1973 when federal funds were made available for the initial study and development of HMOs. Those funds were provided as long as those receiving funds included services for preventive care. But possibly the most im-

T A B L E   1 8 - 1
Federal Health Expenditures (Billings): 1964–1986

Fiscal year	% Health expenditures
1986	12.6
1984	12.1
1982	11.7
1980	11.2
1978	10.6
1976	10.2
1974	9.3
1972	8.4
1970	7.5
1968	6.1
1966	3.6

(Adapted from the United States Budget, Washington, D.C., Office of Management and Budget, 1962–1982 and [ref. 9])

portant facet of the new law was that employers must include qualified HMOs as part of workers' benefit plans, enabling prepaid care to compete with retrospective payments for episodes of care. Today, 60% of the population are covered by HMOs in the workplace. Payments from Medicare for the elderly are as follows:

> *Medicare Part A.* Finances inpatient hospital care, post-hospital stay in skilled nursing facilities, and home health agency visits. There are limits of 90 days on one hospital stay. Payments from the government are direct to hospital facilities and agencies.
> *Medicare Part B.* Physician services and some hospital care are financed through Part B.

An amendment to the Social Security Act in 1972 allowed capitation reimbursement for both parts A and B of Medicare, and HMOs were qualified as providers of care to the elderly. Capitation is a method of health financing and delivery of specified services to an individual for a predetermined payment without regard to type of service. Reimbursement for Medicare patients was alien to HMOs because it was based on year-end assessments, a process against their philosophy of prepayment. Reimbursement for care of the aged was based, in part, on the fear that HMOs would underserve the aged and avoid the sicker Medicare beneficiaries. The Health Care Financing Administration (HCFA) instituted demonstration projects to increase HMO participation in Medicare. In 1985, of 350 HMOs, half were offering other services under Medicare. This is an important change from serving mainly the younger and less sick groups in the community. HMOs must provide evidence of optimal and preventive care services, routine eye examinations, and some services imposed by HCFA to qualify for Medicare funds. Government influence on health care delivery is no longer minimal as the problem of care to the elderly is the nation's problem.

One brief mention of diagnostically related groups (DRGs) is necessary. DRGs are a method of prepayment by diagnosis, which are grouped together. This system was originally intended to apply only to the Medicare system for those 65 years or older; however, it has influenced all third-party payor systems for all age groups. The DRGs were signed into law by yet another amendment to the Social Security Act of 1983, Title VI, and implemented in 1984.[11] The DRGs do not apply to long-term care and rehabilitation facilities nor to home care. The government was established as a "prudent" buyer of services, and the DRG system, developed by Yale researchers in 1970 as an aid to utilization review, is now a mandated method of payment for Medicare services.

The responsibilities for maintaining quality of care is implemented through peer review organizations (PROs), the sequel to PSROs. The law now seems to indicate that each state is a PRO-designated area. Funding is to come from the Medicare trust money, which is separate from the Social Security trust. Medicare funds are authorized by Congress, assigned by the Finance Committees of both Houses, and implemented by the HCFA. This fund is in peril of bankruptcy due to the increasing demands of the aging population.

■ *Epidemiology*

Health care services are an epidemiologic research responsibility and are included in the area of content called health services research. Research in services is concerned with access to care, costs of care, and quality of care in the community. The history of Medicare, the financing of health care to the elderly, is a study of how health policy is used to assure access to care at reasonable costs while maintaining quality of health services. As the growing population of elderly weight the system with the multiple needs of the aged, the government at the federal level has had an increasing impact on protecting the over-65 age group from alienation from needed health services. The public health nurse requires an understanding of payment systems for the aged, as the concern for cost is an overriding anxiety for elderly groups, and costs relate to access and quality of nursing care.

Many public health nurses are employed by HMOs to deliver care in the community for agencies based in outpatient clinics. Hospitals may be viewed as agencies within the health care system, giving care to discharged patients and organizing the rehabilitation of clients to life in the community. It is important for the community health nurse to recognize the impact of health care policies on the counseling needs of the aged in order to assure their best interests. Often it is the nurse in the home who is expected to be a resource for discharged patients. Epidemiologic facts also influence the nurses' understanding of aged populations. The group over 45 years of age has an average of two diagnostic categories, and multiple diagnoses increase as age increases. This relationship is called, epidemiologically, a direct relationship, that is, one variable increases in relationship to increases in another variable. Suicides in the age 65 population are more frequent in males than females, especially in single males.[12] Females live longer and are less prone to coronary artery disease although this is, in part, a corollary of smoking habits, as women have smoked less than men in the past. The aged who consider themselves happy live longer, but the spectre of ill health and loneliness are their major concerns.

Other facts of interest to the community health staff nurse are that increases in diastolic blood pressure correlate with memory loss, and people aged 65 to 75 years old are now more likely as a group to function like 55 to 65 year olds.[13] In the area of health promotion and prevention, nurses should be aware that despite the numerous diagnoses of the older people, prolongation of effective living and quality of life is a primary objective of nursing care. The longer the nurse can maintain current health status and delay disability, the more effective are nursing services. Predictors of longevity are diet, exercise, smoking, retirement from work, marital status, and social activity. These are called nurture variables; they are facts that can be modified by nursing intervention. Heredity, race, and intelligence are fixed: these are nature's variables. The predictors of longevity are SES, socioeconomic factor—good housing, good diet, good care—the nurture variables.[14] The debate over the influence of nature versus nurture on the elderly influences health policy perceptions and values that affect decisions.[15]

The impact of Alzheimer's disease is a significant factor that removes large numbers of the elderly from the community into institutions. But, and this is a significant caveat, the role of the community health nurse is to maintain the aged in their own environment through the judicious use of community support systems, often of a multidisciplinary nature. This role demands an understanding of the scientific basis of the process of aging as well as considerable skills in communication and coordination of services.

The proportion of aged will increase in the forseeable future. By the year 2010, three workers will have to contribute to the support of one nonworking elderly person; and in 2030, the ratio may be 2:1. The projected rise in the proportion of elderly is shown in Figure 18-1.

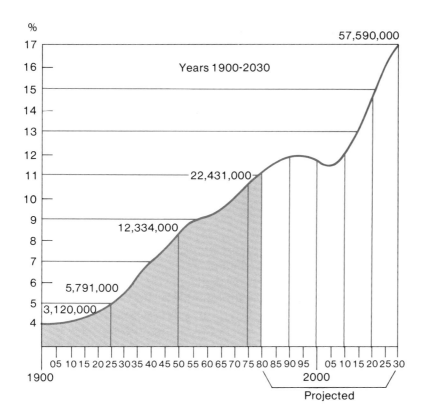

%

17 ┌ 57,590,000
16
15
14
13
12
11   22,431,000
10
9
8   12,334,000
7
6   5,791,000
5
4   3,120,000

Years 1900-2030

05 10 15 20 25 30 35 40 45 50 55 60 65 70 75 80 85 90 95   05 10 15 20 25 30
1900   2000
                                                        Projected

FIGURE
1 8 - 1
The percentage of the American population 65 and older from 1900 to 1975, with predictions for 1980 to 2030. (U.S. Census Bureau)

The care of the aged is a societal responsibility and is a problem of the nation. Its solution involves health policies of the United States. Community health nursing has an important role, which will increase with time, to maintain the quality of life of the elderly and promote their active participation in community living for as long as possible. It is clear that health policy and perception of priorities are of great concern to the well-being of the aged population. Promoting access to care and understanding how the system affects access is an important part of staff nurse responsibilities. Intervention for elderly care includes affecting the health policy as a community responsibility as well as promoting independence and delaying disabilities for the aged as long as possible.

Summary

*H*ealth policy is a method of meeting the needs of groups, especially when local resources are inadequate. Care of the elderly can be traced through the legislative process. Since 1935, the Social Security Act provides income for the elderly after age 65. Although social security originally was designed to supplement income for the unemployed, it also included funds for the unemployable that was justified politically as a method of returning the poor and needy into the work force. Until this time, involvement of government in health care has been paternalistic and minimal. In 1950, the Social Security Act was amended to include the permanently disabled; then, in 1960, Medicare included some payments for health needs for the elderly. In 1965, Title XVIII (Medicare) and Title XIX (Medicaid or welfare) was added to the Social Security Act. In so doing, the Act was split between federal control for Medicare and state rights for Medicaid. This duality affects services, especially for the elderly aged 65 and over. Hospital services are reimbursed for the elderly through Medicare Part A and physicians services through Medicare Part B based on reasonable costs for service. Since 1970, health costs escalated until they threatened to bankrupt the system. Prepayment systems were introduced for Medicare through the DRGs and HMOs. The latter delivered services traditionally for the working well, but were also given incentives to include the elderly in their programs.

Epidemiology of health services provides information on costs, quality of care, and access to care—all the data required for changing nursing services to an aging population. The demographics indicate that there will be three working people for each person over 65 by 2010. Community health nurses are dedicated to delivering services to the elderly in nursing homes and in the community. One of the chief concerns of the aged is payment for health care needs, and the nurse is a resource for information to alleviate these anxieties. Moreover, epidemiologic information on groups is of assistance in counseling and helps to define methods for promotion of health and the maintenance of the quality of life for the elderly in the community.

References

1. NCOA, National Conference: Mauskch I: Keynote Speech, 1986
2. Litman TJ, Robins LS: Health Politics and Policy. New York, John Wiley & Sons, 1984
3. Mustard HS: Government in Public Health. New York, Commonwealth Fund, 1941
4. Witte EE: The Development of the Social Security Act. Modern Univ (at Wisconsin) Press, 1962
5. Sagan JC (ed): Role of state and local governments in relation to personal health services. Am J Public Health #71 (Suppl) Jan 1981
6. Brown GD: Federal Funds and National Supremacy. Amer Univ Law Rev 28:3:Spring 1979

7. Anderson UW: The Uneasy Equilibrium. Private and Public Financing of Health Services in the U.S. 1875–1965. New Haven College and University Press, 1968
8. The United States Budget. Washington D.C., Office of Management and Budget, 1962–1982
9. BOT Report D (I:84) AMA
10. Medicare and Prepaid Health Plans New Directions for HMOs OP196 AMA, 1985
11. AMA DRG's OP #230, 1986, Chicago
12. Atchley RC: Aging and Suicide: Reflection of the Quality of Life Epidemiology of Aging, NIH 80–969, July 198
13. Wallace RB, Lenke JH, Morris MC et al: Relationship of free-recall memory to hypertension in the elderly. J Chronic Dis 38(6):475–481, 1985
14. Palmore E: Predictors of longevity. In Haynes SG, Feinleib M (eds): Epidemiology of Aging. USDHHS NIH 80–969, July 1980
15. Kannel WB, McGee D, Gordon T: A General Cardiovascular Risk Profile. Am J Public Health 38:46–51, 1971

Community Health Nursing in the Home

LEARNING OBJECTIVES

After reading and understanding the contents of this chapter, the student will be able to:

1. Differentiate between a home visit and home health care.

2. Identify the different kinds of nursing services delivered in the home.

3. Identify the population at risk for home health care.

4. Compare and contrast the structure of the health care system denoted by structure to the system denoted by the need for level of nursing care.

5. Relate the nursing goals for families receiving home health care.

6. Understand the impact of Medicare and Medicaid on access to care in the home.

7. Identify the entitlement programs under the Social Security Act and their impact on delivery of care in the home.

8. Relate the eligibility requirements of families receiving nursing care in their homes.

9. Identify the relationship between quality nursing home care and quality home care and the impact of federal reports on health policy.

10. Relate the epidemiologic model to community health nursing care in the home.

11. Interrelate and apply epidemiologic methods with nursing process for home care.

12. Identify how the epidemiologic perspective contributes to the unique role of the community health nurse in the delivery of care.

Introduction

*R*uth Freeman has stated that the home visit, a call upon a family in the home by the community health nurse as a "professional guest," is the heart of nursing in public health.[1] In today's health care scene, delivery of services in the home is changing: home care will play an important role in the future of community health nursing. As the nursing profession makes progress in a changing world, it is useful to distinguish between the home visit and home care. The difference between a home visit and home care is like the difference between a governmental agency nursing role and the role of the Visiting Nurses Association (VNA) in delivery of community services. Both involve public health. Both are guided by the same concepts of community service, prevention and control, surveillance, outreach, and a multidisciplinary approach, which are the guiding principles of public health work. However, home care delivers complex, skilled nursing services.

■ *Home Visit Versus Home Care*

What is different between a home visit and home health care? A home visit is associated with a primarily government agency follow-up of a well group of people. It emphasizes primary prevention nursing techniques.[2] Home visits are made for well baby care, for teaching and counseling, and other health maintenance work.[3] Today, home care delivers skilled nursing care for the sick and needy at home. It is an extension of VNA services delivered almost exclusively through non-profit private sector organizations and is also delivered through proprietary home health agencies (HHAs) including health maintenance organizations (HMOs). Home care emphasizes secondary and tertiary prevention in contrast to the home visit for primary prevention.

There are other differences between the home visit and home health care. A home visit emphasizes the assessment skills in the nursing process. Evaluation of nursing interventions for health promotion are often difficult to apply and may require further epidemiologic research to estimate effects on the community, as Birkauskas indicates.[4] On the other hand, home care utilizes all the steps in the nursing process. Implementation and evaluation are part of the on-going activities for immediate as well as long-term concerns, although evaluation of community effects of home care may require more sophisticated epidemiologic approaches. Typically, home care employs medical–surgical nursing skills in the context of community health principles and epidemiologic skills to deliver services to the chronically ill, the sick elderly, and the disabled. Part of home care nursing is family support and counseling for maintaining the ill in their own environment. During delivery of nursing care of the sick, health promotion is stressed and gains credibility and compliance from family members through competencies displayed for the sick member. If home care is restricted only to medical-surgical nursing activities, the quality of care will be compromised. The family will be isolated from community protection, and coordination of community resources will, by default, fall to other professionals. The era has arrived when home care as well as the home visit is the heart of public health nursing.

With the emergence of home care, the epidemiologic perspective becomes indispensable as a distinguishing characteristic of community health nursing. Epidemiology assures that public health concepts are in full play during the delivery of nursing services in the home. These concepts view any family in its community setting and assess the impact of the family's problems on the community at large. For the community health nurse, an epidemiologic view assures the family of constant surveillance and supplies a method of evaluating services that enhance quality control. Epidemiology is an indispensable part of the way family care is perceived by the nurse. This perspective provokes hypotheses for new methods of delivery of care to the community of families using multidisciplinary resources available to support care in the home (health services research). Epidemiology assures constant vigilance for prevention and control of hazards other than the immediate problem that has precipitated care in the family's own environment and provides risk estimates (risk ratios) to aid counseling and preventive activities.

▮ *The Growth of Home Health Care*

For many years, public health nurses delivered skilled nursing care to communities, mainly through the VNA. In the 1900s, a public health nurse could, and did, carry all necessary equipment in a small black bag for delivering care in the home; but this bag became obsolete in the 1970s except with the VNA nurses. After World War II, funds were legislated for hospital construction through the Hill–Burton Act and improved access to hospitals even in rural areas. The health care system delivered skilled nursing care, mainly through institutions and hospitals. Public health nursing became managerial and educational— a fact that precipitated a crisis in the 1980s when government agencies cut back nursing programs and staff.[5] Education is still difficult to reimburse under government policies.

The field of home care did not expand significantly until 1965, when the Medicare and Medicaid amendments to the Social Security Act (Titles XVIII and XIX) took place.[6] HHAs were formed to meet the needs of the chronically ill at home, mainly, to tend needs for skilled nursing services. In the 1970s and 1980s when costs of health care rose dramatically, the prospective payment system such as diagnostically related groups (DRGs) and health maintenance organizations (HMOs) were perceived as mechanisms to cut the rising costs of care. Hospitals reduced the length of stay of inpatients, and outpatient surgical clinics and ambulatory care centers also contributed to changes in hospital practices. Fixed payments through DRGs assigned before delivery of care promoted close scrutiny of the utilization of all federally reimbursed services, especially services in hospitals. Group averages have been developed through epidemiologic methods. These averages are compared to the care of an individual patient, an approach that is similar to the comparison of empirical norms of a geographic area to a single hospital by the Professional Activities Survey mentioned in Chapter 10 on evaluation of nursing services. Using similar methods, the length of stay in hospitals has been averaged for each DRG. This makes it comparatively easy to question prolonged stay of any patient in a hospital when the stay is not within the "average" limits. Consequently, patients are now discharged earlier, to their homes—some say too early—before adequate stabilization can occur and in poorer health.

The high-tech industry has influenced the growth of home care services. The President of the National Association of Home Care, Val Halamandaris, stated at the 1986 convention that the industry has progressed so much that any kind of technologic care can now be delivered in the home setting.[7] The acutely ill finish their convalescence at home, and the chronically ill can be maintained on life-support systems for long periods without institutionalization. Critical care has entered the family bedroom.

Another contributing factor to the increase in use of home care is the hospice movement.[8] It has long been known that dying patients are more comfortable in their own surroundings. Children with terminal illnesses such as cancer are a special challenge for nursing and often are cared for at home. Chronic pain that often accompanies the terminal cancer patient can also be managed in the patient's own environment. Unfortunately the epidemic of acquired immune deficiency syndrome (AIDS) has increased the numbers of terminally ill that are served in the home, and more and more hospice services are shifting from the hospital to the home.

The pressure of society on costs of health care and improvements in delivery of complex care requiring highly technical systems for administration have enabled hospice patients and the acute and chronically ill to receive services at home.[9] A list of procedures now available for home care include:

A. Intravenous therapies
   1. Central and peripheral parenteral nutrition
   2. Chemotherapy

   3. Antibiotic therapy
   4. Cardiac pressor agents
 B. Ventilators
 C. Apnea monitors
 D. Skeletal traction and therapy
 E. Rehabilitation aids and devices

Facts to support the phenomenal rise in home care services are found by examining expenditures for health care and the numbers of certifications for HHAs for Medicare, called deemed status. Since 1980, Medicare home health expenditures have doubled (as did Medicaid) but still remain at about 5% of the total expenses of Medicare. The increase in home health costs of the period 1974 to 1980 was 47.5% compared to a total Medicare increase of 9.9%.[10] Home health products and services grossed about $9 billion in 1985, and it is predicted that costs will increase to $16 billion for 1990, of which 70% is for services.

HHAs exist as Medicare and non-Medicare agencies. They are also divided into proprietary and not-for-profit categories. Today the proportion of proprietary compared to non-profit agencies is over 30%. Many nurse entrepreneurs give specialized services, such as rehabilitation, through private sector HHAs, and the types of providers of home care are proliferating. The number of HHAs receiving deemed status (certification to qualify for Medicare reimbursement) increased by more than 50% between 1982 and 1984. By 1986, there were at least 6000 HHAs. According to the American Home Care Association, nearly two thirds of the nation's hospitals operate HHAs and/or adult care centers and nursing homes.

■ *The Population At Risk for Home Care Nursing*

The population at risk of home care nursing has changed since the 1960s. The population then consisted of the chronic ambulatory, the well, and the near well. Now it has changed to the chronically ill, long-term patients, the terminally ill serviced through the hospice movement, and the acutely ill, early discharged, stabilized patient. These populations used to be sent to institutions and ambulatory care centers for care, and the population at risk of any nursing care could be determined by the locations or settings where care was delivered. In general, the settings for nursing care are hospitals, ambulatory care centers such as offices and clinics, nursing homes, and the home.[11] Hospitals are used for acute care and critical care. Long-term care facilities include psychiatric hospitals for the retarded and for the chronically, emotionally ill, and nursing homes for the elderly and totally disabled. Ambulatory care centers and the home were traditionally for health maintenance and the walking sick, with some exceptions (Fig. 19-1).

To view care in a more contemporary fashion in keeping with the real world, the system may be viewed as groups labeled by acuity level or severity of the illness or problem. This perception adapts more realistically to allocation of nursing services. The structure of the delivery system for organizing nursing care by need allows flexibility of referral because it is guided by patient/client problems. For instance, unstable chronic conditions requiring day and night skilled nursing care usually require institutionalization unless the home support system is exceptionally strong and coping levels are high. Critical or "high-tech" care usually requires hospitalization to attain stability, once stabilized, patients can be referred for high-tech care in the home for both acute and chronic conditions. This view of the system suggests the setting but allows discretionary judgment of nurses to prevail in order to diagnose the most appropriate safe and effective environment for patient care. This kind of referral system demands that the home be regarded as part of a continuum of care, *not* as an alternate setting for care, and greatly facilitates reimbursements based on level and type of nursing care required rather than the place where nursing occurs (Fig. 19-2).

Viewed from the conceptual framework of a community system of acuity levels, the most appropriate setting can be chosen according to the familial support available to the individual. Hospitals become community agencies that operate 24 hours a day. They no longer restrict their business to acute care but are agents for continuity of care.[12] In summary, the population at risk of home care are those with stabilized conditions, acute or chronic, who have family systems

F I G U R E
1 9 - 1
Structure of health care delivery system by setting.

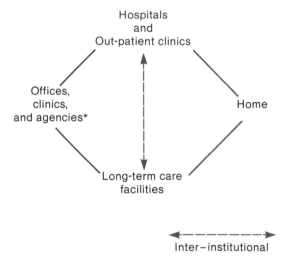

Hospitals
and
Out-patient clinics

Offices,
clinics,
and agencies*

Home

Long-term care
facilities

Inter–institutional

*Home health care agencies are included.

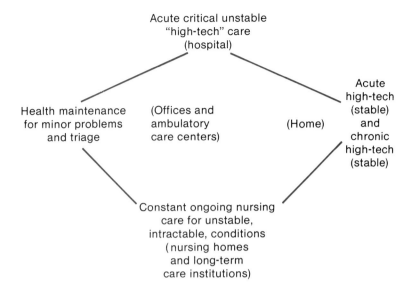

Acute critical unstable
"high-tech" care
(hospital)

Health maintenance
for minor problems
and triage

(Offices and
ambulatory
care centers)

(Home)

Acute
high-tech
(stable)
and
chronic
high-tech
(stable)

Constant ongoing nursing
care for unstable,
intractable, conditions
(nursing homes
and long-term
care institutions)

*FIGURE
19-2*
*Structure of health
care delivery system
by acuity of care.*

that can utilize the community resources and have access to a method
of payment to pay for care.

Another way to approach defining the population at risk of
home care is by age group; however, all ages receive care in the
home, and it is a mistake to consider home care as exclusively for the
elderly. Although the elderly over 65 years of age require home care,
the child with cystic fibrosis, the adolescent with kidney failure, the
young adult with hemophilia, the person with terminal cancer or
AIDS comprise 30% of the home care population. Rehabilitation and
maximizing independency can be applied to all regardless of age or
physical and mental condition.[13] It is estimated that there are 5.4 million elderly in the community.[14] It is true that the elderly in the home
do not use as much high-tech services as they use rehabilitative and
social services to maintain independence; but the younger population
often requires intensive care that demands high levels of specialized
nursing care based on medical-surgical skills and knowledge. For instance, randomized trials indicate that very low birth weight infants
(about 2200 gms) can be nursed safely and effectively in their own
homes.[15] Many children are on life-support systems as are older, end-
stage COPD patients.[16] More epidemiologic research is needed to verify the demographics of the home care population. Meanwhile these
proportions are indicators of the distribution of the population at risk.
It is known that the largest single group served in the home are people over 65 years of age. Home care is regarded as a method of delaying institutionalization for as long as possible.

It is necessary for the community health nurse to know some epidemiologic facts to assist the elderly and have some idea of the likelihood of need for services by age. The prevalence of limitations of ac-

tivity rises dramatically with age. The elderly are 4.5 times more likely to suffer from reduced ability to cope with the activities of daily living than those under 65.[16] Fifty percent of those who are 75 years and older face serious limitations; 22% are dependent on others for assistance.[17] Rates of disability are different depending upon the medical diagnosis. Heart disease and arthritis are rare in the under-30 population; hypertension and impairment of the lower extremities, even if they occur early in life, make slow progress. Senile dementia is the only major chronic condition reported by the National Center for Health Statistics that is exclusive to the over-65 age group.[18] In short, 50% of home care recipients are over 65 years of age, and 71% of all patients requiring long-term care live and receive services in the community.[19]

The goals of home care are generally the same across age groups. These objectives are to maintain the patient and the family as independent units within the health care system as long as possible and to optimize their capabilities to function at all levels. The goals now include prevention of hospitalization and the administration of highly technical, post-hospital care.

■ Cost and Access to Home Care

The areas of concern or substantive content for epidemiology of health services is cost, access to care, and quality of care. Costs of care, or the ability to pay for services, influence access to care; and the relationship between access and cost is very clear when home services are needed—the poor are denied care due to inability to pay. Another denial of access is through the lack of trained personnel and available facilities to deliver care. Because of costs of care, the elderly population is a societal concern; and health policy has been focused on the provision of funds for this population in particular. The other population in danger of denial of access to care through financial problems are the poor population, called the medically indigent. Unfortunately this is often synonymous with the chronically ill impoverished through the need for ongoing or long-term care.[20]

Public health nurses have traditionally given care to underserved groups and the indigent. Medicaid is the largest welfare program subsidizing care to the poor. Under Medicaid law, the program of Aid for Families with Dependent Children (AFDC) is administered. AFDC is the principal program that supplies cash funds as supplementary income for those who are neither sick nor disabled, but are below the poverty line (cited in 1986 as $10,989 for a family of four[21]). In 1935, AFDC was a little-known adjunct to the Social Security Act. The objective for AFDC was to tide over widows and their children until they qualified for social security. During the 1980s, the AFDC program has spent $15.8 billion a year for 3.7 million people. Almost half the families have mothers who have never been married, and 40% of the husbands have abandoned their families. The program is run by the states, and 50% of the costs are subsidized through the federal government through "block" grants. AFDC pays cash monthly to support the family. Many welfare mothers are of the hard-core "underclass." The modern goal for this program is to form a new contract between the federal government and the state to encourage work and discourage the illegitimacy that occurs in order to stay on the welfare roles. This population receives home visits to ensure health promotion for women and children.

The Medicaid program is also most frequently used for nursing home and home health care when private funds are exhausted and Medicare coverage expires. Medicaid has the option to pay for health care for the poor and disabled under its categorically needy program. After prolonged illnesses, the elderly may become poor after using their benefits under Medicare. They then resort to Medicaid to meet their health care costs.[22] Anxiety about meeting the financial burden of chronic illness interferes with families seeking care until the situation is irreversible. The community health nurse must be aware of the differences between the two programs so that she can counsel families and secure needed services for clients under the health policies of their states, which administer Medicaid. In home health care, Medicare and Medicaid reimbursement are important means of access to care—particularly Medicaid, which is not restricted by age. Essentially there are few ways, if any, for the chronically ill, long-term care persons to finance their care.

Medicaid (Title XIX) was introduced in 1965 with the Social Security Act amendment for Medicare (Title XVIII), but has little in common with Medicare. Medicare is a federal program targeted for the elderly: Medicaid is a state program for the indigent of all ages. Medicaid rules and regulations vary from state to state. Under the conditions of the 1980s, at least five states (Iowa, Kentucky, Missouri, Utah, and Washington State) no longer participate in Medicaid. Kansas and Ohio have dropped services for the medically indigent, the unemployed, and the disabled.[23] The impact of their decisions on the health and mortality of these communities can only be assessed through epidemiologic studies. For instance, in Massachusetts the infant mortality increased from 9.6 infant deaths per 1000 live births to 10.1 deaths per 1000 in 1982, the first increase in 9 years. Unequal access to prenatal care was established in some components of the system in Massachusetts and finally, in 1986, $1 million was assigned to delivery prenatal care to uninsured teenagers.[24]

Medicare and Medicaid are the principal sources of payment for home care, although there are some other entitlement programs such as the Older American Act, which emphasize housing, and some social services under Title XX. HMOs and the new social HMOs (SHMOs) provide home care through hospital-based agencies mostly.

Some private insurance carriers influenced by government policies are beginning to pay for home care. All payments are made retroactively on a "reasonable and current cost" basis (Table 19-1).

Some of the most important requirements for receiving care in the home, reimbursable under health care policies, are:

- HHA services prescribed by a physician
- Part-time or intermediate nursing care supervised by registered nurses
- Physical therapy, occupational therapy, or speech therapy prescribed for home services
- Medical supplies *other than* drugs and biologicals such as antibiotics
- Durable medical equipment such as hospital beds, wheelchairs, and oxygen equipment

Eligibility requirements for a person receiving health care are:

- The patient/client must be homebound,
- The patient must be under a physician's care
- The patient must need skilled nursing care, physical therapy and/or speech therapy.
- Home care must be provided in accordance with the physician's plan of treatment.

T A B L E   1 9 - 1
Sources of Reimbursement for Home Care

Entitlement Programs Under Social Security Act

Title III . . . . The Older American Act Program (includes housing)

Title XVIII . . . . Medicare
- Part A—Inpatient hospital care—funded through Social Security
- Part B—Voluntary physician care, skilled nurse care, outpatient care

Title XIX . . . . Medicaid "Categorically Needy Program"

Title XX . . . . Some social services

Federal government . . . . Public Health Service, Veterans Armed Forces, Indian Health Service

Private Sector

Self-pay

Private insurance carriers

HMO's and SHMO's

Examples of levels of reimbursement per visit by multiple providers are shown in Table 19-2.

■ *Some Historical Notes on Health Policy for Home Care*

Care of the disabled and dependent poor in their homes had traditionally been part of the responsibilities of public health nursing. Costs of care and health policies to fund care are irreversibly linked to the problem of access to care.[25] Before the historic year of 1965, HCAs were reimbursed for nursing services through a combination of patient fees and client contributions. HCAs were almost exclusively a VNA responsibility, and the main reason for physicians prescribing home care was for nursing care in the home. After the amendments to the Social Security Act (1965) greater than 50% of home care was through Medicare, indicating that the delivery of nursing services was focused on care to the elderly.

Between 1965 and 1975, many services that had already been provided were denied retrospectively. Claims for reimbursement were unfulfilled. As a result, many HHAs dropped "deemed status"—their certification as Medicare providers. This also meant that access to care for the elderly was unavailable for many areas. In 1977, the Medicare and Medicaid Antifraud and Abuse Amendment, PL. 95-142, addressed home health and made clear the potential growth of the service. The law requested the Department of Health, Education, and Welfare to (1) review its home health program (principally Medicare, Medicaid, and Title XX); and (2) propose changes to improve quality

T A B L E   1 9 - 2
Base Section 223 Medicare Payments: Limits for HHAs

Type of service	Per visit limits for urban areas			Per visit limits for rural areas		
	Total	Labor portion	Non-labor portion	Total	Labor portion	Non-labor portion
Skilled nursing	$53.54	$41.99	$11.55	$62.15	$50.99	$11.16
Physical therapy	50.91	39.91	11.00	61.26	50.17	11.09
Speech therapy	56.88	44.42	12.46	71.47	58.33	13.14
Occupational therapy	54.76	42.82	11.94	73.23	59.71	13.52
Medical social service	85.01	66.17	18.84	89.18	73.14	16.04
Home health aid	35.97	28.18	7.79	39.87	32.64	7.23

and efficiency. To meet this imperative, the Health Care Financing Administration (HCFA) was organized to administer the programs. Fiscal intermediaries were appointed to settle claims against Part B Medicare for HHAs. There are ten regional intermediaries.

The Omnibus Budget Reconciliation Act of 1981 made home care more accessible by removing some of the limits of previous laws, such as the three-day-stay hospital requirement to qualify for Medicare Part A funds. The subsequent Tax Equity and Fiscal Responsibility Act of 1982 required a single cost limit for all health agencies based on the experiences of free-standing (proprietary) agencies. Essentially, these two Acts attempt to control length of stay in hospitals and control home care costs. At present, in those states where a medically needy program exists and clients are entitled to nursing home care, home health care must be available.

Association Between Nursing Homes and Home Care

As has been seen, care for the elderly and the indigent affects laws for financing their care. This includes care in nursing homes as well as primary care, and some state laws mandate the availability of home care for those eligible for nursing home care. Restrictions on length of stay in hospitals is affecting health policy for reimbursement for care in the home environment. Nursing home care is usually regarded as the last, irreversible resort, although some demonstration projects show this is not necessarily true.[26] Both initiatives are based on the goal or policy to reduce institutionalization through delivering care in the home. But the association between nursing homes and home care is more direct than provision of care in the home setting. The issue of quality of care in the home has been compared to quality of care in nursing homes. It is generally accepted that the elderly prefer to stay in their own environment as long as possible. The growth in the population of the chronically ill and the elderly, as well as the growth in chronically ill pediatric and adult populations, ties concern for quality in institutional care with concern for quality of care in the home. This is especially true as complex, high-tech services are available for the family environment.

Influential Reports on Quality of Nursing Care

Two reports concerning quality of care focused on nursing homes, and another report on long-term care for the elderly influenced the concern for quality of care in the home setting.[27] The first report is an Institute of Medicine (IOM) study on nursing home regulation that began in 1982.[27] It was initiated in response to a suggestion from the HCFA to regulate the quality of care in non-hospital institutions through voluntary agencies such as the Joint Committee on Hospital Accreditation (JCAH). The report dismissed the suggestion of voluntary accreditation as an ineffective method of cost control even though the JCAH program has been successful in practice and financially for hospitals.

The multidisciplinary committee of the IOM reported that the quality of care was based on paper compliance, and federal sanctions for inefficient nursing homes were insufficient and unsatisfactory; in other words, standards of care were inadequate and enforcement was lax. The committee saw little difference between nursing homes labeled as skilled nursing facilities and intermediate nursing facilities—a federal categorization. The committee found that financing for nursing home care was mainly through the Medicaid program for indigent populations and advocated private insurance for long-term care of the chronically ill. They recognized that care in nursing homes is labor-intensive and there was a lack of professionally trained nurses to ensure quality; also, transfer between nursing homes and admission to nursing homes was impeded by lack of bed availability. They advocated converting acute hospital beds, vacant through reduced length of stay, to long-term care beds. The conclusions of the IOM committee were made by a group of experts based on their professional judgments, not on scientific assessments of epidemiologic surveys.

The next study on quality was even less scientific and was labeled by some critics as over-dramatization and hyperbole. The Heinz Committee on Aging, a Senate committee, reviewed quality of care in nursing homes and found roughly the same results as the IOM committee.[28] They too, recommended enforcements of standards of care and advocated that the HCFA expand the hospital survey bed program so that reimbursement for long-term elderly care could be made for care in acute care facilities. They recommended that the Medicaid system of reimbursement should relate to case-mix or severity of needs of patients in the nursing home and called for a bill of rights for "residents." They reported that 61% of nursing homes had no registered nurses around the clock, and 75% had no physician supervision. They recognized that any financing system placing almost 50% of the elderly with private funds in jeopardy of impoverishment within 1 year of any health·catastrophe was seriously flawed.

The last report in this review is an IOM effort to study a national strategy for long-term care, which focused mainly on the needs of the aged.[29] This report was, in part, a response to a task force convened by the American Nursing Association and the American Medical Association on care for elderly populations.[30] The IOM called for the elimination of a distinction between skilled nursing facilities and intermediate nursing facilities, and stated that any standards of care for quality should apply to patients' outcomes or the need of patients for medical and nursing care. Patients' rights were viewed as a natural condition rather than a standard of care; funds for research were advocated to test models of care for the aged and the development of viable financial strategies. These reports have been used to relate the quality of nursing home care to concern for the quality of care in the home.

■ *Quality of Care in the Home*

Epidemiologically, any public policy issues in health include references to cost of care and its corollary, access to care; but epidemiology is also the method of choice for evaluating quality of care. Quality issues are now a matter of public concern to assist society in protecting groups that are vulnerable to misuse. Many avenues influence policy, and the reports on nursing homes exemplify the impact of experts' opinions when investigating an issue. These reports on nursing homes have formed the foundation for recommendations for quality of care in the home.

In 1986, under the auspices of the American Bar Association a select committee published a report that stated that quality of care in the home was an unknown quantity, a "black box" that could explode into litigation for malpractice.[31] Protocols for home management and guidelines for standards of care have yet to be produced for general acceptance. Home care services are intended to enhance the opportunities for longer and more satisfactory lives of the disabled and chronically ill; but there is little accountability under the present system and still fewer studies of the extent of the problem. The fear is that the problem of quality of care that has been occurring in nursing homes for the past 20 years may be repeated for home care.

Congress has responded to these reports and political pressure from several organizations, including nursing associations, by introducing a Bill for Quality Assurance in Home Care, HR 5680.[32] The Bill incorporates many of the recommendations made in the reports on quality of care in nursing homes. For political reasons, the Bill was introduced primarily to meet the needs of the elderly. It is important for nurses to clarify to local governments and to their clients that home care is not confined to or reserved for the elderly, but applies to children and adults requiring acute and long-term care, and hospice care. The Bill incorporates a "bill of patients' rights" in the home and requests peer review of care delivered in the home by HHAs. Community health nurses have a great responsibility for delivering home care of distinctive quality. An epidemiologic perspective will add to the quality of care and assure that the community health nurse makes a viable and rewarding contribution to families requiring home care services.

The Community Health Nurse's Visit for Home Care—an Epidemiologic Perspective

When the community health nurse makes a visit for home care, the nursing process is applied using several roles: the role of the psychiatric nurse, the role of the medical surgical nurse, the role of the obstetrical nurse, and so forth. The community staff nurse may have to call one or all of these skills into operation, but the role of the community health nurse requires unique components of care that identify the use of public health concepts that place the home within the broader environment of societal needs.

The operationalization of the unique functions of community health nursing is facilitated by adapting the epidemiologic model to the nursing process for family assessment. Within the epidemiologic framework or model, the host is the family, the environment is the home, and the agent is a stressor of a physiological, psychological, and/or sociological nature. The nursing process takes place within the context of the epidemiologic model, and nursing measures for acuity of needs are applied within this context. Examples of acuity measures to assess the levels of complexity of community services required by a family (originally designed to assist community staffing needs) are exemplified by Regenry's levels of community care (Appendix G, Chapt. 19).[33] Another measure of acuity of need for education of the family unit is "A Family Learning Needs Assessment" (Appendix H, Chapt. 19). The epidemiologic model adapted for home care is shown in Figure 19-3.

Within the general context of the epidemiologic model, the family can be perceived as a group at different conceptual levels. Within the unit of concern (the family), the agent or stressor is the elderly patient or chronically ill child; the host is the family coping with the sick individual; the environment is the home. Through applying nursing process using a medical-surgical approach (mainly), the patient receives individually centered care. Applying the nursing process to another group level defined by the epidemiologic model, the family requiring home care is defined as the agent or stressor, the group of families requiring home care is the host, and the community from which resources are drawn is the environment. Using the perspective of an epidemiologic model assures the application of concepts of aggregates or community.

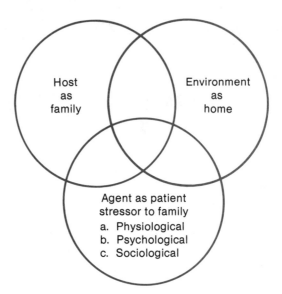

F I G U R E
1 9 - 3
The epidemiologic
model applied to home
care.

The epidemiologic method can now be applied as an extension of the nursing process to assess the interaction between agent, host and environment. Applying the epidemiologic method within the context of the epidemiologic model will ensure that the principles of public health, of surveillance for prevention and control of hazards, of outreach, of multidisciplinary teams and resources will be incorporated into nursing care. It will also allow quantifications to be estimated, and a nursing diagnosis to be made by time, place, and person. For instance, a physiologic stressor such as a nosocomial infection brought into the home will put all members and family contacts at risk for the same infection. In such a case, the epidemiologic methods may provide a hypothesis that prevention methods within another community, a nursing home or a hospital from which the patient has been transferred for home care have failed. Nursing intervention would be directed to the intramural environment that was putting many families in jeopardy. These epidemiologic dimensions bring to nursing care in the home an enlarged community perspective and suggest methods of nursing diagnosis, planning, and intervention that affect local methods of prevention and may require influencing the power structure of the state and ultimately the nation. Epidemiology suggests and substantiates alternative methods of systems of nursing care to protect all families in the community. It also suggests methods of prevention and control that impact the individual family as well as other families by using resources that never enter the home, but nevertheless assure the safety and efficacy of care to families.

▋ *Epidemiologic Method and Nursing Process*

Assessment

The epidemiologic method augments the nursing process. The first step, nursing assessment, integrates steps from the epidemiologic method (1) to establish a problem at community level; (2) to verify the nature of the problem by diagnosis; and (3) to make a quick community survey. In home care, nursing assessment will use the community health nurses' knowledge of other families receiving home care and home visits and invoke community nursing skills to identify commonalities at a neighborhood level. Assessment reviews the clinical knowledge of the nurse to assess the similarity of physiological and psychosocial problems or hazards. For instance, it is reasonable to expect that the community health nurse delivering home care should know how to compute the number of families that are anxious about access to care or the number of families that have respiratory infections from the same microbe. The steps in the epidemiologic process are used to expand the nursing assessment to raise awareness that a problem can be causing concern for more than one family in the community.

Nursing Diagnosis

Nursing diagnosis uses a thinking process similar to hypothesis formulation. It uses observations to form or hypothesize relationships about patients' problems. When this formulation is patient-centered rather than community centered, its process is more suitable to a medical-surgical nursing assessment or other specialty nursing care. In a visit for home care, nursing diagnosis is not confined to a single patient within a family context. The nursing diagnosis should also include an epidemiologic hypothesis about clustering of similar observations by time, place, and person. Epidemiologic thinking will change the nursing plan and its intervention from a plan revolving around the single patient's need to a plan involving group participation.

The nursing diagnosis also depends on considerable knowledge of family dynamics and the ability of the nurse to diagnose the strength of the family to use community resources to support the patient. A plan based on family strength to maintain its sick member outside the community is of utmost importance in home health care. The use of nursing assessment tools will enhance the diagnostic process for the community nurse (Appendices G and H, Chapt. 19).

Plan

The nursing plan depends on the hypothesis or the nursing diagnosis of the public health nurse. The plan will depend on the problem identified during assessment and may involve other community agencies such as nursing homes and hospitals, or community structures such as the local and state legislatures. The plan may require the mobilization of public health agencies for sanitation or for epidemiologic follow-up of a communicable disease hazard, or it may require contacting industries in the area to understand waste management and its effect on families. It is clear that plan mobilizes the resources in the community and may involve accessing care determined by other disciplines. To use epidemiologic method to plan intervention involves a knowledge of community resources and strengths that interact with family support systems and require considerable skills in communication and coordination.

Implementation

Implementing the nursing plan depends on the hypothesis or diagnosis. Analyzing the information to test the hypothesis requires intervention strategies for prevention and control of the problem. Similarly, nursing intervention depends on the plan and the nursing diagnosis. Due to cost-containment needs in the delivery of home care, the community staff nurse may be called upon not only to coordinate skilled nursing care to the index case (a pediatric patient on a ventilator, or the rehabilitation of an elderly stroke victim), but also to implement community initiatives. In home care, implementation is more complex rather than less complex as high-tech care escalates in the home. Referral of critical patient care to clinical nursing specialists is an intervention that is highly appropriate in some circumstances. Influencing political processes, regulations, and political action are community interventions that may be part of long-term planning in the community, just as putting control measures into operation is part of nursing intervention.

Evaluation

Because of the dynamic nature of the nursing process and epidemiologic method, testing the hypothesis (like testing nursing diagnosis) may be used as an evaluation procedure. Evaluation of community intervention plans vary from health services research and intervention studies to simple observations of family care givers attending respite programs. It may be an evaluation of the decrease of the spread of nosocomial infections into homes. All evaluations using epidemiologic approaches should include the outcomes recommended by Donabedian affecting disease rates, such as family satisfaction and reduced cost for the same quality of care within family units. These outcomes affect the way the families view nursing services and are valuable guidelines for quick estimates for ongoing evaluation of the quality of care in the home. Evaluation can also include estimating the effects of nursing care on the agent or stressor, the host, the family, and the community or the environment where families reside. The association between the epidemiologic method and the nursing process are diagrammed in Figure 19-4.

Barriers to Home Care

Home care is an industry within the health care system. Care in the home is family care, and families are the unit of concern for community health nursing. But modern home care emphasizes the weakness of the present system, and several barriers to home care must be overcome if society is to care for the elderly and those requiring long-term care. Policymakers agree that there is a need to create a better balance between public support for institutionalized and noninstitutionalized settings for the entire long-term care population.

A comprehensive national strategy is required to accomplish reorganization and reconceptualization of the system. The financing and delivery system is unstable and inconsistent, and incentives for using the system are absent. Third-party payers enter the home care market with a caution that can only be described as gingerly. Claims denial (the denial of reimbursement for services rendered) make it difficult for proprietary and non-profit agencies to survive. The complexity of a reimbursement system that functions differently at the federal and

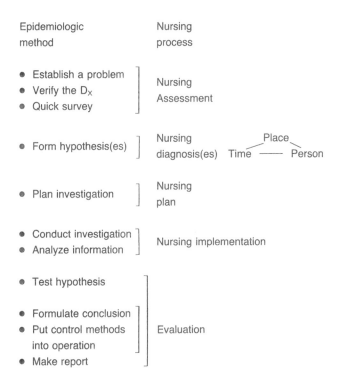

FIGURE 19-4 Summary of association between the epidemiologic method and nursing process.

state levels renders the paperwork required by the bureaucracy as burdensome in the extreme.

Quality of care issues may increase costs of home care but, to date, they have not been adequately addressed. The specter of malpractice in home care has been raised, but litigation has been inconsequential. Record-keeping for home care is particularly challenging; the problem of coordination to assure communication between many providers and retaining privacy of information has been recognized. The view of the system as episodic care delivered from alternate settings hampers change to a system in which need, not setting, is the deciding factor for delivery of care. A reimbursement system based on acute, episodic care must give way to a system providing care on a continuum according to acuity level, and obsolete regulations must give way to enlightened public policies. Community health nurses have the knowledge and the experience to influence these changes and overcome the barriers to future home care.

Summary

*H*ome care has been the traditional role of the public health nurse. Since World War II, the home visit has been used mostly for primary prevention through counseling and health promotion. Home care emphasizes secondary and tertiary prevention and requires new responsibilities for delaying institutionalization and deterioration of family members. Epidemiology provides surveillance and risk estimates for counseling and nursing care for home visits and for home care. Epidemiology promotes a perspective that assures the use of public health principles to enhance the quality of care in the home.

Since 1965, home care has gradually expanded until today it has become the fastest growing health care industry in the system. Many factors have influenced this change including cost-containment policies, the influence of high-tech procedures and techniques on the critical care of patients at home, and the growing population of elderly. For these reasons a shift in the population at risk in home care has occurred. Seventy-one percent of the chronically ill can now be cared for in the home environment and acute care once thought to be only available in hospitals can be stabilized for care at home. Hospice care is a home care prerogative, and rehabilitation services for both young and old can be delivered in their own environment.

Costs, access to care, and quality of services in the home are relevant concerns. These issues are the focus of epidemiologic studies in health services research. Costs of home care impede access to care for the poor and the elderly made indigent when their resources are exhausted through illness. Quality of home care is a "black box," and lack of standards of care may produce a crisis in quality similar to the nursing home dilemma. An epidemiologic perspective enhances community health nursing services. Epidemiologic method applied with the nursing process and guided by the epidemiologic model assures that families receiving care are oriented to community needs and resources. An epidemiologic framework protects the family system from hazard. This perspective allows the nurse to plan and use community services and implement strategies to influence health policies to improve family care.

At present, the home care system requires a dramatic change to accommodate societal needs for cost-effective, quality care. Home care is a method of meeting these needs, but must be perceived as part of a continuum of care to be effective. Reimbursement policies should be based on acuity of ongoing patient/client needs rather than on the present methods of assessing episodic acute hospital needs. These desirable changes will go far towards meeting care needs of the elderly and the chronically ill who have proportionately higher requirements for nursing care in the home. Community health nurses have an important, if not critical, role to play in effecting changes for the betterment of care for patients and clients in their own environment.

References

1. Freeman RB, Heinrich J: Community Health Nursing Practice. Philadelphia, WB Saunders, 1981
2. Mundiger M: Home Care Controversry. Rockville, Md, Aspen, 1983
3. Buhler–Wilkerson K: Public health nursing in sickness and in health. Am J Public Health 75:10:1155–61, 1985
4. Birkauskas VH: Effectiveness of public health nurse home visits to mothers and their infants. Am J Public Health 73:5, 1983
5. Chavigny K, Kroske M: Public health nursing in crisis. Nurs Outlook Nov–Dec 1984
6. Trubo R: Home health care encounters growing pains. Med World News Feb 10, 1986
7. Val Halamandaris: Keynote Address. NAHC Convention, New Orleans, Sept 9–13, 1986
8. Martinson IM, Nesbit ME, Kusey JS: Physician role in home care for children with cancer. Death Studies 9:283–293, 1985
9. Koren MJ: Home care—Who cares? N Engl J Med 314:14:917–919, Apr 3, 1986
10. General Accounting Office, HRD #85-110. September, 1985
11. Chavigny K: Home health care for the chronically ill, presented at Emory University School of Nursing, April, 1986
12. Broady, SJ: American Geriatric Society (quote). Am Med News: Dec 5, 1986
13. Byrne M: Med Trib Nov 5, 1986
14. Isaacs JC, Tam S, Health LK: National Health Council XII:4 August, 1986
15. Brooten DB, Brau LP, Betts P, et al: A randomized clinical trial of early hospital discharge and home followup of very low birth weight infants. N Engl J Med 315:934–9, 1986

16. Goldberg A: Home Care for Life Supported Persons. New Challenges for Physicians. Chic Med 340–341, 344, 365, 1984

17. American Medical Association: Long Term Care for the Chronically Disabled, BOT Report D (I–84) Chicago

18. Bureau of Census: Projection of the Population of the USA, 1982–2005, Series P. 25 #922, October, 1982

19. National Health Council: Long-Term Care: In Search of National Policy, Wash Report, Vol XII:4, 1986

20. Grazier KL: The impact of reimbursement policy of home health care. Pride Inst J of LT Home Care 5:1:12–16, 1986

21. Medicaid and AFDC. Time, January 16, 1987

22. Nordheimer J: Aging of Florida's population burden. New York Times Monday, July 14, 1986

23. Braun R: Health care for the indigent. J Nat Med Assoc 78:5:35, May, 1986

24. Bailus W: The role of statistics in state health policy decisions: The Massachusetts experience. J Public Health Policy 7:1:12–20, Spring, 1986

25. Bernstein LH, Grieco AJ, Dete MK: Primary Care in the Home. Philadelphia, JB Lippincott, 1987 (to be published)

26. O.T.A. Staff Presentation at the APHA meeting on Health Services Research 1986 Project on "Channelling"

27. IOM Committee on Nursing Home Regulations: Improving the Quality of Care in Nursing Homes. Washington DC, National Acad Press, 1986

28. U.S. Senate Task Force on Aging, John Heinz Chairman: Nursing Home Care: The Unfinished Agenda. May, 1986

29. Institute of Medicine: Towards a National Strategy for Long Term Care of the Elderly. April, 1986

30. AMA–ANA Task Force Report on Care for the Elderly. Kansas City, ANA, 1983

31. American Bar Association: The Black Box of Home Care Quality, Select Committee on Aging, House, Pub #99–573. Washington, U.S. Printing Office, 1986

32. Roybal ER: The Homecare Quality Assurance Act of 1986, HR 5680, October 9, 1986

33. A Family Nursing Needs Assessment. J Geriat Nursing 12:4, 1986

34. Regnery G: Patient Care Needs—An Index for Community Staffing. Nurs Admin Quarter 1:4:79–89, 1977

Epidemiology for Community Health Nursing: Research and Roles

LEARNING OBJECTIVES

After reading and understanding the contents of this chapter, the student will be able to:

1. *Describe the recommendations of the Pan American Health Organization Advisory Committee and the Centers for Disease Control for the use of epidemiology in nursing.*

2. *Identify the context in which research becomes a community health nursing concern.*

3. *Differentiate descriptive, analytic, and intervention studies.*

4. *Explain how epidemiology applies to both the generalist and specialist roles in nursing.*

Introduction

*I*n the early 1970s, the Pan American Health Organization (PAHO) Advisory Committee for the practice of community health nursing recommended that epidemiology be incorporated into programs of nursing. In 1975, a committee was convened at the Centers for Disease Control (CDC), in Atlanta to implement the recommendations of PAHO. The committee was composed of nurses with epidemiologic background and nurses representing services and education. Their final report discussed specific aspects of epidemiology in nursing and its application for delivery of nursing care.[1] Their chief concern was to provide a theoretical and practical background for nurses to expand their roles in health care delivery and to utilize the nurse in improving the delivery and the supervision of all health services. As part of the way to accomplish these objectives, the methods and concepts of epidemiology were suggested for the curriculum.

The CDC report outlines several ways to use epidemiology for nursing. It recommends (1) the use of patterns of events relating to health in populations; (2) the assessment of the community; and (3) the study of rates and epidemiologic methods to solve communicable disease problems. The report emphasizes the recent advances in epidemiology that enabled this science to be used for monitoring and surveillance of health care services and for evaluating the results of programs of community care. The report acknowledged that in the past the nurse had applied epidemiologic concepts in a very limited fashion in practice, acting only in a passive role or as an unequal partner in multidisciplinary efforts. New societal needs required expansion of the responsibilities of the nurse in community health, and in the planning, delivery, and evaluation of health services. It recommended the community health nurse become active in surveillance, screening, and case finding through the application of methods and concepts to practice settings, extramurally and intramurally. The theoretical concepts of public health were recommended as the basis for the use of epidemiology in practice. Epidemiology was of special importance to the practice of nursing to ensure a safe environment for patients and clients, and to ensure a community approach within which the needs of the family are met.

This book is consistent with the recommendation of PAHO and provides an approach to assist in the application of epidemiologic principles and methods for community health nursing practice and roles. Epidemiologic methods do not replace more qualitative theory or behavioral or sociologic frameworks; instead epidemiology provides an umbrella of theoretical conceptualizations unique to community health nursing. Within these concepts, other approaches indispensable to nursing care may be augmented and enhanced. The epidemiologic perspective provides techniques and processes for the community health nurse who is a generalist and for the public health nurse who is a specialist.

In order to illustrate the generalist role, the text will be summarized with special reference to the public health model. To provide evidence of the contribution of epidemiology to specialty nursing practice, two models for community health nursing, the Betty Neuman model and Marla White's model, will be detailed. Some studies illustrating the applications of epidemiology to nursing practice will be discussed briefly. The recent research of nursing practice utilizing epidemiology, its methods and research designs, will be reviewed. Epidemiology as a research method in nursing can be applied to assessment and community diagnosis using descriptive epidemiology, seeking causal associations for nursing care using analytic studies, and to evaluation of the effects of nursing services using epidemiologic intervention studies.

▌ *Community Health Nursing Research*

Community health nursing research focuses on the assessment of needs and evaluation of services to communities. Research in public health estimates the impact of health promotion, or primary prevention; the screening and surveillance, or secondary prevention; and rehabilitation, or tertiary prevention in communities.[2-6] The factors differentiating community health nursing research and other research in nursing are the theoretical concepts or principles of public health that provide the conceptual framework for research in public health. These constructs are identified in the public health model and guide community health nursing research into families as units of society and population based research. Using the public health model as a theoretical basis for nursing care, aggregates such as industries and hospitals become the focus for nursing research in these populations.[7,8]

Reference is made to many of these concepts in the nursing literature, usually as a single premise rather than collectively as an interacting model. The idea of multidisciplinary cooperation and collaboration can be researched to estimate the contribution of nursing's impact on the team. Other principles from the public health model are the concept of family within the community, and the impact of health promotion and prevention of illness.[9,10] In a trenchant article on the coming of age of nursing research, Jacox says that nursing research provides information on health promotion as well as information on how to provide care for people who are ill.[11] Therefore pain, decubiti, incontinence, prevention of complications, and alleviating mental confusion "are all the purview of nursing research." When these problems are researched within the context of all the principles contained in the public health model, then the research becomes a community health nursing concern. Jacox adds that without the knowledge of how to care for people who are ill, the prevention of illness and promotion of health is incomplete. In epidemiologic terms, without the outcome of illness as well as health, in accordance with the singular outcomes that characterize epidemiology (the case and non-case), community health nursing research denies its responsibility to conduct research at all levels of prevention for the sick and the well.

Epidemiology cannot be separated from the concepts of public health. Epidemiology and nursing process operationalize—put into action—the concepts of public health. The principles of epidemiology, such as agent–host–environment interaction and the scientific method (especially hypothesizing unknown relationships), contribute to a theoretical framework for community health nursing. As with any conceptual framework, all concepts must be used interactively with each other in order to apply to nursing practice. For instance, if the concept of family is separated from community home health, then care cannot be justified as a public health nursing role and the family will lie outside community nursing responsibilities and research. The inclusion of family as community health also influences policy. If the family is denied as a community health nursing responsibility, then a policy to disenfranchise community health nursing from delivering home care might occur.[12] Similarly, the claim that public health concepts are not applicable to nursing practice raises the question of the need to integrate any science into nursing theory.[12,13,14]

Public health research for nursing may be defined as population-based research initiated and/or implemented by nurses. This definition, however, is incomplete. Research in community health nursing addresses the mandated services of public health, such as child and maternal care. Epidemiologic research in community health nursing addresses environmental impacts, screening services using public health laboratory techniques, and statistical assessments of community needs. The use of rates and the use of epidemiologic research designs, such as case comparison and cohort studies, obviously define epidemiologic research. When studies use the methods and designs of epidemiology and apply these methods to nursing assessment, implementation, and evaluation of nursing services in communities, the inquiries may be called epidemiologic nursing research. For this review, other studies will be included that are undeniably community health nursing, but the linkage between their approach and epidemiology are not acknowledged. The reason for their inclusion is to establish that qualitative methods also are useful for community health nursing research.[15,16] It is important to support the integration of all methods of nursing research with epidemiologic approaches for the prevention and control of disease and promotion of health in the community.

▋ *Epidemiology and Education*

The use of epidemiology in education is insufficiently researched. There are, however, several reports of the effects of epidemiology as part of undergraduate education. Epidemiology was used to teach senior nursing students in a baccalaureate program how to assess the community. Faculty used epidemiology as a systematic approach to study muscular dystrophy as a community health problem.[17] The objectives of the course were to introduce the student to epidemiologic methodology and techniques, not only to assess community problems but to illustrate how community health nurses can apply epidemiologic concepts to family nursing care and community program planning. The effects were evaluated as a student experience. Epidemiology offered the students a way to synthesize knowledge and to make the community nursing experience dynamic and relevant. The students used descriptive epidemiology to describe the problem in the community and, based on their findings, to plan and implement nursing services.

Powers integrated epidemiology into community health nursing by class participation in a screening program for lead poisoning.[18] Children living in pre-1960 housing in an inner-city housing project participated in the Childhood Lead Poisoning Prevention Program. The survey was conducted (in uniform) by senior baccalaureate students. It sought to identify asymptomatic children ages 1–6 years at high risk for lead poisoning. The survey was conducted by a door-to-door request for permission to take erythrocyte protoporphyrin capillary screening samples. Screening is not considered a diagnostic activity. Positive results were forwarded to the local department of public health and community health nursing for continued intervention. The evaluation of the experience by faculty and students was that the host–agent–environment epidemiologic model was easily understandable within this context. Screening and subsequent statistical evaluation were labeled as research process. The family assessment in most cases did *not* predict the degree of blood lead levels in the child. Although intervention and implementation of nursing services to control the problem were not included in the report, the research focus of epidemiology was appreciated by the students and faculty.

In England, the crowded curriculum was blamed for the difficulties in integrating some research awareness into community health nursing or district nursing.[19] A small project evaluating six types of accommodations for the elderly was conducted by students. Epidemiology was identified as the research approach for handling and interpreting data. The integration of research methods associated with behavioral sciences was also used to heighten student awareness of the application of research to practice and policy decision-making.

∎ *Descriptive Studies*

The use of descriptive epidemiology is probably the most accepted application of epidemiologic research for nursing practice. Descriptive epidemiology is community assessment. This process is under-utilized in community health nursing possibly because it is sometimes perceived as an alternative approach rather than a method of amplifying and unifying several methods used by the nursing community. In 1978, a prevalence survey of chronic illness was completed in South Africa.[20] Nurses were heavily involved in this research. It is used here to illustrate nursing outcomes and the use of behavioral sciences to interpret information gleaned from a community assessment. The objectives of the survey were to determine the prevalence of chronic illness in a defined area in Cape Town to identify whether primary, secondary, and tertiary levels of comprehensive care could or should have been implemented and to advance hypotheses for more effective control of chronic illness. The definitions of chronic illness were nonmedical: these definitions concentrated on lack of mobility, dependency, and abnormal development—outcomes where nursing services would be of prime concern. What was not defined were the racial categories of black versus colored versus white. This is unfortunate because psychosocial and cultural factors would influence nursing services designed to meet the needs of these groups. Of the "colored" population, 15.2% were defined as requiring services to supplement function that were not diagnosed by medical personnel as "having a chronic illness". The prevalence of chronic illness was highest in the "colored" community.[19] Knowledge of behavioral and nursing sciences would be necessary for planning and implementing nursing care to this population.

Other description surveys are, of course, exemplified by the National Interview survey data. Surveys of the aging, their social situation as well as their health statistics are used to influence not only service delivery but also budget allocations by the government to fund services.[21] Some descriptive epidemiology is used for pilot studies such as a survey of the nutritional status of men attending a soup kitchen in Alabama.[22] In this study, laboratory evidence of nutrient deficiency was present in 94% of the 50 subjects or volunteers. The control group consisted of university students and staff. These smaller studies are sometimes referred to as community needs assessment or program planning studies. This may be due to the definition of community being reserved for national projects rather than small groups or aggregates.[23] Again the concept of what constitutes a community is crucial to epidemiologic applications. A community does *not* depend on size, but on communal need and communal hazard.

■ *Analytic Studies in Nursing*

Analytic epidemiology tests hypotheses to establish causal association. An example of an analytic study would be to hypothesize about nursing techniques in home care for the frail elderly and their effect on delaying institutionalization. Some of the literature refers to analytic studies as evaluation studies when they mean evaluating hypothesized association in which the outcomes are consistent with epidemiologic events such as rates, patient satisfaction, costs, or any of the quantitative outcomes recommended by Sheps and Donabedian. A more appropriate definition is that analytic studies investigate cause. In the application of nursing process, the assessment and diagnosis made for individual needs seeks to describe and then to associate the reason for patient need with direct nursing intervention. The assessment and diagnosis use known associations to arrive at an effective nursing plan. In epidemiology, the association is hypothesized, that is, it is not based on previous knowledge but seeks new knowledge on which to base nursing judgments; importantly, research in public health nursing seeks answers from looking at the group experience. Hypotheses are logical associations that require testing and substantiation. The function and the focus of analytic epidemiology is to identify causal associations on which to base nursing intervention in the community.

According to Bronstein and coworkers, the stroke data bank could be used to study nursing questions such as how does depression impede recovery of the stroke patients, and what are the factors likely to be associated with life-threatening complications.[24] The answers to these questions not only influence nursing care at the bedside but also influence the organization and delivery of community care of the chronically ill at home. As more and more sick patients are being served in the community, the need for nursing research to be conducted in the family setting will increase. Traditionally little research has been done in the home, although the VNA reports a clinical trial of the effects of different dressings on venous stasis ulcers.[25]

The contribution of epidemiologic approaches for research in oncologic nursing is documented in the literature. The use of descriptive epidemiology to discover problems using the variables of time, place, and person, is well demonstrated.[26] It is, however, the analytic study of patients with cancer that is promoted as a method of answering questions so that nurses can institute health promotion to prevent the occurrence of this disease. The discussion of causality, the theory underlying hypothesis generation for analytic studies, is also documented as indispensable to epidemiologic study.[27] Causality employs the concepts of rational thought to examine evidence so that hypotheses can be formulated that justify investigation. The hypothesis is integral to epidemiology, and it is the formulation of testable hypotheses that is part of epidemiologic thinking. Epidemiology studies biologic, behavioral, and environmental factors in disease and health promotion. These factors are essential components of community health nursing responsibilities. Establishing causal associations for analytic studies to establish the effects of these variables is an important part of nursing research.

Intervention Studies

In 1977, Highriter published an erudite review of community health nursing research.[28] The controversy about titles and definitions of public/community health nursing made the identification and labeling of research specific to community nursing a difficult task. Several studies had evaluated the impact of health knowledge of the behavior of families and health education given to clients by public health nurses. Nursing performance versus performance of other disciplines were compared, although epidemiologically this type of evaluation is programmatic and more appropriately called intervention research. In Highriter's review, many studies had methodologic problems, and the difficulties of random sampling in communities received comment. Although the aggregate approach was mentioned in an overall comment on evaluation studies, the application of epidemiologic research methods was omitted. Epidemiology is designed specifically to overcome the methodologic problems identified in the review of community health nursing research.

In a more recent survey of studies in community health nursing, Highriter includes intervention studies with evaluation studies.[29] This is justifiable because analyzing causal associations is a form of evaluation, such as whether pregnant mothers with influenza have more problems in rearing their children. In epidemiology, the hypothesized association in intervention studies is based on results of analytic studies that then can be used for planning programs of care. Once it has been established that the association exists, then the service can be organized as an intervention. Overlap between analytic and intervention studies occurs when the intervention is also the hypothesized cause and there is no reason to believe that administrative or organization variables will change the outcome.

The interventions reviewed by Highriter are identified as maternal and child care, home health, chronically ill patients, the elderly, and quality assurance. These areas have already received considerable attention in this text as community health nursing concerns. Besides the relevance of topics, what is also evident in the review of the literature from 1977 to 1981 is the gradual acknowledgment of epidemiologic methods in the studies. Highriter notes that studies dealing with collaborative interventions between physicians and nurses in public health had dramatic results.[30] A 6-year follow-up of counselling by doctor–nurse teams of normal, first-born infants showed significantly better results than those randomly allocated to clinics. In Britain, a study of sleep problems in the home improved the sleep patterns of children when the psychiatrists gave group instructions on this topic to district nurses.[31] In New York City, a multidisciplinary health education program reduced morbidity and mortality from children's falls from tenement windows.[32] Other studies of hypertensive control in the community found that nurse-run clinics were more effective than physician care; however, rehabilitation could be performed by disciplines other than nursing with equally beneficial results.[33,34] Highriter cites a successful demonstration of nursing effectiveness in 75% of the nursing research reviewed in her article. Barkauskas notes that the assessment skills are much better than the intervention skills of the public health nurse.[35]

In summary, the use of epidemiologic methods, variables, and techniques is increasing in nursing, although many times the linkage between epidemiology and behavioral research methods is not acknowledged. There is a growing awareness that epidemiology is useful not only for teaching research to community health nurses but also for educating community health nurses. As competition increases in the health care system, it will become imperative to teach intervention and to evaluate the effects of intervention through valid research.[36] Epidemiology has an essential part to play in practice, in education, and in research in community health nursing.[37]

▌ *Roles*

The purpose of this book has been to introduce the community health nurse to a general overview of the principles and methods of epidemiology. This perspective for the generalist role is inseparable from the public health theory for which epidemiology was designed. Epidemiology provides a perspective for nursing in groups that is necessary for the assessment, diagnosis, planning, intervention, and evaluation of nursing care needs in the community. Once this perspective is attained, once this framework for looking at group needs is integrated into the thinking of the community health nurse, it can never be erased. The viewpoint becomes part of the nursing process for care of aggregates.

For the generalist at the staff nurse level, epidemiology augments the practice of the community health nurse. It provides a language and a method of quantification that can be understood by all workers in the field. It provides methods that have been developed over many centuries to diagnose community needs and evaluate the effectiveness of intervention. In the modern world, it provides tested research methods in risk assessment and in evaluating the improvements in the quality of life of families and of groups. The scope of this work is broad because it is intended to provide the vocabulary for the staff nurse to read public health literature and interpret epidemiologic quantifications to serve clients and families. The breadth of epidemiology provides a framework into which all nursing sciences and behavioral sciences may be integrated; all the skills and knowledge of the nurse may be synergised and activated within its process and methods. Moreover this public health science provides an understanding for the staff nurse of the rigor required for documentation of exposures, of the care that must be exercised when providing facts for community decision making, and of the contribution of case finding to the total welfare of all who have needs and hopes in common.

Epidemiology provides highly specialized skills and knowledge essential for the specialist roles. As a research method developed for public health, it is a prerequisite for the nurse epidemiologist researcher. This role can be applied within intramural environments. In the hospital, the nurse epidemiologist is the research arm of infection control practice and the identifier of hazards to patients in hospitals.[38] In industry, the specialist role of the nurse is to provide ongoing information for risk assessments and to identify hypotheses for research. Nurses with epidemiology specialist education serve in state health departments and county departments.[39] Home health care will continue as an essential part of the delivery of service in the community: the nurse epidemiologist researcher in home health care will be developed to work with nurse researchers with a behavioral science background.

Epidemiology cannot be separated from public health theory; however, public health theory can be separated from epidemiology. The Neuman model was originally designed to assist in curricular development. The theoretical framework is systems theory, but epidemiologic principles and methods and the theory of causality for hypothesis formulation is notably absent. However, the public health principles of prevention and control and community are included. In the Neuman model, the community experiences stressors that nursing care has to address to relieve problems in groups. This model is useful in planning services as a director of nursing in public health.[40] Neuman's model shows the application of sociologic theory to the executive role and is a most useful orientation at the specialist level.[41]

Another model for specialist roles illustrates how part of the public health model can be integrated into nursing theory to guide the role of the specialist in public health. Marla Salmon White introduced a model to assist in prioritizing community health nursing practice.[42] This model is useful for the executive in community health nursing and for planning of delivery of services to the community. The White model is based on a sociologic framework invoking mores and social values. The values are used to evaluate biological, environmental, medical, and social determinants of health in communities. As in the public health model, the nursing process activates the system for application to practice situations. This is a most helpful approach to assist the nurse manager to determine where and when to use scarce resources for the benefit of the greatest good. Both the Neuman model and the White model, illustrated in Figures 20-1 and 20-2 would enhance the specialist role through the integration of epidemiologic scientific principles and methods. The implications of theoretical models in nursing and, for want of a better term, epidemiologic "theory" for clinical practice will be addressed in a subsequent text.

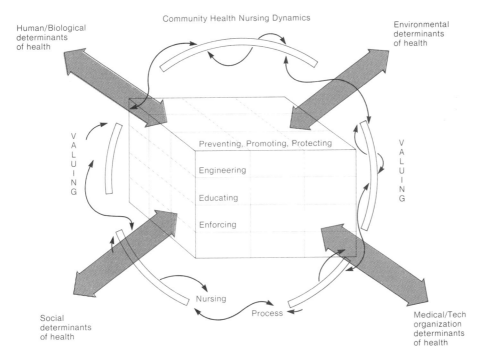

FIGURE 20-1
A community health nursing conceptual model.

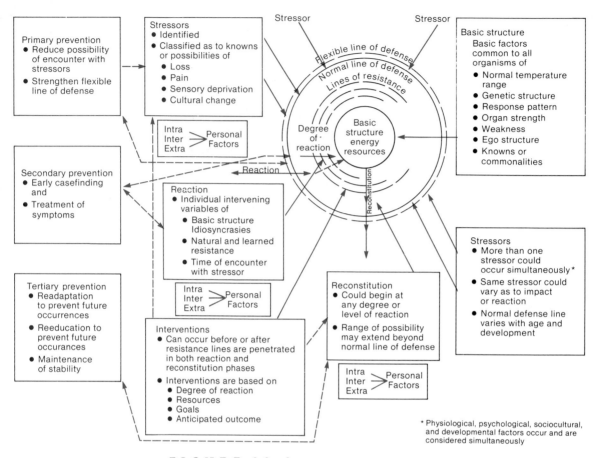

F I G U R E   2 0 - 2
The Betty Neuman Model: a total person approach to viewing patient problems.

Summary

*T*here is a surge of interest in the applications of epidemiology to nursing practice in the community. The American Nurses Association (ANA) officially defined community health nursing as a "synthesis of nursing practice and public health practice . . . for the health of populations" as early as 1974.[43] In 1980, the ANA corroborated this statement and stated that the focus of "community health nursing practice was the population as a whole."[44] The community health nursing section of the American Public Health Association defined public health nursing in similar terms with special emphasis on nursing care to populations at risk.[45] Archer has said that all specialty practice in nursing is a combination of nursing science and other sciences that are appropriate to the specialty area.[46] The public health model is consistent with these definitions and congruent with Archer's recommendations. Epidemiology is the public health science that operationalizes the public health model and identifies and quantifies populations at risk.

Epidemiology underlies public health theory and practice. In spite of this, and in spite of the recognition of the use of epidemiology for community health nursing, a survey of schools of nursing that teach community health showed that just over one half required their students to take epidemiology courses, and rarely was the course over three credits in length.[47] If the recommendations of PAHO are to be heeded, if the recommendations of the Milbank Memorial Study are to be taken seriously[48] and if the definitions of the nursing profession are to be operationalized, then the future of epidemiology for community health nursing is assured.

The world is increasingly competitive. Community health nursing must use all methods and all approaches to evaluate the impact of nursing care and to establish and maintain quality of services. The opportunity for nursing to reestablish its traditional role in the community and expand its services to meet new needs has arrived. An epidemiologic perspective will assist and enhance the contribution of the profession of nursing to promote the health and welfare of the public and the communities in which they live.

References

1. PAHO Report: Epidemiology and nursing. Bull Pan Am Health Organ 10:30:258–265, 1976
2. Laffrey SC: Health promotion: relevance for nursing. Top Clin Nurs 7:2:29–38, 1985
3. Chen SC, Sullivan JA: Chapter 2, School Nursing 26–46. Annual Review of Nursing Research. Sills GM, Goeppinger J. New York, Springer & Co, 1984
4. Robertson C: Evaluation and screening: an epidemiologic approach. Health Visitor Part 1: 54:1:20–21; Part 2: 52–57, Part 3: 104–105, 1981
5. Faden RR, Chu Walow Quaid K, et al: Prenatal screening and pregnant women's attitudes toward the abortion of defective fetuses. Am J Public Health 77:3:288–290, 1987
6. Williams CA, Beresford SAA, James SA, et al: The Edgecombe County high blood pressure control program: III. Social support, social stressors, and treatment dropout. Am J Public Health 75:483–486, 1985
7. Chavigny KH, Lewis A: Team or primary nursing care. Nurs Outlook 32:6:322–325, Nov/Dec, 1983
8. Chavigny KH, Nunnally DM: A comparison of methods for collecting clean catch specimens in a clinic population. Am J Obstet Gynecol 122:5:34–42, 1975
9. Olds DL, Henderson CR, Chamerlin R, Tatelbaum R: Preventing child abuse and neglect: A randomized trial of nursing home visitation. Pediatrics 78:1:65–78, July, 1986
10. Whall AL: The family as the unit of care in nursing: a historical review. Public Health 3:4:240–249, Dec, 1986

11. Jacox A: The coming of age of nursing research. Nurs Outlook 34:6:276–280, 1986
12. Birkauskas VH: Public health nursing practice: An educator's view. Nurs Outlook 30:7:384–389, July/Aug, 1982
13. Williams CA: Making things happen: Community health nursing and the policy arena. Nurs Outlook 31:4:225–228, 1983
14. Combs T, Reis J, Ward LD: Effectiveness of home visits by public health nurses in maternal and child health. Pub Health Rep 100:5:490–497, 1985
15. Cunningham R: Participant observation: A research technique in public health nursing. Can J Public Health. 69:2:101–106, 1978
16. Ruffery-Rahal MA: Qualitative methods in community analysis. Public Health Nurs 2:3:130–137, 1985
17. Roybal SE, Bauwins E, Fasla MJ: Community-assessment: An epidemiologic approach. Nurs Outlook 23:6:365–368, 1975
18. Powers KA: Epidemiology: First hand study by community health nurses. Issues Comp Ped Nurs 5:4:211–217, 1981
19. Rumbold G: Community forum district nursing. The role of research. Nurs Mirr 155:3:2–5, 1982
20. Dick B, Spencer IW, Watermeyer GS, Bourne DE, et al: Chronic illness in non-institutionalized persons. Prevalence and epidemiology. S Afr Med J 53:22:892–904, 1978
21. Kovar MG: Aging in the Eighties. National health interview survey. US. Jan–Jun 1984. NCHS 116:1–7, May 9, 1986
22. Laven GT, Brown KC: Nutritional status of men attending a soup kitchen: A pilot study. Am J Public Health 75:8:875–878, 1985
23. Sills GM, Goeppinger J: The community as a field of inquiry in nursing. Annu Rev Nurs Res, Springer Publishing Co. 3–23, 1984
24. Bronstein K, Murray P, Licata–Gehr, et al: The stroke data bank. Implications for nursing research. J Neurosci Nurs 18:3:132–134, 1986
25. Kendrick VM, Sullivan JH: Nursing research at VNA. Home Health Nurse 2:5:44–46, 1984
26. Brown LM, Pottern LM: Epidemiological approaches to cancer research. Semin Oncol Nurs 2:3:146–153, 1986
27. Senie RT: Assessment of carcinogenesis through epidemiologic and experimental investigation. Semin Oncol Nurs 2:3:154–160, 1986
28. Highriter ME: Status of community health nursing research. Nurs Res 26:3:183–192, 1977
29. Highriter ME: Public health nursing evaluation, education and professional issues. Annu Rev Nurs Res, Springer Publishing Co, 165–189, 1984
30. Gutelius MF, Kirsch AD, MacDonald S, et al: Controlled study of child health supervision. Behavioral results. Pediatrics 60:294–304, 1977
31. Sanger S, Weir K, Churchill E: Treatment of sleep problems. Health Venture 54:421–424, 1981
32. Spiegel MA, Lindaman FC: Children can't fly. A program to prevent childhood morbidity and mortality from window fall. Am J Public Health 67:1143–1147, 1977
33. Logan AG, Milne BJ, Achber C, et al: Worksite treatment of hypertension by specially trained nurses. Lancet 2:1175–1178, 1979

34. Andersen E, Andersen TP, Koltke FJ: Stroke rehabilitation: Maintenance of achieved gains. Arch Phys Med Rehabil 58:345–352, 1977

35. Birkauskas VH: Effectiveness of public health nurse visits to primiparous mothers and infants. Am J Public Health 73 (5): 573–580, 1983

36. Chen SC, Sullivan JA: School Nursing. Ann Rev Nurs Res, Springer Publishing Co, 25–48, 1985

37. Ryan MN: The epidemiologic method of building causal inference. ANS 5:2:73–81, 1983

38. Chavigny KH: The changing role of the infection control practitioner. Am J Infect Control, September, 1985, 183–188

39. Drusin LM, Marr JS, Lambertsen EC, et al: The New York City nurse epidemiology program. Bull NY Acad Med 53:6:569–585, 1977

40. Benedict MB, Sproles B: Application of the Neuman model to public health practice. 223–237, 1986

41. Neuman B: A total person approach to viewing patient problems. Nurs Res 21:3:264–269, 1972

42. Salmon White M: Constructs for public health nursing. Nurs Outlook 527–530, Nov, 1982

43. ANA Standards of community health nursing practice. Kansas City, 1974

44. ANA: A conceptual model of community health nursing. Kansas City, 1980

45. APHA Public health nursing section. The definition and role of public health nursing in the delivery of care. 1980

46. Archer SE: Synthesis of public health science and nursing science. Nurs Outlook 30:442–446, 1982

47. Kornblatt ES, Goeppinger J, Jagger J: Epidemiology in community health nursing education: Fit or misfit? Public Health Nurs 2:2:104–108, 1985

48. Milbank Memorial Fund Commission 1976 Higher education for public health. Prodist New York

Appendices

Outline of the Natural History Model*

Four Stages in the Natural History of Disease

A. *State of Susceptibility:* Here the disease has not yet developed, but the groundwork has been laid by the presence of factors that favor its occurrence. These factors that are associated with an increased likelihood that disease will develop at a later time are called "risk factors," and can be categorized as host, agent, and environment.
   1. The host-agent-environment (HAE) triad should be identified when known. If the specific causative agent is unknown, that should be so stated.
   2. Where risk factors can be identified, they should be eliminated under the concepts of primary prevention.
      a. Specific protection
      b. General health promotion

B. *Stage of Presymptomatic Disease:* Here through the interaction of HAE, pathogenic changes have started to occur even though those changes are not yet detectable via signs and symptoms or diagnostic technology.
   1. Prediction of host outcomes is made depending on what is known about the natural history. Host outcomes can be
      a. Recovery
      b. Chronicity
      c. Immunity (in the case of some communicable diseases)
      d. Disability or irreversible physical or psychosocial change
      e. Death
   2. The incubation period, if known, should be stated.

C. *Stage of Clinical Disease:* Here there are recognizable symptoms that initiate contact with the health care delivery system, or in the absence of symptoms, disease can be detected either through physical signs or other diagnostic procedures such as x-rays, sonograms, or laboratory work.
   1. Nursing management is centered around the components of secondary prevention strategies.
      a. Early diagnosis and treatment
      b. Disability limitation

D. *Stage of Disability:* If this stage is entered at all, it is because there have been irreversible physical changes or limitations of the client's psychosocial roles such as parent, wage earner, and so forth.
   1. Client is viewed holistically throughout the natural history.

*Adapted from Mausner and Kramer, 1985

2. Nursing management is based on precepts of tertiary prevention.
   a. Rehabilitation/restorative goals

Appendix B

Exercise on Calculation of Rates

A. Instructions to the Learner

1. Review Chapter 4, Epidemiology and Community Health Nursing
2. Review Objectives of the exercise.
3. Review Definitions of Rates by two numerator and denominator in Chapter 4.
4. Review the concepts of relating to the selection of denominator for specific rates.

B. Objectives

1. To assist the students to calculate the most frequently used rates.
2. To show the calculation of specific rates.
3. To assist the student in learning how to calculate properties.
4. To enable the generalist staff nurse to use simple epidemiologic measures to prioritize professional learning for quality nursing care.

C. Calculation of Rates

The following information is from an imaginary census tract served by a nursing agency. A community assessment has revealed these statistics for 1980.

Total midyear population	60,000
Population 45 years of age and older	10,000
Number of infants born alive	1,200
Fetal deaths (reported)	16
Maternal deaths	1
Total deaths	324
Deaths of infants under 1 year of age	12
Deaths of persons 45 years and older	200
From heart disease	45
From cancer	30
From accidents	13

1. Using the above data, calculate the following indices of health for the community served by the nursing agency applying the usual constant (10^x) where applicable. Show all calculations.
    a. Crude or summary birth rate
    b. Crude or summary death rate
    c. Infant mortality rate
    d. Maternal mortality rate
    e. Age specific death rates for persons   45
    f. Age cause specific death rates for   ≥45 years for:
        (1) Heart disease
        (2) Accidents
    g. Proportion of elderly in this population
2. As a staff nurse in community health nursing, which problems in this census track would guide your selection of topics for study for delivery of nursing care to this population.

Answers

1. a. $\dfrac{1,000}{60,000} \times 10^3$ for 1980 = 16.7/1,000 for 1980

    b. $\dfrac{324}{60,000} \times 10^x$ for 1980 = 5.4/1,000 for 1980

    c. $\dfrac{16}{1,200 \text{ live births}} \times 10^3$ for 1980 = 13.3/1,000 live births for 1980

    d. $\dfrac{1}{1,200} \times 10^4$ for 1980 = 8.3/10,000 live births for 1980

    e. $\dfrac{200}{10,000} \times 10^4$ for 1980 = 20/1,000 persons ≥ 45 years for 1980

    f. Age cause specific death rates for 45 years for:
        (1) $\dfrac{45}{10,000} \times 10^3$ for 1980 = 4.5/1,000 persons ≥ 45 years for 1980
        (2) $\dfrac{13}{10,000} \times 10^3$ for 1980 = 1.3/1,000 persons ≥ 45 years for 1980

    g. $\dfrac{10,000}{60,000} = 0.17$

2. There is a fairly large proportion of elderly in the census track. Nursing care for elderly would be the highest priority, with special focus on cardiac nursing care and reduction of accidents. Well-baby care and prenatal services would also be of interest. Oncological nursing could be reviewed.

Appendix C

Exercise in the Application of Epidemiologic Method

A. Instructions to the Learner

1. Review Chapter 11, Applied Epidemiology
2. Read about the transmission of Hepatitis B from the literature such as MMWR Dec 30 1977, vol 25, #52.
3. Complete the pre-test.
4. Read the problem.
5. Answer the questions.
6. Write report.
7. Read objectives of this exercise.

B. Objectives

1. To assist the student to learn the principles of applying epidemiology to hospital infection control practice.
2. To adapt the epidemiologic method for hospital infection control practice.
3. To assist the student to identify the steps in the epidemiologic method.
4. To illustrate the activities which are associated with the epidemiologic method.
5. To allow the student to practice hypothesis formation using practical examples.
6. To assist the student in relating the needs of hospital environment to the needs of the community.
7. To assist the student to relate hospital infection control to responsibilities of prevention and control.

Pre-Test

1. A person-to-person outbreak is the same as a propagated epidemic.

    True _____   False _____

2. In a common-source outbreak, the characterization of an epidemic by periods of time is adequately done using the following facts. Select the most appropriate answer.

    _____ a. Relating the suspected propagated (common-source) cases to the known propagated cases to periods of time; the beginning, end, and duration of the epidemic; the peak of the epidemic.

_____ b. Periods of time relating the peak of the outbreak; the beginning, end, and duration of the epidemic; the probable period of exposure of the cases to the source.

_____ c. Periods of time relating to the place of exposure; the beginning, end, and duration of the outbreak; the probable period of exposure of the cases.

3. When you have a small number of cases in an epidemic, the best way of presenting a graph is one of the following:
   _____ a. A histogram
   _____ b. A polygon
   _____ c. Case plots or case charts
   _____ d. Time-line
   _____ e. c and d above

Answers to Pre-Test

1. True
2. b
3. e

Problem Set:
Hepatitis B—An Occupational Health Hazard

In distress, the director of nursing services at a large university hospital telephones the hospital epidemiologist. One of the nurses, Ms. Elizabeth Caron, R.N., is claiming work compensation for contracting hepatitis B while on duty. At this time, Ms. Caron is so ill that she has been admitted to the hospital. The director asks the infection control nurse to follow up the case to establish if the workplace had exposed this nurse to the occupational hazard.

Case History of Elizabeth Caron, R.N.

Ms. Caron is admitted on August 31 to the university hospital with a diagnosis of hepatitis B. SGOT is raised; Hb_sAg is positive. She is jaundiced. She is 34 years old, married, with three children aged 7, 6, and 5 years. She is a part-time nurse at this same hospital and is placed wherever she is needed (*i.e.*, she is a "floating nurse").

The epidemiologist reviews the hospital record and interviews Ms. Caron. The nurse-patient claims that even though she works only part-time she has not worked in any other clinic or hospital where she could have contracted the disease. Moreover, she cannot recall ever having worked on any floor with a patient who had a diagnosis of hepatitis B nor has she worked in the dialysis unit.

A review of all hospital charts for the last 6 months does not disclose the occurrence of any patient or staff cases of hepatitis B. Ms. Caron's schedule (part-time) for the approximately 4 months pertaining to incubation period is retrieved from nursing service. She always works days from 7:30 AM to 3:30 PM. A summary of the work schedule is as follows:

Work Schedule

Date	Floor	Date	Floor	Date	Floor	Date	Floor
April 1	12A (Neuro)	May 3	PAR	June 8	CRR	March 3	7A
2	7A (Surg)	5	PAR	9	CRR	9	8A
5	PAR	6	PAR	12	7A	10	8A
6	7A	7	8A	18	7A	12	8A
14	7A	10	8A	19	8A	15	8A
15	12A	11	8A	10	12A	16	7A
16	8A (Med)	12	10A	VACATION		17	7A
19	8A	14	PAR			21	PAR
21	8A	17	7A			24	CRR
23	CRR	18	7A			25	CRR
27	12A	19	7A			26	12A
29	8A	25	12A			30	12A
30	8A	27	12A				

Key
PAR: post-anesthesia room   Adult floors: 12A, 12 (renal), 8, 7, 5C (psych)
CRR: cardiac recovery room   Pediatric floor: 12B (prem), 13B, 13A, 14

This schedule is reviewed with Ms. Caron. She still denies having had contact with a known hepatitis case or having had any incidental injury that might have resulted in a puncture wound. Ms. Caron is discharged from the hospital on September 12.

Six days later, another case of hepatitis B is admitted to the same hospital. The nurse interviews the new case, Mr. Charles Riley, aged 52 years, who does not admit to any contact with a person with hepatitis outside the hospital. He has no explanation for his present illness. A review of his voluminous chart does not reveal a history of drug addiction; however, it reveals a previous admission to the hospital. His hospital history is reviewed and summarized as follows:

Case History of Charles Riley

Mr. Riley is admitted to the university hospital with a diagnosis of hepatitis B. SGOT is raised; Hb$_s$Ag is positive. He is jaundiced. Mr. Riley is 52 years old and is divorced. He lives alone. He has two married daughters who live out of state and whom he has not seen for the past year. He is a carpenter by trade.

Hospital Course

He was admitted to the university hospital April 17, Floor 7A Surgical Service.

> Discharged May 21
> Diagnosis: Cholecystitis
> Readmitted to university hospital September 18
> Diagnosis: Hepatitis B

Operation 1: Cholecystectomy, April 23, performed by Dr. Brantam and Dr. Niel.

> RNs Riegel and Campbell
> LPN Johnstone (nurses in attendance at the operation)
> Received whole blood as follows:
> > #21 J.15.485 (exp. date April 29)
> > #21 J.15.929 (exp. date April 29)
> > #21 J.15.966 (exp. date April 19)

Operation 2: End-to-end anastomosis for intestinal obstruction—surgical emergency, May 4, performed by Dr. Mack and Dr. Brown.

> RN Collins and LPN Johnstone in attendance
> Received whole blood as follows:
> > #21 G.15933 (exp. date May 14)
> > #21 G.19536 (exp. date May 14)
> > #21 G.15941 (exp. date May 14)
> Diagnosis: cholecystitis
> Readmitted to university hospital September 18
> Diagnosis: hepatitis B

The epidemiologist phones Ms. Caron at home to inquire if at any time Ms. Caron had nursed Mr. Riley. She is told that Ms. Caron does not recall the patient and has had no contact with Mr. Riley at all.

Answer the following questions using the information given:

1. Is this a person-to-person case occurrence? Justify your answer.
2. a. Is there any logical hypothesis that might connect these cases?
   b. Make a time-line drawing to substantiate your answer.
3. Outline the activities that coincide with each step of the epidemiologic method (*i.e.,* identify the activities with which epidemiologists must be involved during this investigation that illustrate *each* step of the epidemiologic method).

Answers

1. This is not a person-to-person (or propagated) problem. The onset of the disease in both Mr. Riley and Ms. Caron are within 2½ weeks of each other, September 18 and August 31, respectively. Exposure must have occurred before the minimum incubation period 2 months earlier.

2.   a. The most likely hypothesis is one of a common source exposure to the same hazard.
b. Time-line graph (Fig. App-C-1)

An examination of the time-line or individual case charting
graph puts the two cases in possible contact on May 17, 18, and
19. This is just previous to Mr. Riley's discharge and 2 weeks after his last operation, when the patient was most likely to be
ambulating. Recall that Ms. Caron denies any contact with this
patient.

Another more likely hypothesis is that the two cases were
exposed around the time of the operation. However, no direct
contact is indicated on the time-line chart of cases. The surgery
was performed on May 14, and Ms. Caron was in the postanes-
thesia room (PAR) the following day. These dates are very close
together and indicate proximity, and an hypothesis that she contacted equipment used in the operation is tenable. For instance,
the intravenous equipment after the emergency operation during
the night might have required clean-up, during which a puncture wound with contaminated blood was possible. This hypothesis is testable through direct inquiry from Ms. Caron and the
OR supervisor.

3.   *STEP 1—Establish the existence of a problem (or epidemic).* The nurse
is part-time and young. It is possible that she or her husband
has an unadmitted drug problem, but this is unlikely in view of

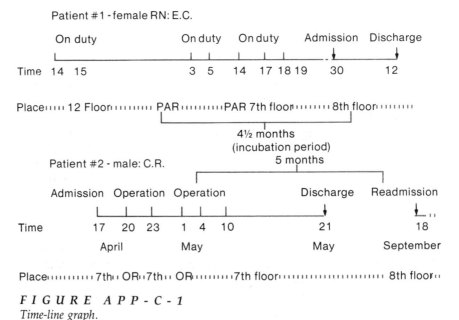

FIGURE   APP-C-1
Time-line graph.

the family responsibilities. Also, it is possible that because she is only part-time, contact has been from a source other than this hospital. Because hepatitis B is a known occupational hazard of nurses, the problem is to establish exposure within the hospital. The occurrence of the second case substantiates the need for investigation.

STEP 2—Verify the diagnosis. Laboratory tests and medical diagnoses confirm that these cases are, in fact, cases of hepatitis B. The Hb_sAg is pathognomonic for this disease. There is no evidence given to assume that either Ms. Caron or Mr. Riley are chronic carriers of the antigen. In view of the presence of acute liver disease (jaundice), it is unlikely that either case is "old."

STEP 3—Quick survey of cases and the community situations. A quick survey of the two cases reveals no age or sex association (*i.e.*, no "clustering"). We know from experience that cases of Hepatitis B occur mostly in young adults (WHO). We also know that cases increase in hospital workers such as physicians and nurses (WHERE). It will be necessary to establish some TIME relationship and PLACE of occurrence for the two cases to establish hypotheses about causation (HOW).

The community situation is defined as follows. The hospital community hires Ms. Caron as a float. Records of her floor assignment are available from nursing services and so is access in the case histories from charts.

The natural history of the disease shows an incubation period of 2 to 6 months (WHEN), a virus that uses blood as a reservoir, such as a chronic carrier (WHERE), and attacks people and primates (WHO). The virus resists freezing and (to a degree) acids, and ultraviolet irradiation. Only a very small dose is required to produce illness (WHAT). The route of transmission is parenteral, although traumatized mucous membranes such as bleeding gums, skin punctures and abrasions provide portals of entry for the virus (HOW).

STEP 4—Formulate hypothesis. The immediate hypothesis using the incubation period as evidence is that a common source exposure of both cases is postulated. This implies that the two cases have been associated with the same place at the same time.

STEP 5—Plan the investigation. The investigation plan is to gather information concerning Mr. Riley's experience in the hospital and compare this by time and place with the nurse's experience. The patient's chart and interview is a source of information. The nursing office supplies the time schedule for Ms. Caron. Personal interview and telephone contact are corroborating sources.

STEP 6—Conduct the investigation. Information is collected as planned. Time schedules are correlated with chart information. Appropriate people are interviewed.

STEP 7—Analyze the data. Data is analyzed through a time-line drawing which graphically displays the observations, and permits the formulation of new hypotheses when necessary.

STEP 8—Test hypothesis. Testing of hypothesis must be preceded by restating the postulated relationship, which is then correlated by a thorough examination of the data. In the present discussion there are two relevant hypotheses:

H_{01}: The two cases were exposed to a mutually shared reservoir of hepatitis B pathogen such as a blood product and transfusion equipment while patient was on the same ward, 7A, at the time the nurse was assigned to that floor. Testing of this hypothesis may be accomplished through reiterating that the nurse had no recollection of contacting this patient. It is also unlikely that Mr. Riley would have been receiving blood and blood product transfusion this late in his hospital course. His chart does not indicate blood transfusions on these dates. The first hypothesis is unsupported.

H_{02}: The next hypothesis is that they were in close proximity in the operating room (OR) and PAR and were exposed to the same reservoir. Review of Mr. Riley's chart shows that the end-to-end anastomosis was an *emergency* operation and was unscheduled. Even though the date was the 4th, it is reasonable to assume that the emergency took place late in the day of the 4th. Mr. Riley received many transfusions. The IV equipment could have remained in the OR until Ms. Caron came on duty at 7:00 AM. (This problem is a real occurrence. In fact, an interview with Ms. Caron substantiated that often after a busy night in surgery she would assist in cleaning up and discarding used IV equipment.)

STEP 9—Formulate conclusions. The conclusion is that there is enough epidemiologic evidence to put Ms. Caron and Mr. Riley in the same place at the same time with the same possible exposure to risk of hepatitis B through an infected blood product.

STEP 10—Put control measures into operation. Prevention and control measures include:

    a. Advocating the use of rubber gloves when handling used IV equipment.

    b. Care of the skin, particularly the hands, to avoid abrasions.

    c. Reporting of accidents, particularly puncture wounds.

    d. Informing the blood bank of the results of the investigation and the blood batch numbers used.

    e. Reporting the cases to the public health agencies, with the results of the investigation.

    f. In-service education to all disciplines on the occupational health hazards of hepatitis B and precautions that are necessary to prevent and control the spread of the disease.

STEP 11—Report. Three reports should be written. The first is a synopsis of the investigation to be sent to the director of nurses. The second is a similar report sent to Ms. Caron to substantiate her claim for compensation. The third is a full and detailed report similar to this outline to retain for the records of the infection control program.

Guidelines for Safe Sex*

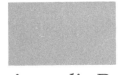

Appendix D

Many diseases may be transmitted during sexual encounters between homosexual, bisexual, or heterosexual partners. Examples of diseases that can be transmitted include syphilis, gonorrhea, herpes, hepatitis, acquired immune deficiency syndrome (AIDS) as well as lesser known infections such as Chlamydia. By following the safe sex guidelines outlined in this pamphlet, one can greatly reduce the chances of becoming infected with any of these debilitating and sometimes fatal diseases.

1. Having fewer different partners and knowing one's partner and his or her state of health and lifestyle reduces the risk. Avoid sex with persons who use intravenous drugs or who have multiple sex partners. From a communicable disease standpoint, the safest sexual partner is a monogamous one.
2. Engage in sex in a setting conducive to cleanliness. When both partners shower together as a part of foreplay, there is an opportunity to check for sores and swollen lymph glands, and bodily cleanliness is a prelude to enjoyable and safe sex. Don't share personal hygiene items such as toothbrushes and razors.
3. Kissing, as long as oneself and one's partner have no open sores on the lips, mouth, or tongue, also has a low risk of transmitting disease (with the possible exception of mononucleosis). Sexual experience is not limited to penile penetration. One should be creative with other types of body contact that do not involve exchange of body fluid, such as cuddling, massaging, and mutual masturbation. Information to date indicates that AIDS is not transmitted by casual kissing.
4. Exchanging body fluids has a high risk of transmitting disease. Oral contact or swallowing semen, urine, stool particles, and menstrual flow increases the risk of transmitting disease and should be completely avoided. Oral sex should be avoided when cuts or sores are present in the mouth.

*These guidelines were adapted with permission from pamphlets by the Gay Men's Health Crisis, Inc., New York City and AID Atlanta, Georgia. Copyright.

5. Some sexual practices are quite hazardous. Rimming has a very high risk of transmitting disease, especially in nonmonogamous situations. Fisting is extremely dangerous under any circumstances.

6. Lubricants should be water-soluble (not oils or greases). Not only is saliva a poor lubricant, but it may be loaded with germs. The lubricant should not be in any open container nor shared with others. Use one that is packaged in a pump, squeezer, or other closed container that dispenses one application at a time. Use non-perfumed lubricants.

7. Data at this time indicate that use of quality condoms prevents the spread of most sexually transmitted diseases when used appropriately.

8. Anal intercourse causes tiny tears through which germs from both partners can enter the body. Use of a water-soluble lubricant helps reduce friction and tears and should be used even with a condom. Anal or vaginal douching before or after sex increases the risk of acquiring some infections because it removes normal barriers to infection.

9. Urinating after sex may reduce the risk of acquiring some diseases.

10. Reduce or eliminate use of toxic substances such as alcohol, cigarettes, marijuana, poppers, and non-prescription drugs. These substances affect judgment and tend to decrease the body's ability to fight off infection.

11. Maintain the body's immune system by eating well, exercising, and getting adequate rest. Sex should not be used as one's only means of stress reduction. Other stress reduction techniques should be learned such as self-hypnosis.

Symptoms of sexually transmitted diseases vary, but if any of the following are experienced, one should see a local health care provider for evaluation.

1. Extreme fatigue
2. Fever and night sweats
3. Unexplained weight loss
4. Enlarged lymph glands
5. Unexplained discharge from penis or vagina
6. Sores on or around genitalia
7. Painful urination or chronic diarrhea
8. Heavy, dry cough, and/or shortness of breath
9. Unexplained bruising or purplish patches

Home Care of Persons with Aids: Infection Control Guidelines

Health care providers should be familiar with current epidemiological information on AIDS including modes of transmission of HIV.

Patient Care Precautions

Handwashing: Hands should be washed before and after direct client care and after contact with blood, body fluids, or other body excretions.[1]

Gloves: Gloves should be worn when direct contact with clients' blood, body fluids, excretions or secretions, or direct contact with surfaces or articles contaminated with blood or body excretions is expected.[1]

Gowns: Gowns should be worn if soiling of clothing with clients' blood or body excretions is anticipated.[1]

Masks: Although not routinely needed, masks have been recommended for care providers having close contact with clients with a productive cough.[2,3]

Needles and syringes: Needles should not be bent or recapped after they are used, and the syringe and needle should be disposed of in a puncture-proof container.[1] Contact the local health department for information on disposal of containers.

Treatments: Gloves should be worn, and the double-bagging technique should be used for dressing changes.[4]

Waste disposal: Body wastes should be flushed down the toilet. Dressings or other materials contaminated with blood or body excretions should be collected in a plastic-lined trash can. Contaminated waste and other household trash may be disposed of in a garbage can lined with a plastic bag. The can should have a tight-fitting lid. Contact the local health department for further information about waste disposal.[4,5]

Blood spills: Promptly clean up all blood or body fluid spills with an appropriate disinfectant solution, such as 1:10 dilution of household bleach (5.25% sodium hypochlorite) in water.[1]

Client Precautions

Sex: A variety of sexual practices have been associated with an increased risk of transmission of HTLV-III (HIV).

Good hygienic practices by the client and other household members, such as regular bathing and handwashing after toileting and before meal preparation, should be encouraged.[5]

Personal hygiene items that may become contaminated with blood or body fluids, such as razors and toothbrushes, should not be shared with other household members. Towels and washcloths should not be shared between launderings.[5,6]

Laundry: Soiled linen should be kept in a plastic bag separate from other household laundry. Clients' laundry should be washed separately in hot, soapy water. Household bleach can be added to cottons and colorfast materials. A phenolic disinfectant, such as Lysol, can be used with noncolorfast fabrics. A second wash and rinse without the phenolic assists in removing chemical residues.[4]

Dishes: Dishes, glasses, and eating utensils may be run through the dishwater using the hot water cycle or washed in hot, soapy water and air dried.[4,5]

Food: Due to the risk of salmonella infection, only pasteurized milk or milk products should be eaten. Fruits and vegetables composted with manure should be peeled or cooked before being eaten.[5]

Living areas should be well ventilated. This decreases the risk of airborne diseases.[4,5]

Housecleaning: Routine housecleaning procedures in the kitchen and bathroom should be followed to prevent the growth of bacteria and fungi that may cause infections. The inside of the refrigerator should be kept clean to prevent growth of molds. The kitchen counter and sink used for food preparation should be scoured and rinsed prior to food preparation. *Kitchen and bathroom floors* should be mopped at least weekly, with any spills cleaned up as they occur. A 1:10 strength bleach in a water solution can be used as a disinfectant in mop water and for cleaning up blood and body fluid spills. Dirty mop water should be flushed down the toilet. Mops and sponges used to clean floors or spills or blood or body fluids should not be rinsed out at the sink used for food preparation. A 1:10 bleach solution may be used to disinfect sinks. Full-strength bleach may be added to the toilet bowl as a disinfectant. Mops and sponges may be soaked in the 1:10 bleach solution for 5 minutes to disinfect them.[5] Mops and sponges used to clean the bathroom and blood and body fluid spills should be separate from those used to clean other parts of the house.[4]

Pets: Pets may pose potential infection risks. Gloves and masks should be worn when cleaning birdcages, due to the risk of psittacosis, and cat litter boxes, due to the risk of toxoplasmosis. Since fish tanks may harbor mycobacterium species, which have caused serious infections in persons with AIDS, someone other than the client should clean the tank.[4,5]

References

References for Appendices D and E

1. Centers for Disease Control: Acquired Immune Deficiency Syndrome (AIDS): Precautions for Clinical and Laboratory Staffs. MMWR 31:577–580, 1982
2. Conte JE Jr, Hadley WK, Sande M, and the University of California, San Francisco, Task Force on the Acquired Immunodeficiency Syndrome: Infection Control Guidelines for Patients with the Acquired Immunodeficiency Syndrome (AIDS). New Engl J Med 309:740–744, 1983
3. American Hospital Association: Recommendations of the Advisory Committee on Infections Within Hospitals. In Acquired Immune Deficiency Syndrome: An Educational Packet, Mundeleen, IL, Educational Committee of the Association of Practitioners in Infection Control, 1984
4. Dhundale K, Hubbard PM: Home care for the A.I.D.S. patient: Safety first. Nursing 86 16(9):34–36, 1986
5. California Public Health Services: Public Health Nursing Standardized Care Plan: Acquired Immune Deficiency Syndrome, San Francisco, CPHS, 1985
6. Centers for Disease Control: Provisional Public Health Service Interagency Recommendations for Screening Donated Blood and Plasma for Antibody to the Virus Causing Acquired Immunodeficiency Syndrome. MMWR 34:1–5, 1985

Two Tools for Functional Assessment of the Elderly

Appendix F

Mini-Mental State Examination

	Maximum Score	Score
Orientation		
1. What is the (year) (season) (day of week) (date) (month)? Give one point for each correct answer.	5	___ 48
2. Where are we (state) (county) (city) (hospital) (floor)? Give one point for each correct answer.	5	___ 49
Registration		
3. Repeat these objects: **chair, tree, cigarette.** One second to say each. Then ask the patient all three you have told them. Give one point for each correct answer. Repeat them until he learns all three. Count trials and record number. Number of trials _____.	3	___ 50
Attention and Calculation		
4. Begin with 100 and count backwards by 7 (stop patient after five answers). One point for each correct response. Alternatively, spell "world" backwards. 100 93 86 79 72	5	___ 51
Recall		
5. Ask for three objects repeated above. Give one point for each correct answer.	3	___ 52
Language		
6. Show a pencil and a watch and ask patient to name them. Give one point for each correct answer.	2	___ 53
7. Repeat the following: **No if's, and's, or but's.**	1	___ 54
8. A three-stage command, **"Take a paper in your right hand, fold it in half, and put it on the floor."** Give one point for each correct answer.	3	___ 55
9. Read and obey the following: (show patient the written item). **CLOSE YOUR EYES.**	1	___ 56
10. Write a sentence. **SEE THE DOG RUN.**	1	___ 57
11. Copy a design (complex polygon as in Bender-Gestalt).	1	___ 58
Total Score		___ 59–60

Katz Index of Independence in Activities of Daily Living

The Index of Independence in Activities of Daily Living is based on an evaluation of the functional independence or dependence of patients in bathing, dressing, going to the toilet, transferring, continence, and feeding. Specific definitions of functional independence and dependence appear below the index.

A   Independent in feeding, continence, transferring, going to toilet, dressing, and bathing.

B   Independent in all but one of these functions.

C   Independent in all but bathing and one additional function.

D   Independent in all but bathing, dressing, and one additional function.

E   Independent in all but bathing, dressing, going to toilet, and one additional function.

F   Independent in all but bathing, dressing, going to toilet, transferring, and one additional function.

G   Dependent in all six functions.

Other   Dependent in at least two functions, but not classifiable as C, D, E, or F.

Independence means without supervision, direction, or active personal assistance, except as specifically noted below. This is based on actual status and not on ability. A patient who refuses to perform a function is considered as not performing the function, even though he is deemed able.

BATHING (Sponge, shower or Tub)

Independent: assistance only in bathing a single part (as back or disabled extremity) or bathes self completely

Dependent: assistance in bathing more than one part of body; assistance in getting in or out of tub or does not bathe self

DRESSING

Independent: gets clothes from closets and drawers; puts on clothes, outer garments, braces; manages fasteners; act of tying shoes is excluded

Dependent: does not dress self or remains partly undressed

GOING TO TOILET

Independent: gets to toilet; gets on and off toilet; arranges clothes, cleans organs of excretion; (may manage own bedpan used at night only and may or may not be using mechanical supports)

Dependent: uses bedpan or commode or receives assistance in getting to and using toilet

TRANSFER

Independent: moves in and out of bed independently and moves in and out of chair independently (may or may not be using mechanical supports)

Dependent: assistance in moving in or out of bed and/or chair; does not perform one or more transfers

CONTINENCE

Independent: urination and defecation entirely self-controlled

Dependent: partial or total incontinence in urination or defecation partial or total control by enemas, catheters, or regulated use of urinals and/or bedpans

FEEDING

Independent: gets food from plate or its equivalent into mouth; (precutting of meat and preparation of food, as buttering bread, are excluded from evaluation).

Dependent: assistance in act of feeding (see above); does not eat at all or parenteral feeding.

(Katz S, Ford AB, Moskowitz RW et al: Studies of illness in the aged. The Index of ADL: A standardized measure of biological and psychosocial function. JAMA 185:94, 1963)

Regnery's Assessment Tool for Acuity of Community Services*

T A B L E 1
Patient Care Classification LEVEL I

DEFINITION: This category of care includes those patients and/or families requiring intensive public health nursing service. This category comprises patients who demand a high degree of nursing skill in utilizing knowledge of the physical and behavioral sciences, in in-depth analysis of the patient's needs and problems, in formulation of the nursing care plan and in therapeutic treatment of the patient and family.

Family Situation	*Psychological Component*	*Therapeutic Competence*	*Knowledge of Health Conditions*
This category includes criteria which broadly describe the family and how it is coping as a unit with its developmental tasks.	*This category includes criteria relating to the emotional health of the family as a whole and/or of the individual members.*	*This category includes criteria pertaining to treatments, procedures and medications prescribed for the care of illness.*	*This category includes criteria relating to the acquisition of information about the particular health condition that is the occasion for care.*
Disorganization in all areas of family life.	Family/patient have deep seated emotional or behavioral problems or such problems are suspected.	Family/patient either not carrying out procedures or treatments or are not doing it safely.	Family/patient totally uninformed about health condition or health problem.
Family does not meet its needs for security and physical survival.	One or more family members reactions to illness, disability and stress need professional intervention.	Family/patient giving or taking medication as prescribed.	Family/patient has lack of knowledge about the disease or disability as it relates to cause and effect.
Family has inability to secure adequate wages or to budget money.	Family/patient does not recognize their obvious and serious health and/or social needs or problems.	Family/patient fail to keep scheduled medical appointments and/or appointments with other professional services (P.T., O.T., social services) as prescribed.	
Members of family not working; dependent on public assistance or fixed income.	Family/patient does not face reality		
Family expresses alienation from the community—lack of trust of outsiders, hostile, resistant			

*Reprinted with permission from Regnery G: Patient care needs—an index for community health staffing. Nurs Adm Q pp 77–89

Appendix G

Health Attitudes	Principles of General Hygiene	Environmental Milieu	Community Resources
This category includes criteria which describe the way the family feels about health care in general.	*This category includes criteria which describe activities of daily living such as personal care, personal hygiene, nutrition, sleep, and relaxation and which relate to completing needed immunizations.*	*This category includes criteria concerned with the condition of the house and the type of neighborhood in which the patient/family lives.*	*This category includes criteria which describe the degree to which the family knows about and uses area agencies and facilities.*
Family/patient resents or resists all health care providers.	Necessary immunizations not secured for children and/or adults.	House in poor condition—lead or safety hazards exist.	No community activities exist or are participated in; family/patient has no hobbies or outside interests.
	Family members unkempt, dirty, inadequately clothed, diet grossly inadequate or unbalanced; children and adults getting too little sleep.	Overcrowding exists. Neighborhood deteriorated	Family/patient unaware of and unwilling to utilize community resources.
	Family fails entirely in providing required personal care to one or more of its members.	Community environment is totally unsatisfactory or unsafe, alcoholism or drug abuse problems suspected or known.	
		Rodent or insect problem known or suspected.	

T A B L E   2
Patient Care Classification LEVEL II

DEFINITION: This category of care includes those patients and/or families requiring regular public health nursing service. This category comprises patients who need nursing care to achieve a higher level of independence and who need continuous evaluation of their health status.

Family Situation	Psychological Component	Therapeutic Competence	Knowledge of Health Conditions
This category includes criteria which broadly describe the family and how it is coping as a unit with its developmental tasks.	*This category includes criteria relating to the emotional health of the family as a whole and/or of the individual members.*	*This category includes criteria pertaining to treatments, procedures and medications prescribed for the care of illness.*	*This category includes criteria relating to the acquisition of information about the particular health condition that is the occasion for care.*
Family life may be less disorganized in many areas.	Family must struggle to provide for emotional health and social functioning of family members.	Family-patient is carrying out some but not all of prescribed procedures or treatments; PHN support and encouragement required.	Family patient has the information concerning the health condition or health problem but actions do not indicate that the information is being applied in the situation.
Family barely meets its needs for security and physical survival.	One or more family members expresses anxiety, guilt, depression or inability to cope with stress.	Family/patient giving or taking medications correctly but does not understand purposes of the drug or symptoms to be observed.	Family/patient has some general knowledge of the disease or condition but fails to grasp the underlying principles or is only partially informed.
Family finances are able to meet expenses of daily living but cannot meet any type of crisis.	Family/patient usually recognizes their obvious health or social problems or needs but need help in identifying the less obvious needs or problems.	Family/patient not consistently following through with scheduled medical appointments and/or appointments with other professional services or only following through with PHN assistance or effort.	
Members of family are forced to work beyond reasonable limits (household head holding two or more jobs)			
Although still alienated from the community, some beginning trust is evident in the family.			

Health Attitudes	Principles of General Hygiene	Environmental Milieu	Community Resources
This category includes criteria which describe the way the family feels about health care in general.	*This category includes criteria which describe activities of daily living such as personal care, personal hygiene, nutrition, sleep, and relaxation and which relate to completing needed immunizations.*	*This category includes criteria concerned with the conditions of the house and the type of neighborhood in which the patient/family lives.*	*This category includes criteria which describe the degree to which the family knows about and uses area agencies and facilities.*
Family/patient accept health care only in crisis situations or in case of serious illness, no preventive health care is sought.	Some initial immunizations secured but follow up immunizations not pursued.	House in fair condition—safety hazards exist but family could rectify if identified	Few community activities to participate in; family/patient has few hobbies or outside interests.
	Family/patient generally meeting hygiene needs of sleep, nutrition and cleanliness but need reinforcement, reminders and on-going teaching and help with these measures.	Overcrowding exists but house livable.	Family/patient know some community resources but no help to use appropriate resources.
	Family is providing partially for personal care needs of its members or is providing personal care for some members but not for others.	Neighborhood poor.	
		Some juvenile or adult delinquency among neighbors known or suspected.	

T A B L E   3
Patient Care Classification LEVEL III

DEFINITION: This category of care includes those patients and/or families requiring occasional public health nursing service. This category comprises patients who require nursing care for therapeutic purposes and for being maintained in their homes or to avoid institutionalization.

Family Situation	*Psychological Component*	*Therapeutic Competence*	*Knowledge of Health Conditions*
This category includes criteria which broadly describe the family and how it is coping as a unit with its developmental tasks.	*This category includes criteria relating to the emotional health of the family as a whole and/or of the individual members.*	*This category includes criteria pertaining to treatments, procedures and medications prescribed for the care of illness.*	*This category includes criteria relating to the acquisition of information about the particular health condition that is the occasion for care.*
Family situation is essentially normal but it has more than a healthy amount of conflicts and problems.	Family/patient reached its highest level of functioning within its resources and environment but may need PHN intervention to keep from deteriorating	Family/patient demonstrates ability to carry out procedures and treatments may need some PHN support and encouragement to continue.	Generally family/patient knows and accepts health condition or problem but may need PHN teaching support and supervision to avoid lapses into old patterns.
Members are beginning to meet their need for security and physical survival.	One or more family members may be lacking in emotional control	Family/patient giving or taking medications as prescribed with fairly good understanding of the purposes for and symptoms to be observed but needs some PHN supervision.	
Family finances are adequate for most situations except long term or disastrous types of conditions.	Family/patient recognizes problem but their problem-solving approach needs improvement	Family/patient following through with scheduled medical appointments and/or appointments with other professional services but may need PHN reminders and encouragement.	
Members of family working above normal limits.			
Family demonstrates a greater trust in people and the community, limited alienation may persist.			

Health Attitudes	Principles of General Hygiene	Environmental Milieu	Community Resources
This category includes criteria which describe the way the family feels about health care in general.	*This category includes criteria which describe activities of daily living such as personal care, personal hygiene, nutrition, sleep, and relaxation and which relate to completing needed immunizations.*	*This category includes criteria concerned with the condition of the house and the type of neighborhood in which the patient/family lives.*	*This category includes criteria which describe the degree to which the family knows about and uses area agencies and facilities.*
Family/patient understand and recognize need for medical care in illness.	Immunizations generally complete for children and adults.	House in good repair but safety hazards may be present that need PHN evaluation.	Community Activities provided but access may present some problems; family/patient has some hobbies and outside interests but need encouragement to continue participation.
	Family/Patient able to apply most general principals of hygiene.	Overcrowding not a problem although living space may be small and cramped.	Family/patient knows and uses community resources but may need PHN intervention to continue to follow through.
	Family providing personal care needs of its members but only with PHN encouragement and support.	Neighborhood borderline to respectable.	
		Some undesirable social elements exist but able to protect children from poor social influences.	

T A B L E   4
Patient Care Classification LEVEL IV

DEFINITION: This category of care includes those patients and/or families requiring limited public health nursing service. This category comprises patients who require nursing care in times of crisis or on a short-term basis for resolving health problems or for referral to other agencies.

Family Situation	*Psychological Component*	*Therapeutic Competence*	*Knowledge of Health Conditions*
This category includes criteria which broadly describe the family and how it is coping as a unit with its developmental tasks.	*This category includes criteria relating to the emotional health of the family as a whole and/or of the individual members.*	*This category includes criteria pertaining to treatments, procedures and medications prescribed for the care of illness.*	*This category includes criteria relating to the acquisition of information about the particular health condition that is the occasion for care.*
Family is normal, stable, and healthy with a fewer than usual number of problems which they are normally able to handle as they arise.	Crisis may immobilize the family but they have the ability to adapt and change, enjoy the present and plan for the future.	Family/patient is able to demonstrate that they carry out the prescribed procedures safely and effectively with an understanding of the principles involved and with a confident willing attitude.	Family/patient knows salient facts about the disease or problem well enough to take necessary action at the proper time.
The family's physical survival and security needs are met.	All family members are able to maintain a reasonable degree of emotional calm.	Family/patient giving or taking medications as prescribed and knows purposes for and symptoms to be observed with each.	Family/patient understands the rationale of care and are able to observe and report significant symptoms.
Family finances are usually not a problem.	Family/patient recognizes its problems and develops solutions.	Family/patient giving or taking medications as prescribed and knows purposes of and symptoms to be observed with each.	
Members of family working at a normal limit (household is not working more than one job). No alienation exists.	The family faces reality realistically and optimistically.	Family/patient following through with medical appointments and with appointments with other professionals.	

Health Attitudes	Principles of General Hygiene	Environmental Milieu	Community Resources
This category includes criteria which describe the way the family feels about health care in general.	*This category includes criteria which describe activities of daily living such as personal care, personal hygiene, nutrition, sleep, and relaxation and which relate to completing needed immunizations.*	*This category includes criteria concerned with the conditions of the house and the type of neighborhood in which the patient/family lives.*	*This category includes criteria which describe the degree to which the family knows about and uses area agencies and facilities.*
Family/patient understands, recognizes and accepts the need for health care.	Immunizations complete for all children and adults according to standard recommendations.	House in good repairs—no safety hazards identifiable.	Many opportunities for community activities; family/patient has hobbies and outside interests which they enjoy.
	Personal Hygiene excellent; family meals well selected and well balanced; habits of sleep and rest adequate to needs.	No Crowding exists; adequate living space is present providing for privacy of all family members.	Family/patient use available resources and suitable facilities as needed
	All family members whether or not there is infirmity or disability in one or more of its members are receiving the necessary personal care.	Neighborhood respectable.	
		Neighborhood free from undesirable social elements.	
		Home is free of rodent and pest problems.	

Appendix H

Family Learning Needs Assessment

Primary caregiver _____ age _____
Family members _____ age _____
               _____ age _____
               _____ age _____

Check Off   *Comments*

1. *Present knowledge level, is aware of:*

   • Diagnosis
   • Symptom progression
   • Duration of disease

2. *Wants to know*

   • Problem management techniques
     — Wandering
     — Aggression
     — Memory loss
   • Communication techniques
   • Diagnostic procedures
   • Care options
   • Support groups
   • Disease
     — Possible causes
     — Duration
     — Symptom progression
   • Community resources

3. *Stressors:*

   • Health status
   • Financial
   • Household reorganization
   • Internal family conflicts
   • Aging produced changes, *e.g.,* hearing,
     visual, or memory deficits

4. *Readiness:*

   • Expresses desire to learn
   • Asks questions
   • Provides for teaching time
   • Requests learning experiences
     — Reading material

Glossary of Epidemiologic Terms

Adjusted rates: Summary rates that are standardized, so that they control for effects of the distributional differences of a confounding variable (like age or sex) between groups.

Antibiograms: A series of susceptibility responses of a pathogen to several antibiotics are called antibiograms. This profile is used to prescribe the most effective antibiotic for the infected patient. Antibiograms are used as epidemiologic markers to identify quickly probable strains of bacteria as similar strains. They can be used to plan nursing interventions in communities.

Bacteriophages: Pieces of chromosomal material, similar to a virus that multiplies in bacterial cells. Phages spread by lysing bacterial cells. Phage typing is an epidemiologic marker used to verify similar bacterial strains in an epidemic.

Bar graph: A distribution of values using classes of discrete or nominal variables, illustrated by separate columns or bars.

Biocin typing: Biocins are antibiotic-like substances secreted by strains of gram negative bacteria that may be used as epidemiologic markers to verify cross-infection by the same strain.

Case comparison study: A research design, unique to epidemiology, that compares a group of identified "cases" to a comparison group selected because they have experiences similar to the "cases" but have no disease or negative characteristic. Information is collected retrospectively from both groups.

Case control study: Another name for case comparison study.

Case fatality ratio: A measure of virulence that is calculated by relating the number of deaths from a given disease to the number of cases of that same disease.

Case finding: Systematic activities aimed at uncovering new cases or instances of a given health problem.

Clinical trials: A small, carefully controlled intervention study, applied in a clinical situation. Clinical trials are always cohort studies, and the independent variable is usually a new technique or therapy.

Cluster theory (theory of commonalities): Used during the application of the epidemiologic method for hypothesis formulation. Groups of observation are reviewed according to time, place, and person to theorize the probable cause of a problem or epidemic hazard.

Cohort study: The epidemiologic research design that applies to a prospective study. The cohort or group experiencing the same phenomenon or exposure, (also called propositii) is compared to another cohort who do not have the exposure experience. Both cohorts are followed prospectively over time to compare observed results.

Common source epidemic: Refers to the instance in which all the sick people in an epidemic got their illness from the same source (although not necessarily at the same time), rather than from one another.

Community health nursing: A field of nursing practice that blends knowledge and skills from nursing and public health sciences and applies them toward the promotion of optimal health for the total population.

Conceptual model: A perspective or framework consisting of interrelated principles, constructs, and concepts that form a general frame of reference for application to reality, such as nursing practice and research.

Control group: The group that receives no treatment or manipulation from the independent variable.

Cross-sectional: A prevalence study.

Crude rates: A summary rate that counts events in a total population, p.a.r., and has not been subject to any further definition, computation, or constraint.

Deductive process: A logical method of thinking that starts with a premise and is logically supported by argument. This process is usually defined as going from the general (idea) to the specific (facts) using accepted logical inference.

Demographics: Characteristics that all human beings hold in common, which then can be used to describe the group or community, such as age, race, sex, socioeconomic status, etc.

Diagnostically related groups: Represents an amendment to the Social Security Act that is a method of prospective payment based on groups of medical diagnoses.

Distribution: A table, graph, or mathematical expression giving the probabilities with which a random variable takes different values or sets of values.

Endemic: Expected levels of health phenomena in any given setting. Used in contrast to epidemic.

Epidemic: The occurrence of a disease or health anomaly in excess of normal expectation; exceeding endemic levels.

Epidemiologic markers: Methods of identifying a group of cases caused by the same strain of organism, viruses, fungi, and bacteria. Usually requires complex laboratory tests to verify strains.

Epidemiologic tools: Used in the application of epidemiologic methods for prevention and control of disease in populations. Statistics, laboratory tests for screening populations, epidemiologic markers, and scientific observations and research and sophisticated methods of comparison are all epidemiologic tools.

Epidemiology: The most often used definition is the following: The study of the frequency and distribution of the determinants of an infective process, a disease, or a physiological state and their precursors in a community.

Experimental group: The group in a cohort study that is manipulated or receives treatment; or the group designated as ill in the instance of a case control study.

Extramural communities: Communities not confined within walls (*e.g.,* a neighborhood).

Graph: A method of illustrating a distribution of values.

Hypothesis: A statement of *expected* relationships between variables that are measurable and therefore testable.

Incidence: A measurement of the number of new cases of a disease or other event occurring during a given period.

Incidence rate: The statement of probability of the risk of becoming or experiencing new disease or change of state within a defined time period.

Incidence study: A cohort study.

Inductive process: The scientific process in which observations are used systematically to arrive at a conclusion. Also referred to as the process of going from particular (discrete facts) to the general (conclusion).

Longitudinal study: A cohort study.

Minimum inhibitory concentration (MIC): Used in serial dilution tests to indicate the least amount of antibiotic needed to inhibit growth of a susceptible bacterium *in vitro*.

Morbidity: Refers to illness or morbid condition.

Mortality: Refers to death.

Natural history model: A Public health model utilized to describe the natural sequence of disease when not altered by the levels of prevention.

Noscomial infection: Those infections not present or incubating at the time of admission to an inpatient care facility.

Odds: Probability or likelihood.

Odds ratio (OR): A risk ratio derived from case-comparison studies. The odds ratio quantifies risk of exposure to a hazardous behavior or event relative to the unexposed group from information gathered retrospectively from groups. It is an estimate of relative risk (RR).

Pathogens: Microbes capable of causing disease.

Phage typing: An epidemiologic marker that consists of a method of identifying bacteria using specific strains of bacteriophages.

Pica: The consumption of nonfood items such as dirt, clay, and ashes.

Polygon: A linear configuration used in graphs to express continuous or interval level data.

Population at risk (p.a.r.): The population at risk is (usually) quantified in the denominator of the rate. It refers to a population at risk of the event in the numerator of a rate. The p.a.r. identifies a group that is susceptible to attack from a hazardous event.

Population at high risk: A population at *high* risk is a group with characteristics or behaviors that are known to be associated with high rates of disease and/or mental and social problems.

Prevalence: A measurement of all cases of disease or other phenomena, new or old, existing at any given time.

Prevalence rate: The statement of probability of risk of experiencing or being either a new or old case of disease or change of state at one particular point in time.

Prevalence study: A cross-sectional survey of a community conducted at one point in time to estimate the prevailing level of diseases or status. A community assessment is a prevalence study.

Primary prevention: Preventive strategies that occur before actual disease occurs; may involve general health promotion or specific disease prevention such as active immunizations.

Propagated epidemic: An epidemic in which person-to-person or vector-to-person transmission occurs.

Proportionate mortality ratio (PMR): Expressed as deaths from a specific cause over a denominator that includes death from all causes. The PMR is not a statement of probability, but is useful to estimate the number of lives that could be saved from a specific cause of death through the modification or eradication of factors contributing to that death.

Proprietary agency: Agencies that exist to make a profit, as opposed to voluntary agencies.

Prospective study: A cohort or incidence study.

Public health policy: A process of decision making that helps ensure government use of power for health care needs.

Quarantine: Period of isolation from public communication following onset or exposure to a contagious disease.

Rate: Probability statements concerning the risk of occurrence of an event or state. A measure of the likelihood that a special event or characteristic occurs to or is possessed by a "typical" member of the population.

Ratio: An expression of the relationship between two quantities that refer to different events. A risk ratio is a comparison of two rates expressing two different likelihoods.

Relative risk: A risk ratio derived from a cohort study. The relative risk ratio quantifies the risk of exposure to a hazardous behavior or event relative to the unexposed group from information gathered prospectively from groups.

Reliability: The degree of consistency with which any given instrument measures the attribute it is designed to measure.

Retrospective study: A case control or case comparison study.

Risk factor: A characteristic or exposure that is associated with increased rates of disease, antisocial behavior, or disability.

Risk ratio: Comparison of rates computed from two groups where one group has been exposed to a given risk factor, and the control group is not exposed. In essence, risk ratios measure the risk of the effects of exposure to any given risk factor.

Secondary attack rates: The rate of second generation of infectious disease occurrence occurring within a family with an infected person(s).

Secondary prevention: Preventive strategies occurring in the clinical stage of the natural history model that are aimed at early recognition and treatment and disability limitation. Early case finding is included in secondary prevention.

Serial dilution: A laboratory method of diluting aliquots of specimen or therapeutic substances in carefully measured doses, to compare with a standard.

Specificity: The ability of a test to identify and exclude all negative cases.

Specific rates: A conditional statement of probability of the risk of hazard; the risk is conditional upon the presence of a characteristic, such as age or sex, or an event, such as level of exposure to radioactivity. The conditional events are used for high-risk profiles for populations.

Surveillance: Activity aimed at monitoring the level of health hazards in the community. An ongoing mechanism to collect information.

Territorial bonds: Those physical boundaries that define the parameters of any given community.

Tertiary prevention: Strategies aimed at maximizing health potential and/or rehabilitative efforts in the disability stage of the natural history.

Validity: The degree to which data or study results are correct or true.

Variable: Any characteristic or attribute that has changing values (*i.e.,* is not a constant).

Variolation: The first rudimentary form of active immunization that involved innoculation with a live smallpox virus.

Vector: A carrier, usually an insect, that transmits the causative organisms of disease from infected to noninfected individuals. A biological vector is one in which the disease-causing organism multiplies or develops prior to becoming capable of infecting susceptible hosts.

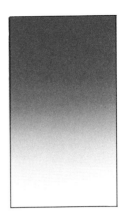

Index

Page numbers in italics denote figures; page numbers followed by "t" denote tables.

ISBN 0-397-54658-0

90000